THE WOMAN PATIENT

MEDICAL AND PSYCHOLOGICAL INTERFACES

Volume 1
Sexual and Reproductive Aspects
of Women's Health Care

WOMEN IN CONTEXT: Development and Stresses

THE WOMAN PATIENT — *MEDICAL AND PSYCHOLOGICAL INTERFACES*
Volume 1: Sexual and Reproductive Aspects of Women's Health Care
Edited by Malkah T. Notman and Carol C. Nadelson

THE WOMAN PATIENT
MEDICAL AND PSYCHOLOGICAL INTERFACES

Volume 1
Sexual and Reproductive Aspects of Women's Health Care

EDITED BY

MALKAH T. NOTMAN, M.D.
AND
CAROL C. NADELSON, M.D.
Harvard Medical School

PLENUM PRESS · NEW YORK AND LONDON

Library of Congress Cataloging in Publication Data

Main entry under title:

Sexual and reproductive aspects of women's health care.

(The woman patient, medical and psychological interfaces; v. 1) (Women in context)
   Includes bibliographical references and index.
   1. Gynecology—Psychology—Psychological aspects. 2. Pregnancy—Psychological aspects. 3. Gynecology. 4. Sexual disorders. 5. Women's health services. I. Notman, Malkah T. II. Nadelson, Carol C. III. Series. IV. Series: Women in context. [DNLM: 1. Gynecology—Collected works. 2. Delivery of health care—Collected works. WP100.3 W872]
RG103.5.S49   618   78-17972
ISBN 0-306-31151-8

First Printing — September 1978
Second Printing — August 1979

© 1978 Plenum Press, New York
A Division of Plenum Publishing Corporation
227 West 17th Street, New York, N.Y. 10011

Printed in the United States of America

Contributors

Ann B. Barnes, M. D. ● Assistant Clinical Professor, Obstetrics and Gynecology, Vincent Memorial Hospital (Gynecology Service, The Massachusetts General Hospital); Harvard Medical School, Boston, Massachusetts

Pauline B. Bart, Ph. D. ● Associate Professor of Sociology, Department of Psychiatry, Abraham Lincoln School of Medicine, University of Illinois, Chicago, Illinois

Jessica G. Davis, M. D. ● Associate Clinical Professor, Department of Pediatrics, Cornell University College of Medicine; Director, Child Development Center/Genetics Program, North Shore University Hospital; a teaching affiliate of Cornell University College of Medicine, Manhasset, Long Island, New York

Emanuel A. Friedman, M. D., Med. Sc. D. ● Professor of Obstetrics and Gynecology, Harvard Medical School; Obstetrician-Gynecologist-in-Chief, Beth Israel Hospital, Boston, Massachusetts

Elizabeth B. Gaskill, M. S. W. ● Department of Social Service, Peter Bent Brigham Hospital, Boston, Massachusetts

Jean Gillon, B. A. ● Research Assistant to Drs. Nadelson and Notman; Columbia University, New York, New York

Robert M. Goldwyn, M. D. ● Associate Clinical Professor of Surgery, Harvard Medical School; Head of Plastic Surgery, Beth Israel Hospital; Surgeon, Peter Bent Brigham Hospital, Boston, Massachusetts

Marlyn Grossman, Ph. D. ● Psychologist, Madden Mental Health Center, Hines, Illinois; Women in Crisis Can Act, Inc., Chicago, Illinois

v

Gay Guzinski, M. D. ● Assistant Professor of Obstetrics-Gynecology; Director, Division of Women's Health Care, University of Washington, Seattle, Washington

Wilma Scott Heide, Ph. D., R. N. ● Former Chair of Board and President of NOW, National Organization for Women, Inc.; Feminist consultant

Elaine Hilberman, M. D. ● Assistant Professor, Department of Psychiatry, University of North Carolina School of Medicine, Chapel Hill, North Carolina

Martha H. Izzi, B. S. ● COPE, Boston, Massachusetts

Eileen B. Kahan, M. D. ● Instructor, Department of Psychiatry, Peter Bent Brigham Hospital; Harvard Medical School, Boston, Massachusetts

Ruth W. Lidz, M. D. ● Clinical Professor, Department of Psychiatry, Yale University, New Haven, Connecticut

Miriam D. Mazor, M. D. ● Clinical Instructor, Department of Psychiatry, Harvard Medical School; Associate in Psychiatry, Beth Israel Hospital, Boston, Massachusetts

Carol C. Nadelson, M. D. ● Psychiatrist, Beth Israel Hospital; Associate Professor of Psychiatry, Harvard Medical School; Director, Medical Student Education, Department of Psychiatry, Beth Israel Hospital, Boston, Massachusetts

Malkah T. Notman, M. D. ● Psychiatrist, Beth Israel Hospital; Associate Clinical Professor of Psychiatry, Harvard Medical School, Boston, Massachusetts

Johanna F. Perlmutter, M. D., M. P. H. ● Assistant Professor, Department of Obstetrics and Gynecology, Beth Israel Hospital, Harvard Medical School, Boston, Massachusetts

Peter Reich, B. A., Candidate for M. P. H. ● Department of Socio-Medical Sciences, Boston University School of Medicine, Boston, Massachusetts

Nancy C. A. Roeske, M. D. ● Professor, Director of Undergraduate Curriculum, Coordinator of Medical Education, Department of Psychiatry, Indiana University School of Medicine, Riley Hospital, Indianapolis, Indiana

Maj-Britt Rosenbaum, M. D. ● Director, Human Sexuality Center, Long Island Jewish-Hillside Medical Center; Associate Clinical

Professor of Psychiatry, Albert Einstein College of Medicine, New York

Anne M. Seiden, M. D. ● Director of Research, Institute for Juvenile Research, Department of Mental Health and Developmental Disabilities, Chicago, Illinois

Eleanor G. Shore, M. D., M. P. H. ● Assistant to the President and Associate Physician to the University Health Services, Harvard University, Boston, Massachusetts

Caroline B. Tinkham, M. S. W. ● Vincent Memorial Hospital (Gynecology Service, The Massachusetts General Hospital), Boston, Massachusetts

Sigrid Lemlein Tishler, M. D. ● Assistant Professor of Medicine, Beth Israel Hospital, Harvard Medical School; Internist, Harvard Community Health Plan, Boston, Massachusetts

Maureen Finnerty Turner, R. N. ● COPE, Boston, Massachusetts

Preface

This volume presents the knowledge, views, and experiences of experts in the fields of health care that are particularly important to women. Not all of the authors agree on all of the issues, but all share the same concerns about women's health and recognize the importance of providing information to enable women to become active participants in the health care partnership.

The idea for the book evolved from our own work in the field of women's health care. The positive responses we received to several papers and presentations based on our experiences and addressed to patients, physicians, and other health care professionals indicated that there is a growing need for open discussion of women's health care issues as well as a need for developing and implementing new and better ways of dealing with these issues. We were further motivated by the repeated failure of the health care community to integrate new insights and information (that frequently contradict older, established beliefs and practices) into current health planning, education, and practice.

Our focus in this volume is on the two areas of health care—reproduction and sexuality—in which women's experiences differ greatly from those of men. Each chapter discusses one aspect of a specific topic or issue that is in some way related to these two areas. The impact of feminism on the status of women's health care and its important role in bringing about the changes of the past years are discussed. The need for further changes in existing medical hierarchies is stressed, as is the importance of taking humanistic, as well as pragmatic, aspects into consideration when establishing health care priorities. The role of self-help in the therapeutic process is also explored.

Developments in the field of genetics and their effects on pregnancy are examined. The topics discussed include the importance of prenatal influences and genetic counseling, and the ethical questions being raised by the potential uses of techniques such as amniocentesis. Several chapters are devoted to the physiological and psychological aspects of pregnancy. They include discussions of the advantages and disadvantages involved in using the new techniques of pregnancy monitoring, the importance of dealing with the special emotional, as well as physical, needs of the pregnant woman, and the growing interest in maternal control and mastery of both the childbirth experience and postnatal care. In recognition of the special problems and concerns associated with it, we have devoted an entire chapter to teenage pregnancy. Contraception and abortion are discussed from a historical standpoint, in terms of recent technological advances, with an eye to the continued controversies in which these issues are involved. Psychological and physiological consequences are also examined.

In the chapters dealing with gynecology, medical information is provided, and special note is taken of the emotional disturbances that can result when a woman fears that her physical problem will in some way diminish her sexuality. In particular, the psychological effects of a hysterectomy on the woman and her family are considered. Because of the symbolic and sexual connotations of the breast, equal emphasis is placed on the medical and psychological implications of mastectomy and other problems.

The treatment of terminal diseases, the reparative, restorative, and therapeutic aspects of cosmetic surgery, the recent developments in and modern approaches to sexual dysfunction, and the misunderstandings and controversies surrounding rape are all fully discussed in their respective chapters. In the final two chapters consideration is given to the physiological changes that occur during menopause, and to the impact these changes, and the myths surrounding them, have on the woman's perception of herself.

MALKAH T. NOTMAN
CAROL C. NADELSON

Boston, Massachusetts
August, 1978

Contents

Chapter 1

The Woman Patient

Malkah T. Notman and Carol C. Nadelson

The Doctor–Patient Relationship

Women have generally received their health care in settings that have been organized in a hierarchical model, with the physician dominating. The expectation that the doctor, who has usually been male, is informed, helping, authoritative, and protective conforms with the conventional social role of women, who have been seen as compliant, accommodating, and less well informed. This emphasizes the "child-like" position of the woman patient with respect to the "parent" physician. Indeed, in many instances, decisions about a patient's care have been, and still are, based on a paternalistic view, that is, on the doctor's understanding of the best interests of the patient. This is exemplified in decisions about female sterilization and abortion. Until recently, these decisions were made largely on the basis of the physician's assessment of their necessity. Another example is that physician's attitudes about a woman's childbearing plans and potential have influenced recommendations for hysterectomy. Similarly, the physician with a woman patient who has breast cancer has found it difficult to empathize with her or to understand her views or decisions if they are different than his. Often if radical surgery is his choice, he has not given serious consideration to her wishes to retain her breasts.

Changes in women's expectations, increased demands for knowledge, and the growth of self-help movements have affected the doctor–patient relationship. Traditional views of women have been challenged in medical and in feminist literature.

Paternalism, however, is not fostered by the physician alone; it

Malkah T. Notman, M.D. and Carol C. Nadelson, M.D. • Department of Psychiatry, Harvard Medical School, Beth Israel Hospital, Boston, Massachusetts 02215.

1

requires some degree of compliance on the part of the patient. Since, to some degree, all people regress when they are ill, their responses may be at variance with their normal behavior. Some people cannot comfortably accept help without feeling that their self-image is threatened; others depend on a strong figure to cure them.

This regressive response may, in addition, encourage the physician to have unrealistic views. The patient's heightened expectations are then enhanced by the physician's willingness to be regarded as omnipotent. This prevents communication and mutual respect. Later, disappointment and frustration, deriving from an unequal relationship, lead to mistrust and antagonism.

Efforts have been made to remedy the situation by spelling out the dangers and risks to a patient of a particular procedure or medication. Despite efforts to inform the patient in a manner appropriate to her understanding, barriers to communication arise from the authoritarian relationship itself. A doctor's recommendation, whether it is explicit or implicit, can overshadow a cautionary statement. The language may simply not be understood and the implications not heard, or they may be so frightening to the patient that in order for her to agree to a procedure potential problems or complications must be ignored. The authority of the physician may thus prevent the patient from objectively assessing dangers, benefits, or alternatives.

The experiences of being a patient and the situation of needing help do not necessarily have to be accompanied by uninformed submissiveness or by angry confrontation. Although for all patients the support and assurance of a helpful physician are important components of the therapeutic effort, many patients find it particularly appealing to relinquish their care to an authority. Others find that coping with their illness is made easier if they have a genuine collaborative role. In order to do this, they must be informed and aware, and they must understand their options.

THE RESPONSE OF THE CARETAKER

The physician, as caretaker to his/her patient, must differentiate that role from the role of physician as an agent of society. The extent to which these roles may be in conflict, as well as the dilemmas arising from this conflict, is often not considered. This role conflict is evident, for example, in laws requiring that certain illnesses, such as venereal disease, be reported, where protecting the patient's confidential relationship with the physician runs counter to societal concerns. The particular implications for women involve the different standards of morality applied to men and women, particularly regarding sexual behavior. For instance, since greater sexual restraint is expected of women than of men, the woman who contracts venereal disease or who is raped is likely to be condemned and held responsible for what happened, and the physician may contribute, albeit unwittingly, to her exposure to this situation.

As we have noted, concepts of appropriate treatment are in flux since assessments of benefits and risks are not clearly established. It is apparent that changes in conventional views also are occurring. This is particularly true when sexual and reproductive functions are involved. In these areas, physicians as well as patients have complex emotional reactions. Mathis comments:

> Sex, reproduction, and the reproductive system are almost synonymous with emotional reactions in our culture. The emotional charge invested in the genitalia makes that area peculiarly vulnerable to symptoms arising from any conflictual aspect of living. The woman who seeks medical attention for her reproductive system deserves a physician who understands the total significance of femininity as well as he knows the anatomy and physiology of the female. The physician who assumes this responsibility automatically becomes involved in emotional processes unequaled in any other branch of medicine, psychiatry not excepted.[1]

The health professional also is vulnerable to his/her emotional responses to sexuality and reproduction and may avoid these concerns with patients. Physicians often refer emotional problems to nurses or hospital social workers. In medical and nursing schools, students generally have been taught about sexuality while studying anatomy, physiology, and biochemistry, or as a part of obstetrics–gynecology, urology, medicine, and so forth. Human sexuality has rarely been considered a discipline. Much of the information, then, is not integrated to relate to the kinds of problems faced in practice.

In Western culture, women are encouraged to be more expressive of feelings than men. They may demonstrate greater "emotionality," which is often distressing to physicians who are unaccustomed to open displays of feelings and who are trained to repress their own responses. The physician may withdraw or depreciate the patient who makes him/her uncomfortable. Thus, the care of the patient is compromised.

The patient who develops functional symptoms presents a complex and sometimes frustrating problem for the caretaker, who is tempted to dismiss these symptoms as unimportant since they may not be life threatening or associated with organic pathology. Functional symptoms may be seen as manipulative, deceitful, or foolish. The patient's anxiety and pain are dismissed as "in her head" and therefore not deserving of serious attention and concern. This attitude presumes that the physician or health professional can decide what is a valid symptom. This depreciates the patient and the meaning of the symptoms as a communication. Physicians view emotional problems as less important than physical ones, and therefore, psychosomatic labeling has been depreciatory. In 1973, the Lennanes documented the greater prevalence of psychosomatic diagnoses for women.[2] However, if women's symptoms are discounted, doubt is cast on assessments of therapeutic or experimental results based on self-reports of symptoms.

The doctor–patient dyad also carries with it the potential for sexualization. The intimacy of the interaction and the exposure of private information and body parts may in part cause this response. While the statistical incidence is obviously difficult to document, it is a problem that is frequently reported by patients.

Here also, the interaction is important, and the issue is a complex one, although the caretaker clearly bears the responsibility for the resultant behavior.

Women who have learned to sexualize many of their relationships with men bring these patterns into the patient–doctor relationship. In response to the anxiety induced by their illness, they may use coping mechanisms that appear to be seductive. This apparent seductiveness may be unconscious on the part of the patient, who also may not be aware of her anxiety. It may be perceived as seductive by a doctor who is vulnerable because of his own life circumstances, such as loneliness, disappointment in his career, or stresses in his relationships. These problems may lead him to respond inappropriately to a patient who enhances his feelings of importance and effectiveness or who is sexually appealing. Sexualization of a relationship may be brought by the patient or by the doctor into almost any relationship.

Dependency, anger, and homosexual feelings also may be evoked by the intensity of the interaction and by the nature of the expectations between physicians and patients. For the woman physician, these issues also exist, although they are not so prominent, either because there have been too few women physicians or because the nature of the interaction with a "mother" caretaker may be less overtly sexualized.

The emotional responses of physicians provide a source of resistance to the incorporation of new data and understanding. In addition, there is evidence that much of the old data on which these responses had been based are questionable. These new data and concepts may expand the roles of health professionals, but it may cause increased resistance to change. The specific patient problems of obstetrics–gynecology include the social, legal, and ethical implications; that is, family planning, abortion, and sterilization have an impact far beyond the individual patient.

IMPACT OF CHANGE IN REPRODUCTIVE AND SEXUAL PATTERNS

Among the social changes of the past few years many have affected women. Birthrates have declined; families are smaller; and more women choose to remain single, to marry late, or to be childless. An increasing number of young women are seeking sterilization, many of whom are in their early twenties and have never had children.

The pregnant woman now has less social support than she did fifteen or twenty years ago, when prevailing social norms favored larger families and women had fewer nondomestic options. In fact, values have shifted to the opposite pole; women who are having third or fourth children describe outright hostility from peers and occasionally encounter doubts from obstetricians as well.

Many women are postponing pregnancies until their education and training are completed or their careers are established. The older pregnant woman often has difficulty gaining support and clear information from medical people. The physician must keep in mind the changed social realities that are important to the patient.

The fact that sexual mores have changed is by now self-evident. Sexual relations outside of marriage are more widespread; lesbian relationships are more open, some as an expression of political ideology or as an explanation of alternate patterns of intimacy. The gynecologist has had to become accustomed to these new realities—including the possibility of venereal disease in a wide cross section of patients, requests for contraceptive and sexual counseling for unmarried couples, and gynecological care of patients identifying themselves as bisexual or lesbian.

The health professional should be aware of his/her attitudes and responses to patients regardless of the issue involved. The example of teenage pregnancy illustrates this point. Obstetricians delivering babies of teenagers find themselves frustrated by the teenagers' seeming inability to use effective contraceptives, and are uncomfortable in dealing with young women who may have a very different concept of pregnancy and motherhood than their own.

There also has been a move toward home delivery among some women who have stressed their discontent with the institutional atmosphere of a hospital and who have wanted to include husbands and other family members in the delivery. This trend has been accom-

panied by a movement toward self-examination and less reliance on
trained medical personnel and more on peers and self. The presence of
a woman physician often is helpful in understanding the responses of
the patient.

Since the gynecologist–obstetrician is the physician many women
turn to for primary health care, his/her role has necessarily been expanded to include counseling, whether or not this is his/her original
intent. The potential for a preventive approach in both physical and
mental health also is important. It requires complex skills and psychological understanding that have not been part of the traditional training in obstetrics–gynecology.

The full impact of gynecological treatment and procedures on an
individual's self-image and sexuality must be understood. In some
areas, notably, pregnancy, contraceptive counseling, and sexual dysfunction, the illness model may be inappropriate.

Gynecologists have been criticized for their insensitivity to many
of the needs, feelings, and perspectives of their patients. Others, however, have been responsive when communication is attempted. The
sources of these differences are complex and lie within the social relations between doctor and patient, man and woman.

Since gynecology is a surgical specialty, it contains many of the
same patient considerations and approaches that are important to
surgery: schedules are grueling; communication is often minimal because of lack of opportunity; and the special pressures of practice may
encourage compromises that often are antithetical to values that confront conflict differences more directly.

In discussing some of the unique characteristics of obstetrics–
gynecology, Pasnau stresses the wide-ranging nature of the clinical
setting, which demands that the obstetrician–gynecologist function in
multiple roles and situations, causing considerable stress.[3] These factors, coupled with an action orientation and personality characteristics
that may make them less at ease with emotional expression, may contribute to some of the difficulties in communication often reported by
patients.

Hertz stresses the polarization and dissonance often experienced
by the gynecologist,[4] for example, he/she is oriented toward the maintenance of pregnancy, yet aborts it; counsels about contraceptives yet
administers artificial insemination. These demands may evoke unconscious conflict and role conflict in the gynecologist.

The patient is best served if she is able to participate in her own
medical care. Health care professionals must not only be more responsive to patient needs and requests but also must be able to relinquish
some aspects of their authority and power.

We have attempted to highlight some of the more critical issues. The authors in this volume will expand these views and will present important information and perspectives on the health care of women, as it involves reproductive functioning.

REFERENCES

1. Mathis J: Psychiatry and the obstetrician–gynecologist. *Medical Clinics of North America 51* (6): 1375–1380, 1967.
2. Lennane KJ, Lennane PJ: Alleged psychogenic disorders in women—a possible manifestation of sexual prejudice. *New England Journal of Medicine 288* (6): 288–292, 1973.
3. Pasnau RO: Psychiatry and obstetrics–gynecology: report of a five year experience in psychiatric liaison, in *Consultation-liaison psychiatry*. Edited by Pasnau, RO. New York, Grune & Stratton, 1975.
4. Hertz DG: Problems and challenges of consultation psychiatry in obstetrics–gynecology. *Psychotherapy and psychosomatics 23*:67–77, 1974.

Chapter 2

Feminism: Making a Difference in Our Health

WILMA SCOTT HEIDE

This chapter will focus on some of the contributions of feminism to health care, and some of my visions of the differences feminism will make for holistic health care. I expect that health occupations will become increasingly "desexigrated." Not only will more women become physicians but more men will become nurses. Currently, increasingly influenced by feminist consciousness, nurses are not only rejecting the "handmaiden" role but also are assertively redefining the nurse as a humanist who may best guide the total care of the whole patient. In this changing context, physicians often are seen as highly trained technicians, more prepared for instrumental roles, but not the sole decision makers. As nurses and nursing become more powerful and as men become more liberated from sex stereotyping, more men may become interested in nursing, especially as nursing is rewarded financially, commensurate with its value in health care.

In the process, the feminist redefinition of power (i.e., enabling the self to "be" and "become" and *not* to control) portends qualitative changes in the legal and other relationships among health providers and their clients/patients.[1]

DEFINITIONS OF HEALTH CARE

The definitions of health care have been profoundly influenced by feminism. Health care generally is based on relationships between

WILMA SCOTT HEIDE, Ph.D., R.N. • Feminist consultant, 15 Simpson Drive, Framingham, Massachusetts 01701. Dr. Heide was Chair of the Board and President of NOW, National Organization for Women, Inc.

people mediated and augmented by chemical and physical technologies. Instrumental technology and the relative overvaluing of procedures and techniques that are performed on passive people have often dominated the qualitative, expressive components of care. Transcending any medicine, surgery, and/or physiotherapy may be the experiential reality of whether encounters by patients/clients are affectively positive, conducive to healing and/or nurturing of positive self-images of both clients and practitioners. Feminism has generated these ideas and ideals.

Wildavsky states:

> According to the great equation, [available] medical care equals health, but the great equation is wrong. More available medical care alone does not equal health. The best estimates are that the medical system itself affects about 10% of the usual indices for measuring health: i.e. whether you live, how well you live, how long you live. The remaining 90% are determined by factors over which doctors have little or no control: such as individual life style, social conditions, and the physical environment.[2]

Health policy decisions are made in the context of a value system that is white, patriarchal, and capitalist. Medical technologies representing the instrumental approach to problem solving are often funded at the expense of social programs. These affect many of the factors that are important in determining the health status of people, that is, housing, nutrition, employment, and mental health. The expressive component refers to nurturant qualities reflecting the "feminine" (and generally subordinated) values toward which women primarily have been socialized. The instrumental approach represents the "masculine" (and usually dominant) values toward which men primarily have been socialized. Both sexes are being freed to express feminine and masculine behaviors by feminism, which also insists on valuing feminine qualities privately and publicly.

DEMYSTIFICATION

Feminist consciousness now demystifies important knowledge and rejects condescending attitudes toward women, as well as toward the poor and the ethnic and social minorities. For example, the physician or other practitioner who explains the treatment of a woman only to her husband or another male, or who feels his/her social control and power threatened by clients who insist on participating in care and therapy (unless unconscious or completely disoriented), must be re-educated. The implications for children's and men's health in feminist reorientations of all health care are, of course, profound.

Self-Help Movements

Self-help organizations are vital to the women's health movement. They involve "assertive nurturance" based on the discovery and sharing of knowledge and skills so that women and men create their own health destinies. Self-help groups were formed by people sharing common problems to help themselves devise and effect methods of treatment, for example, people suffering from "ostomies" (like colostomies, for instance), or parents of seriously ill children.

Feminist Women's Health Centers [3] are at the forefront of the self-help movement. Other important self-help modalities that are not frankly feminist have developed around the country and often work with or as agents of feminist change. The self-help movement reflects and generates certain values, including the self-confidence and therapeutic value of being expected to help oneself and others and to possess the skills to do so. The process requires active contribution instead of or in addition to passive reception. It is based on the principle that one can learn something by being prepared to teach it. Persuading others first requires self-persuasion and involvement. One thus gains self-confidence, competence, strength, and health.

The professional model of care emphasizes cognitive knowledge, an instrumental approach, and "objectivity" in relation to patients. It also involves systematic and standardized approaches, a controlled environment, the promise of cure (at least of symptoms), and a fee for service.

The aprofessional self-help model emphasizes the intuitive and experiential, spontaneity, and identification with the consumer. It often is free or the fee is based on a sliding scale and with less visibly circumscribed techniques. It stresses the total person. Although both approaches overlap, the relative emphases are important. The feminist approach is closer to the self-help aprofessional model. It therapeutically empowers the consumer and attempts to diminish hierarchies of control and power.

While the self-help potential for health care, especially in a capitalist society, is an important force, there are political risks. These become critical if support for self-help allows public services to be funded inadequately or if it lets ostensible national leaders "off the hook" with respect to their responsibilities to fund health and other important public services. There also is the risk that needed public services will only be provided in lifesaving or emergency situations and that self-help will be relegated to those problems that have traditionally been "blamed on the victims," thereby avoiding societal responsibility to remove the institutional causations of problems. Since professional expertise is often necessary, an important goal is to make it nonauthoritarian.

The National Women's Health Network[4] monitors and participates in national health policy, provides a clearinghouse, and serves an action-generative function that avoids overpersonalization and regionalism. In 1977, a bimonthly academic journal, *Women and Health*,[5] was initiated. The burgeoning of feminist research on health and other human issues portends new insights and potential for unbiased, human problem solving.

MEDIA

In addition to books, articles, and pamphlets, the involvement of the media indicates that a dynamic development of changed consciousness has occurred. For example, the film *Taking Our Bodies Back*[6] brilliantly explores ten critical areas of the women's health movement from revolutionary self-help concepts to informed surgical consent.

WOMEN'S PARTICIPATION IN PUBLIC POLICYMAKING ORGANIZATIONS

The National Institutes of Health have been pressed to include more women in public advisory, research, and administrative functions. Prior to 1972, less than 10 percent of these positions were filled by women, although women comprise over 75 percent of health care providers and over 50 percent of health care users. Sustained attempts to produce change were not persuasive until a 1972 lawsuit began to effect some results.[7]

GENETIC ISSUES

Feminists also are concerned with genetic engineering and manipulation. The demographic characteristics of the researchers influence their judgments about appropriate criteria. Ethical issues are raised by genetic research and manipulation. Genetics is *not* value free, nor is any other area of science and health care. This work occurs in a political, socioeconomic context. Genetic research, policy, and practice do not begin or end with the intrauterine life of the embryo. The allocation of health research funds is profoundly influenced by politics in both the generic and partisan senses.[8]

Mental Health Issues

An example of the abuses of the virtually powerless by the relatively powerful is found in the area of psychosurgery. These procedures were discredited in the late 1940s as being both ineffective and irreversible. Many critics felt that the patients were victimized by powerful physicians.

One major group of subjects was women. The goals of the treatment were to eliminate or modify aggressive behavior supposedly not responsive to other methods. The treatment was deemed "successful" if women returned to passive femininity, willingly performing housekeeping, homemaker "duties." The absence of consent, informed or otherwise, and understanding by these subjects, who were already confined in institutions, often against their will, also was a cause for protest.

Although a moratorium on psychosurgery did result, eternal vigilance appears to be necessary. In 1977, the federal government again allocated funds for lobotomies for a project whose primary "target" was white middle-class, middle-aged women.[9]

A double standard of mental health has been documented by Friedan, the Brovermans et al., Chesler, and other feminists, some of whom are also professionals.[10] Newer data overwhelmingly document the charges, but problems continue to exist in the mental health field.[11] Those who deviate from standards of "appropriate" feminine or masculine behavior are considered not only abnormal but also "unnatural" and "sick." "Masculine" behavior is valued by mental health practitioners more highly than "feminine" behavior and is considered virtually synonymous with ideal behavior for mature adults; "feminine" behavior, while considered "ideal" for allegedly mature females, is seen as immature for adults. Those who deviate have been, and still may be, exposed to therapists who try to adjust them to "their place." Efforts are being made in many fields to educate our colleagues and society to a single standard of mental health for both sexes.

Genesis and Validity of Feminist Changes

An examination of significant societal changes reveals that many of the ideas now considered as truth originated in earlier, activist concerns that were often initially rejected by the professionals and "experts." What programs and proposals might we most progressively support, especially with public funds: the pro-active change agent initiatives or the re-active professional and "experts" or both?

Many feminists are emphasizing a "wholly new science of medicine—one that could integrate objective findings with the subjective experience of health or illness, that is, integrate the *curing* functions with the *caring* and vice versa." [12] This means integrating and esteeming the instrumental and expressive, the quantitative and qualitative, the cognitive and affective, indeed, the "masculine" and "feminine." Assertive nurturance is a concept I use to describe these continuing examples of the healing possibilities of gynandrous (usually called androgynous) visions of people and health care.

INTERNATIONAL PROGRAMS AND POSSIBILITIES

Issues and problems of women were addressed in the 1977 state and national conferences consequent to the International Women's Year (IWY). Four major areas were considered: health rights, health literacy, access to quality care, and women as health consumers. The IWY commission report of 1976 made recommendations in health research, policy, economics, drug abuse, alcohol, cancer, training, mental health, consciousness raising, and women's assertiveness training. The implementation of these recommendations would be a major gain and may become possible as increasing numbers of feminists enter policymaking positions.

International feminists also have taken independent actions on health issues. For example, Fran P. Hosken has been campaigning to end the mutilation of girls (as young as four years old) and women in Africa by infibulation, circumcision, excision, and/or clitoridectomy. These procedures cause many physical and psychological problems, and even death. The purposes are to assure chastity, virginity, and reduced sexual response. Although part of an entire cultural pattern, the decisions are made by and for men. [13]

Health needs in many parts of the world beg for feminist perspectives and actions. One example is the pressures on poor women in developing countries to spend their limited resources on bottle feeding and on prepared baby foods, rather than rely on breast-feeding. This pressure is applied by U.S. multinational corporations that exploit the actual or functional illiteracy of many women so that they spend scarce funds when breast-feeding is more efficient, healthier, and economical.

Other examples are found in India, where women generally receive fewer resources. It is the practice among some groups for wife, mother, and girls to eat only after males of all ages have eaten, and then only whatever is left; marriage and childbearing occur as young as ten years old for girls; less education (if any) is available for girls than boys; and the "neglect and maltreatment of women by society, in-laws or husbands after marriage affects their emotional and mental health."[14]

India is not alone in its misogyny. In March 1976, feminists around the world organized an International Tribunal on Crimes against Women, including those crimes by the medical profession.[15]

OTHER HEALTH PROBLEMS

The tragic case of corporate malpractice can be seen in the use of the Dalkon Shield, an intrauterine device (IUD) that was removed from the market in 1975 after evidence mounted as to its harmful effects and protests increased from feminists and others.[16] Seventeen women had died from its use before 1976, and countless others were infected, but those who profited from its sale have never been prosecuted.[17]

DRUGS: DIETHYLSTILBESTROL

The need for monitoring and constraining is illustrated by the problems arising from the use of diethylstilbestrol (DES). Beginning in the 1940s, DES was prescribed to pregnant women to prevent miscarriages. By 1960, DES effectiveness was questioned, and most physicians stopped using it. "In January, 1973 the Federal Food and Drug Administration, FDA, banned use of DES in cattle feed, judging the .00003 mg remaining in beef to be carcinogenic for human consumption."[17] In March 1975, the FDA approved the use of DES in a 250 mg. dose for use as a postcoital contraceptive, or "morning-after pill," in "emergency situations." Left to the physician's discretions were decisions about what constitutes an emergency and informing patients of possible side effects to the fetus, should the drug be ineffective, and of the possible carcinogenic effects with long-term use.

By April 1975, some daughters of DES-treated women had developed vaginal cancer, which is rare in this age group.

It has been estimated that 80% of the DES daughters will have adenosis, which is an abnormal form of vaginal cellular development which may be a precursor of cancer. There is now an incontestable chain of evidence linking DES given to pregnant women with the possible appearance of adenocarcinoma in their daughters.[18]

NUTRITION

Feminists are concerned with the practices of drug and pharmaceutical corporations, the food industry, as well as physicians, all of whom pay inadequate attention to nutritional needs. Especially in poor countries, but also in the United States, medical schools have failed to emphasize the science of nutrition.

FUNDAMENTAL ISSUES FOR FEMINISTS

A familiar demand of feminists is for control of our bodies and for self-determined reproductive choices. This includes contraception, abortion, and voluntary sterilization. In a world where millions starve each year, compulsory pregnancy is obscene. It is the right of the woman (who still bears the major daily consequences of completed pregnancy) to determine whether or not she will bear children. In two hours, the world spends on armaments what it spends in one year on children.[19]

Control of our bodies, including reproductive choices and childbirth practices, is neither possible nor adequate until women redefine power and share leadership and control of health and other social institutions.

Jean Baker Miller makes some important observations:

> . . . in the course of projecting into women's domain some of its most troublesome and problematic necessities, male-led society may also have simultaneously, and unwittingly, delegated to women not humanity's "lowest needs" but its "highest necessities"—that is, the intense, emotionally connected cooperation and creativity necessary for human life and growth. Further, it is women who today perceive that they must openly and consciously demand them if they are to achieve even the beginnings of personal integrity.[20]

Miller asserts that women have filled in these necessities without portfolio, with little societal support, and even without the dominant culture substantively acknowledging these as essentials or recognizing women's creativity. She correctly emphasizes the strengths of women performing humanity's highest necessities.

This has enormous implications for health care education, policy, and research. For example, the selection of medical students and the education of physicians. Some educators feel that the selection process for medical schools has been weighted too heavily toward those students with scientific ability to the detriment of humanistic qualities. They posit the need for a stable counselor who can listen and be supportive, compassionate, and psychologically sensitive. It has been especially women who develop the feminine "humanistic" qualities and who have been, until recently, limited in medical and other professional schools.

VISIONS OF THE FUTURE

Having shared a sampling of some changes that feminism has initiated or created in health care in little more than a decade, I want to address possibilities for the future. In doing so, I share the risks of others who envision profoundly changed possibilities. Adrienne Rich says:

> . . . any vision of things—other-than-as-they-are tends to meet with the charge of "utopianism," so much power has the way-things-are to denude and impoverish the imagination. Even minds practiced in criticism of the status quo resist a vision so apparently unnerving as that which foresees an end to male privilege and a changed relationship between the sexes.[21]

To envision nonsexist health concepts, policy, and practice, I suggest, first, corrective women's studies and, then, futurist feminist studies as required parts of curricula for all health practitioners.

The elimination of sexist language is basic to all visions. Language is a tool of thought, a powerful method to create or exclude images.

A universal network of quality child care at health care institutions, as elsewhere, is essential. This would have values for children, for parents, and, particularly, for all health practitioners' education. While use of child care opportunities by parents would be optional, their presence and experience would not be optional for educators and students. Nurturance experience is central to health practice and a potentially humanizing experience for all practitioners.

Feminism supports a decrease in the hierarchy of current health practices. I foresee the specialist as more of a physical technician and the generalist–humanist, as the health leader. Some of these generalists will be nurses, some physicians, but all will be educators in the most generic sense. Much health knowledge will be demystified, with greater emphasis on preventive care.

Some women presently are excluded from certain occupations that are deemed dangerous to our health—particularly if we are pregnant. These working conditions are hazardous to men as well. The work situation should be changed for all, rather than "protecting" women to an extent that excludes us from opportunities.[22]

INSURANCE

Changes also are needed in financing health care. Much of the sexism in health insurance is due to mythology, such as inaccurate information that women's absenteeism is greater than men's. Feminists are changing laws and insisting on equitable compliance with laws by civil rights enforcement agencies. For example, in 1973 the Equal Employment Opportunity Commission was prepared to accept the notion that, since women generally outlive men, all women should receive less retirement benefits per month or year than men. The author reminded the commissioners that, since white people generally outlive black people, it follows that white people should receive lower benefits than black people. The inconsistency and double standard became apparent, but change occurred primarily to avoid our promised media campaign and legal action.

As a feminist wanting to translate private compassions into public health policy, I suspect that even the foregoing few sample visions will soon appear myopic. In the human interest, I envision that these and other profound changes in health philosophies, practices, research, policies, and practitioners will become, not questions of if, but questions of when, where, and how. Women and men with changed feminist consciousness and confidence will create the differences—for the health of us all.

REFERENCES

1. NOW Women and Health Task Force and Nurses NOW Task Force, NOW Action Center, 425 13 Street, N.W., Suite 1048, Washington, D.C. 20004. NOW means National Organization for Women, Inc.
2. Wildavsky A: Doing better and feeling worse: the political pathology of health policy. *Daedulus, Journal of the American Academy of Arts and Sciences*, Issue on doing better and feeling worse: Health in the United States, winter, 1977, *106* (1):105. 165 Allandale St., Jamaica Plain Station, Boston, Massachusetts 02130.
3. Feminist Women's Health Center, 1112 Crenshaw Boulevard, Los Angeles, California 90019. Publications include How to start your self-help clinic, $2.50, and other resources written in Spanish and English.
4. National Women's Health Network, P.O. Box 24192, Washington, D.C. 20034.
5. Women and health. New York: State University of New York at Old Westbury.
6. Taking our bodies back. Cambridge Documentary Films, a nonprofit organization, P.O. Box 385, Cambridge, Massachusetts 02139.
7. NOW Legal Defense and Education Fund, 9 West 57 Street, New York, New York 10019; records of case of *Association for Women in Science et al. vs. Elliot Richardson et al.* (HEW Secretary), records of Dr. Julia Apter, spokeswoman for Coalition of Professional Organizations, Rush Medical College, 1753 West Congress Parkway, Chicago, Illinois 60612, and author's own records of change endeavors and the lawsuit and correspondence with attorney Sylvia Roberts and Helen Hart Jones and others.
8. Heide WS: A feminist's perspectives on manipulation of woman (woman includes man and can be generic). Symposium on The genetic manipulation of man (*sic*), University of Wisconsin, Stevens Point, Wisconsin, November 8, 1973. Available from KNOW, Inc., P.O. Box 86031, Pittsburgh, Pennsylvania 15221 or from author.

9. Silver L, Eisenberg E, Kain K, Fern S: HEW ok's federal funds for lobotomies. *Majority report*, May 14–27, 1977, p. 5, 74 Grove Street, New York, 10014.
10. Heide WS: The reality and the challenge of the double standard in mental health. Symposium at Chatham College, May 1969, reprinted by KNOW, Inc., P.O. Box 86031, Pittsburgh, Pennsylvania 15221.
11. Women's Health Conference. 1975 Proceedings, Box 192, West Somerville, Massachusetts 20144, $2.00.
12. Heide WS: Some egalitarian* alternatives to androcentric science. Symposium:What can the behavioral sciences do to modify the world so that women who want to participate meaningfully are not regarded as and are not, in fact, deviant? American psychological convention, Washington, D.C., Sept. 3, 1969, unpublished paper.
13. Hosken FP: Genital mutilation of girls and women in Africa. W.I.N. News, and information in every W.I.N. News since its 1975 initiation, 187 Grant Street, Lexington, Massachusetts 02173, $15.00 per year. Actions people can take in each issue.
14. Kapur P: Myth or reality. Equal rights. *World Health*, WHO, January 1975, pp. 8–11, Avenue Appia, 1211 Geneva 27, Switzerland, $.70 copy.
15. Russell D, Van Ven N: Crimes perpetrated by the medical profession. *The proceedings of the international tribunal on crimes against women*, Les Femmes Publishing, 231 Adrian Road, Millbrae, California 94030, $5.95, 1976.
16. Fatt N: DES—the caucus. *Healthright*. Women's Health Forum, 175 Fifth Avenue, New York, New York 10010, pp. 1, 4.
17. Downie M, Johnston T: A case of corporate malpractice. *Mother Jones,* magazine for the rest of us, November 1976, 1:36–39, 46–50. Foundation for National Progress, 607 Market Street, San Francisco, California 94105.
18. Brudney K: DES, the history. *Healthright*. Women's Health Forum, 175 Fifth Avenue, New York, New York 10010, pp. 1, 4.
19. Heide WS: Feminism for healthy social work. Commencement address, Smith College School of Social Work, August 20, 1975. Taped and transcribed in *Smith College School of Social Work Journal*, 3 (1):1–4, 1976, Northampton, 00160. From UNESCO statement by Danny Kaye, December 1974.
20. Miller JB: Towards a new psychology of women. Boston, Beacon Press, 1976, pp. 25–26.
21. Rich A: Toward a woman-centered university, in *Women and the power to change.* Edited by Howe F. New York, McGraw-Hill, 1975.
22. Stellman J, Daum S: *Work is dangerous to your health, A handbook of health hazards in the workplace and what you can do about them.* New York, Random House, 1973.

*Egalitarian means equality of all men, thus a more appropriate word I would now use is feminist.

Chapter 3

Prenatal Influences on Child Health and Development

Eleanor G. Shore

Every parent hopes that his/her child will start life as a normal, healthy individual with maximum capacity to handle the problems and opportunities that life presents. While the majority of parents are granted this wish, a few are faced with loss of an infant in utero (known as abortion or fetal wastage) or by stillbirth, physical abnormalities detectable at birth, or developmental abnormalities detectable only as the child matures and demonstrates limitations in physical or mental growth. Old wives' tales and superstitions have long held that events in the mother's life during pregnancy may affect the health of the infant, but only in this century has modern science provided the opportunity to study and distinguish among hereditary factors, prenatal influences, and later events that affect the child after birth.

Any woman anticipating pregnancy should become acquainted with those measures she herself can take to assure healthy offspring. She also should be prepared to cooperate in research to find further ways to reduce the possibility of significant developmental abnormalities in yet-to-be-conceived children.

Of particular importance to a woman is knowledge about the range of environmental agents (infections, chemicals, drugs, or radiation) that may be injurious to the developing fetus since their effect on fetal development may be greatest in the early weeks of pregnancy, when the woman is uncertain if she is pregnant and has not yet consulted an obstetrician or other physician. Fortunately, in many instances, the steps necessary to avoid exposure to a teratogen (an agent

ELEANOR G. SHORE, M.D., M.P.H. • Assistant to the President and Associate Physician to the University Health Services, Harvard University, Boston, Massachusetts 02215.

that has an injurious effect on the development of a fetus) can be taken
by the woman herself. (These steps will be discussed later.)

Our understanding of teratogenic infections, chemicals or drugs,
and radiation has increased greatly since the observation was first
made in 1941 that rubella (German measles) in the mother might be
associated with such birth defects as heart malformation, deafness,
and cataracts.[1] One way in which this understanding has been increased has been by the use of animal research. Unfortunately, the
outcome of an intrauterine exposure to a particular agent may be specific to the particular species. For example, a drug fed to a pregnant
mouse may result in no abnormalities in the offspring, while the same
drug fed to a monkey may cause very specific and reproducible defects
in the fetus. Or a drug may interfere with the development of certain
animal progeny but not that of human offspring.[7] In addition, a defect
may occur in offspring of exposed pregnant women without evidence
of fetal damage in animal studies. This variability means that one cannot be certain of the safety of a particular agent until it has been studied in humans. Such human research studies are difficult to perform,
however. Ethical considerations deter investigators from conducting
planned studies in which one group of pregnant women is purposely
exposed and a comparable group (the control group) is not exposed in
order to measure the difference in the developmental abnormalities in
their children.

However, from time to time, certain natural experiments occur to
permit another kind of research, epidemiology, which is the study of
the distribution and determinants of disease in humans. Using epidemiologic methods, scientists can study the relationship between specific prenatal events and subsequent birth or developmental defects,
information that may help to identify specific preventive measures.

Experience has shown that the most likely route to establishing a
clear association between an event during the mother's pregnancy and
later developmental defects in the offspring is by an astute observation, such as occurred in rubella and in thalidomide ingestion, when,
in each case, a physician suspected the relationship between these
events and severe malformations in newborns. The fact that each of
these agents caused an unusual pattern of defects (cardiac, eye, and
ear in the case of the rubella virus; abnormality or absence of limbs in
the case of thalidomide) helped the relationship to be established.
Even so, it took five years and thousands of affected children before
the thalidomide association was made. Random searches for relationships have been less fruitful. However, once the specific relationship has been suggested, then the offspring of the exposed and
the unexposed groups can be compared for the occurrence of the sus-

pected abnormality. This comparison provides the evidence that makes the difference between scientific proof and suspicion or superstition.

The process of epidemiologic investigation sounds simple and straightforward, but it is complicated for a number of reasons.

1. Initially, an astute observation must be made in order to trigger the study of an association between a particular prenatal event and a particular outcome.

2. An unequivocal objective test, such as that done in a laboratory for the development of antibodies to a particular infectious agent, is desirable in order to document the fact of exposure and its exact timing during the pregnancy. The best example is the hemagglutination inhibition test for rubella antibodies, which, when followed over a two- to three-week period, can clarify whether no rubella infection has occurred, whether a recent infection has occurred, or whether there is immunity because of a previous infection. Such information is invaluable when the doctor and patient need to know if a developing fetus might be infected. However, in many instances, no such objective test exists, and the investigator must rely on the mother's verbal account of what happened during pregnancy.

3. In lieu of a specific laboratory test, the history of exposure of a pregnant woman to a particular agent must be as accurate as possible. Studies that are begun after the outcome of a pregnancy is known and that compare affected and unaffected fetuses and children in terms of previous exposure to a teratogenic agent are known as retrospective studies. Of necessity, they incorporate some degree of error because the time between the exposure and the study dims memory and because, with the outcome of the pregnancy known, the feelings of the mother may bias her account of possible exposures to teratogenic agents. She may wish to have an identifiable reason for her infant's developmental problems and, therefore, recall every event in pregnancy. Or she may regard the defect with guilt and deny any exposures. Furthermore, the historical account is of limited value in such infections as rubella, where a rash or other external evidence of infection may or may not be present. Studies that begin before the time of exposure and continue until the final outcome is known, at which time comparisons of exposed and unexposed may be made, are referred to as prospective studies and may be more accurate than retrospective studies. However, they are more time consuming, more expensive, and more dependent on the long-term cooperation of mother and child.

4. The effects of harmful agents need to be easily identifiable if they are to be measured accurately in an epidemiologic study. Some

developmental abnormalities are so clear that there is no mistaking their existence shortly after birth, for example, absence of a limb, blindness, or severe deafness, but others are subtle and may not be apparent until the child is much older, for example, impaired motor coordination, speech defects, language disability, or mild deafness. This range of possibilities means that careful definitions of abnormalities must be agreed on and that the studies, whether retrospective or prospective, must extend far beyond the first one or two years of the child's life.

5. In any study, it is necessary to be aware that there is a variation of outcomes from exposure to a particular agent, depending on the time in the pregnancy when the exposure occurs. For example, in one study, exposure to the rubella virus during the first five weeks of pregnancy was associated with a high incidence of abortion or moderate to severe developmental defects.[2] However, exposure between the fifth and eight week of pregnancy was associated with a variety of outcomes, ranging from death, to severe defects, to mild defects, to normal offspring. With each successive month, the proportion of normal to affected children increased, although there were still some severe defects among the children whose mothers were infected during the second trimester of pregnancy.

6. Great care must be exercised by the investigator to see that the groups (exposed and unexposed) being compared are similar in all respects except for the agent being studied. Also, the outcome of a particular exposure must be measured in a way that eliminates bias due to expectation of that particular outcome. When possible, it is desirable that the observer-recorder not know whether or not the individual was exposed to the agent being studied.

7. Since the cooperation of large numbers of women is essential to epidemiologic research, mothers must be convinced that their participation in any study is important for better understanding of fetal and child development. Even though knowledge acquired in the particular study may come too late to change the outcome of the pregnancy being studied, improved understanding will be helpful to future pregnancies of other women. It is because most developmental abnormalities are rare that it is necessary to study a very large number of mother–child pairs to establish a statistically significant increase in frequency of any particular defect.

Although the above problems of epidemiologic research have all been expressed in terms of mother–child involvement, the father's participation may be as important as the mother's. There are interesting animal studies that suggest that events affecting male spermatogenesis before conception may affect fetal and infant development.

Given the difficulty of doing either animal or epidemiologic research, it is not surprising that prenatal influences on fetal and child development are still not understood completely and that much more research is needed. However, concentrating on environmental factors known or suspected to be associated with abnormalities of fetal and later development will help to focus attention in areas where intervention can occur.

The focus here is on environmental factors and not on the entire range of obstetrical complications and chronic illnesses in the mother. Environmental factors can often be approached with primary or secondary preventive measures. Primary prevention refers to such measures as vaccination to prevent an intrauterine infection or avoidance of a teratogenic drug to prevent a developmental defect. Secondary prevention refers to measures taken after infection or other exposures but before complications have occurred in the fetus, as in the case of penicillin therapy for syphilis early in pregnancy. Because infection of the fetus by syphilis spirochetes (organisms causing syphilis) may destroy certain developing tissues and produce a pattern of abnormalities known as congenital syphilis and because this infectious process can be arrested by penicillin before destruction has occurred, screening each pregnant woman for syphilis and treating those who are infected permits secondary prevention. Most obstetrical complications are ameliorated when the woman is knowledgeable and cooperates in planning her maternity care; in the case of environmental factors, the mother's knowledge may be critical in avoiding teratogenic agents at the outset of pregnancy.

CHEMICALS, DRUGS, AND MEDICINES

The first category of environmental factors contains those chemicals, drugs, or medicines that have been demonstrated to cause fetal abnormalities. Thalidomide, a sedative that was taken between the years 1957 and 1962 with and without prescription (not in the United States) is the classic example. Ingestion between the twentieth and thirty-fifth day postconception was associated with interference with fetal limb development (phocomelia) or, in the most severe cases, with absence of arms and legs (amelia).[3,4] Once the association was confirmed and publicized, thalidomide was no longer produced. As tragic as this episode was, it provided the stimulus needed to intensify the study of the effects of many drugs in pregnant women and underscored the caution necessary in using drugs during pregnancy. Another well-documented but rarely incriminated teratogenic chemical is organic mercury, which damaged nervous tissue and caused cerebral palsy in the offspring of mothers who had consumed fish from Japanese waters containing high levels of mercury from a chemical factory.[5] Folic acid antagonists (drugs used in the treatment of cancer) have been associated with malformations of the head and face when administered during the early months of pregnancy.[6,7] Female sex hormones (estrogens and progestogens) have recently been shown to be associated with an increased incidence of cardiovascular birth defects. A recent report of 1,042 women who received female hormones during pregnancy demonstrated nineteen children with cardiovascular defects (18.2 cases per 1,000 children exposed as compared with 7.8 per 1,000 without this exposure).[8] Tetracycline, when taken during pregnancy, has been associated with hypoplasia (underdevelopment) of teeth and with stained dental enamel.[9]

Beyond these examples of definite association are other drugs that are suspected but not proven to be teratogenic. Some of these are anticonvulsants, anticancer agents, lead, warfarin (an anticoagulant), and amphetamines. The question of whether or not mild tranquilizers and commonly used medicines are teratogenic remains unanswered because, although animal studies are suggestive, confirmation in humans has not been forthcoming. Furthermore, the doses used in animal studies were well above therapeutic levels for the drugs.[7] Clearly, many medications are not injurious to the fetus: in one survey of 1,369 mothers, although 97 percent took at least one prescribed drug and 65 percent took at least one self-administered drug during pregnancy, the great majority had normal children.[10] However, the evidence is not yet available about which of these drugs, taken singly or in combination, are safe for use in pregnancy.

Another kind of long-term effect of a drug taken in pregnancy has been vaginal adenocarcinoma in the daughters of women who took diethylstilbestrol (DES) during pregnancy to prevent abortion.[11,12] The incidence of this developmental abnormality has been low to date, but it deserves mention because it demonstrates the problem of detecting an association between a prenatal medication and an event that occurs many years later. This association was made only because one physician's suspicion was aroused when he found multiple cases of a very rare type of cancer.

To date, the most ambitious effort to gather evidence to clarify some of the associations between drugs and fetal development has been the Collaborative Perinatal Project, in which 50,282 mother–child pairs from twelve centers in the United States were studied between 1959 and 1965.[13] Although hypotheses have emerged from this study, no clear new associations, such as that between thalidomide and subsequent congenital anomalies, were established.

INFECTIONS   ·

A second category of environmental agents that affect the development of the fetus is infectious agents. Viral and bacterial infections have well-demonstrated associations between prenatal exposure and subsequent developmental defects. The first and clearest association was found between rubella and fetal damage or later developmental abnormalities in the child. When the capacity developed to pinpoint the time of infection from specific antibody tests, correlations were made between the kind of developmental defect and the time of infection. Rubella infection very early in pregnancy may result in the death of the fetus. Infections later in the first trimester have been associated with heart lesions, cataracts, deafness, microcephaly (small head size), and mental retardation. Second trimester infections have been associated with mental and motor retardation as well as deafness. Retarded language development may be the presenting symptom in cases of congenital rubella, where deafness and psychomotor retardation have been present but undiagnosed.[14]

According to reports from the Perinatal Research Branch of the National Institute of Neurologic Diseases and Stroke, the frequency of abnormal children following rubella infection in the first month approaches 50 percent; in the second month, 22 percent; and in the third, fourth, and fifth months, 6 to 10 percent.[15] These statistics further demonstrate the significance of the timing of the infection during pregnancy. Multiple mechanisms for the teratogenic effect of this virus have been suggested, including direct cell damage, vascular damage with secondary effects on various organs, and growth interference. The variation in effect on different organs has been attributed in part to the capacity of some tissues to regenerate.[15]

Rubella does not stand alone among the viruses that have been identified as teratogenic. A recent report of a retrospective epidemiologic study of ten measles epidemics in Greenland provided evidence (although the number of cases was small) of an increased incidence of severe congenital defects without a detectable pattern in the offspring of mothers infected in the first two months of pregnancy.[16] Fortunately, the great majority of women in this country are immune to measles by the time they reach childbearing age. Other less well-known viruses associated with damage to the fetus are the cytomegalovirus and herpes simplex virus. Both of these affect individuals of all ages, can involve multiple organs, and may cause an acute infection or remain latent (i.e., without symptoms) for many years before giving evidence of a disease. Both can cross the placenta and infect the fetus. Cytomegalovirus infections in utero have been associated with microcephaly, hydrocephaly (large head size), microphthalmia (small eye size), blindness, seizures, and mental retardation. Herpes simplex infection has been associated with microcephaly and microphthalmia.[17]

Efforts to demonstrate an association between still other prenatal virus infections, such as mumps and chickenpox, and subsequent developmental defects have not been so conclusive and further study is needed.

Treponema pallidum, the infectious agent of syphilis, is the clearest example of a bacterial agent that can affect intrauterine development. With involvement of multiple fetal organs by the infectious process, certain structural changes occur. Infection of the nasal cartilages and bones may cause sufficient damage to flatten the nasal bridge. Permanent teeth also may be malformed.

RADIATION

Radiation constitutes a third category of environmental agents that affect intrauterine development. In the 1920s, evidence was gathered to establish an association between pelvic radiation (for treatment of cancer) and subsequent fetal malformation and abnormalities, which included microcephaly and mental retardation.[18] Further evidence was accumulated in the study of children exposed to radiation in utero at Hiroshima and Nagasaki. Not only was there an increased rate of fetal and infant mortality but also a diminished growth rate in surviving children and a higher incidence of thyroid nodules.[19]

OTHER POSSIBLE TERATOGENS

Although there is much concern about the effects of tobacco and alcohol on fetal development, the evidence is still incomplete. In a study recently reported in *The American Journal of Epidemiology*, lower birth weight and higher perinatal mortality (deaths before and after birth) were correlated with maternal smoking, but no developmental defects were reported.[20] Reports of an increased incidence of developmental abnormalities in infants of heavy-drinking mothers have aroused considerable controversy over whether the alcohol or the socioeconomic conditions associated with alcoholism are the real offenders. However, a study reported in *The New England Journal of Medicine* establishes a strong association between heavy drinking (defined as the consumption of five or more drinks on occasion and an average daily consumption of 45 ml of absolute alcohol) and abnormality of the fetus at birth, including congenital anomalies, neurologic abnormalities, and premature and postmature infants.[21] The congenital malformations did not, however, fall into a recognized pattern, although microcephaly was reported in 12 percent of infants born to heavy drinkers as compared with 0.4 percent in the abstinent or moderate-drinking groups combined. Other factors such as nutrition, drug use, and sociologic conditions were studied as well but did not account for the difference in fetal abnormalities. Because of the frequency of exposure of the fetus to alcohol and tobacco, an accurate perception of their effects on intrauterine development is much needed. Such a perception can be obtained only by continuing research.

WHAT CAN BE DONE?

Given the three pieces of evidence—that the great majority of infants and children are born healthy and develop normally, that certain environmental agents are known to cause specific developmental anomalies in the fetus and child, and that the majority of congenital anomalies are still of unknown cause—what course should the concerned prospective parent follow?

The prudent course would be to avoid as many unnecessary environmental exposures as possible. Although developmental defect is rare, the toll, when it occurs, may be great. Efforts to overcome specific handicaps can extend over a lifetime.

There are several specific measures that every woman who is about to become pregnant may take to maximize the chance of healthy offspring. The first is to assure immunity to rubella, either from the natural disease or from immunization. Because rubella often is inapparent or may be confused with other viral diseases that may have rashes as part of the clinical picture, a history of the disease is insufficient proof. Before pregnancy occurs, a serum antibody test should be performed. If the titer of antibody is low and suggests no previous infection with rubella, a live virus vaccine is available that is thought to be 95 percent effective in producing a satisfactory antibody level. However, because the virus of the vaccine itself can cross a placenta to infect a fetus, a woman must not become pregnant for at least four months after receiving the vaccine. Ideally, this vaccination will have been administered to each child, but in fact, many women reach maturity without vaccination, and assessment must begin then. In some states, a determination of the presence or absence of protective antibodies for rubella is required before a marriage license is issued. The woman may then elect to have a vaccination if she is not immune.

Although the evidence for teratogenicity is less complete for measles than for rubella, the likelihood provides sufficient reason for vaccinating all children against the disease.

All live virus vaccines can cross the placenta to the fetus, although no specific teratogenic effect has yet been proven. Therefore, it is generally advisable, unless the risk of a mother's exposure to a disease outweights any theoretical risk to the fetus, to receive live vaccines against such diseases as measles, mumps, polio, smallpox, and yellow fever before or after but not during pregnancy.

Another precaution is to avoid all but the most essential medicines, drugs, and chemicals during pregnancy. Although evidence is not available to confirm the teratogenicity or lack of it for each drug, there is enough evidence to demonstrate that fetal damage does occur with some drugs so that it seems wisest to hold all drug exposures to a minimum.

Each pregnant woman also should be certain that a serologic test for syphilis is performed early enough in pregnancy so that any infection can be treated before it damages the developing fetus.

Finally, because of the potential risk to the fetus of large doses of radiation, diagnostic X-rays should be avoided throughout pregnancy, except when essential to the health of the mother.

To avoid unnecessary exposure to teratogenic environmental agents, it is important that a woman inform her physician of her earliest suspicion of pregnancy, or even of her intent to become pregnant, in order that drugs, X-rays, or vaccines not be unwittingly administered.

It is important to be aware of prenatal factors in fetal and child development not only because it may help to protect a child now but also because it may encourage mothers to press for and cooperate with long-term studies of fetal and child development. Animal studies already have, for example, provided provocative indications of an association between certain drugs taken during pregnancy and subsequent learning disabilities, as well as suggestions of associations between a wide variety of drugs and infections and subsequent developmental abnormalities. Confirmation in humans is lacking, however, and continuing public pressure on the federal government to support slow and expensive human research is essential if future fetal wastage and child disability are to be prevented. At present, there is a collaborative study of congenital malformations based at the Center for Disease Control of the U.S. Public Health Service, but this project only follows infants through the first one or two years and thus offers little or no opportunity to study speech defects, subtle motor defects, or learning or behavior disorders arising in later years. As expensive as long-term human studies may seem, each lifetime handicap prevented represents such an enormous saving that it offsets in part the expense of research. Only through better understanding of the causative factors in developmental defects can primary prevention be attempted. Clearly, prevention is preferable to treatment, however sophisticated, if the treatment has to be aimed at providing man-made substitutes for an individual's sensory, motor, or other capabilities.

References*

1. Gregg NM: Congenital cataract following German measles in the mother. *Transactions of the Ophthalmological Society of Australia 3:* 35, 1941.
2. Hardy JB: Rubella as a teratogen. *Birth Defects, Original Article Series VII:* 64–71, 1971.
3. McBride WG: The teratogenic action of drugs. *Medical Journal of Austria 2:* 689–693, 1963.
4. Lenz W: Malformations caused by drugs in pregnancy. *American Journal of Diseases of Children 112:* 101–105, 1966.
5. Fraumeni JF Jr.: Chemicals in human teratogenesis and transplacental carcinogenesis. *Pediatrics 53:* 807–812, 1974.
6. Thiersch JB: Therapeutic abortions with a folic acid antagonist, 4-aminopteroylglutamic acid (4-amino P.G.A.) administered by the oral route. *American Journal of Obstetrics and Gynecology 63:* 1298–1304, 1952.
7. Wilson JG: Present status of drugs as teratogens in man. *Teratology 7:* 3–15, 1973.
8. Heinonen OP, Slone D, Monson RR, Hook EB, Shapiro S: Cardiovascular birth defects and antenatal exposure to female sex hormones. *New England Journal of Medicine 296:* 67–70, 1977.
9. Witkop CJ Jr., Wolf RO: Hypoplasia and intrinsic staining of enamel following tetracycline therapy. *Journal of the American Medical Association 185:* 1008, 1963.
10. Nelson, MM, Forfar JO: Associations between drugs administered during pregnancy and congenital abnormalities of the fetus. *British Medical Journal 1:* 523–527, 1971.
11. Greenwald P, Barlow JJ, Nasca PC, Burnett WS: Vaginal cancer after maternal treatment with synthetic estrogens. *New England Journal of Medicine 285:* 390–392, 1971.
12. Herbst, AL, Ulfelder H, Poskanzer DC: Adenocarcinoma of the vagina. Association of maternal stilbestrol therapy with tumor appearance in young women. *New England Journal of Medicine 284:* 878–881, 1971.
13. Heinonen OP, Slone D, Shapiro S: The teratogenic role of drugs in humans, in *Birth defects and drugs in pregnancy.* Edited by Kaufman DW. Littleton, Mass.: Publishing Sciences Group, chapter 1, 1977.
14. Weinberger MM, Masland MW, Asbed RA, Sever JL: Congenital rubella presenting as retarded language development. *American Journal of Diseases of Children 120:* 125–128, 1970.
15. Sever JL: Viruses and embryos. Congenital Malformation, Birth Defects, Amsterdam, Excerpta Medica, 1969, p 182.
16. Jesperson CS, Littauer J, Uffe S: Measles as a cause of fetal defects. *Acta Paediatrica Scandinavica 66:* 367–372, 1977.

* Two other books for suggested reading: Beard RW, Nathanielsz PW, eds. *Fetal physiology and medicine.* London, W. B. Saunders Company Ltd., 1976, Chapters 3, 18, and 21; Turnbull AC, and Woodford FP, eds. *Prevention of handicap through antenatal care.* Amsterdam, Associated Scientific Publishers, 1976.

17. Sever, JL: Virus infections and malformations. *Federation Proceedings* 30:114–117, 1971.
18. Yamazaki J: A review of the literature on the radiation dosage required to cause manifest central nervous system disturbances from in utero and postnatal exposure. *Pediatrics* 37:877, 1966.
19. Yamazaki J: A review of the literature on the radiation dosage required to cause manifest central nervous system disturbances from in utero and postnatal exposure. *Pediatrics* 37:894–896, 1966.
20. Meyer MB, Jonas BS, Tonascia JA: Perinatal events associated with maternal smoking during pregnancy. *American Journal of Epidemiology* 103:464–476, 1976.
21. Ouellette EM, Rosett HL, Rosman NP, Weiner L: Adverse effects on offspring of maternal alcohol abuse during pregnancy. *New England Journal of Medicine* 297:528–530, 1977.

Chapter 4

Decisions about Reproduction: Genetic Counseling

Jessica G. Davis

Recent advances in human genetics and medicine have increased our understanding of genetic disorders and have enabled us to participate in reproductive decision making and behavior. The chemical structure of DNA and the underlying biochemical mechanism for many hereditary disorders are understood. Tissue culture techniques permit cells to be grown and analyzed, both biochemically and cytogenetically, in laboratories. Many genetic disorders that result in birth defects are amenable to surgical correction. Specific chromosome abnormalities, many inborn errors of metabolism, and some birth defects can now accurately be detected in utero, with little risk to mother or fetus. Genetic counseling services have expanded, and the ability to detect genetic defects in asymptomatic carriers of mutant genes has increased. Genetic screening programs, implemented in many communities, have gradually increased public awareness of problems of heredity. This cumulative increase in theory and practice constitutes a quantum leap in knowledge.

Progress in medical genetics has occurred as public attitudes and practices toward reproductive behavior, abortion, and population control undergo radical change. Available techniques, whether or not used, for genetic intervention pose complex ethical, social, religious, and economic issues. For example, should known carriers of severe genetic disorders be allowed to bear children? Should all pregnancies

JESSICA G. DAVIS, M.D. • Associate Clinical Professor, Department of Pediatrics, Cornell University College of Medicine; Director, Child Development Center/Genetics Program, North Shore University Hospital; a teaching affiliate of Cornell University College of Medicine, Manhasset, Long Island, New York 11030.

be monitored for chromosome abnormalities? What criteria should be met for genetic screening programs? Can an individual's genetic makeup be altered? Should these questions even be asked? And by whom?

In order to weigh such issues and to recognize both the potential good and the inherent danger, it is important to understand basic genetic principles and how such knowledge is applied in medical practice today.

A REVIEW OF CURRENT MEDICAL GENETIC PRINCIPLES

There are three major groups of genetic disorders: chromosome disorders, Mendelian (single-gene) disorders, and multifactorial (polygenic) disorders.

CHROMOSOME DISORDERS. The cells of all living organisms contain a fixed amount of genetic material in their nuclei. The genetic material is arranged in distinct units called chromosomes (Fig. 1). Each chromosome is believed to contain hundreds, if not thousands, of genes. In humans, most cells contain 46 chromosomes, or 23 like(homologous) chromosome pairs. Important exceptions are the reproductive cells, the ovum and the sperm, which each contain 23 unpaired chromosomes, or half the number allotted to humans.

Of the 23 chromosome pairs, 22 pairs are called autosomes. The remaining pair are called sex chromosomes and are identified as the X and the Y chromosomes. A normal human female is designated 46,XX because her total chromosomal number is 46, consisting of 44 autosomes and 2 X chromosomes. A normal male is designated 46,XY because his total chromosomal number is 46, consisting of 44 autosomes and a single X and a single Y chromosome.

Chromosomal analysis is usually performed on special preparations of peripheral blood leukocytes. Similar studies also can be done on cells derived from bone marrow, skin biopsy, and amniotic fluid. The recent development of fluorescent staining or banding techniques enables precise chromosome identification and permits analysis of smaller chromosomal segments. Chromosomes are counted and arranged in pairs according to size, shape, and banding patterns. Each pair is then numbered according to a uniform system of identification (Figs. 2,3).[1]

In 1959, an extra chromosome, number 21, was found in white blood cells obtained from individuals with Down syndrome, or mongolism.[2] Affected individuals were said to have Trisomy 21, or 47,XY + 21 or 47,XX + 21. This was the first time a specific chromosomal anomaly was linked to a constellation of clinical findings. Other

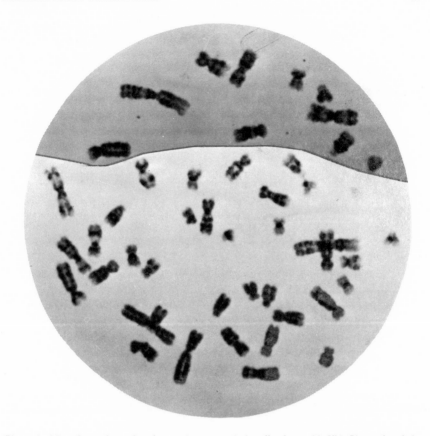

Figure 1. Metaphase plate taken for a primary amniotic cell culture, 46, XY. Giemsa banded.

human chromosome abnormality syndromes were reported, usually associated with either a structural rearrangement of chromosomal material or a deviation in the number of sex chromosomes or autosomes. The initial discoveries were made in persons exhibiting problems of sexual differentiation, physical malformation, mental retardation, or chronic myelogenous leukemia. Subsequently, laboratory studies on cells have uncovered gross chromosomal deviations in patients showing no evidence of physical or cognitive problems.

Chromosome disorders are classified as genetic because there is either excessive or deficient chromosomal DNA. Cytogenetic abnormalities are seldom familial, or inherited, and usually occur as isolated events in any one family's history. Chromosomal surveys of live-born infants show that approximately 1 in 200 newborns display a major chromosome variation. The most frequently seen autosomal chromo-

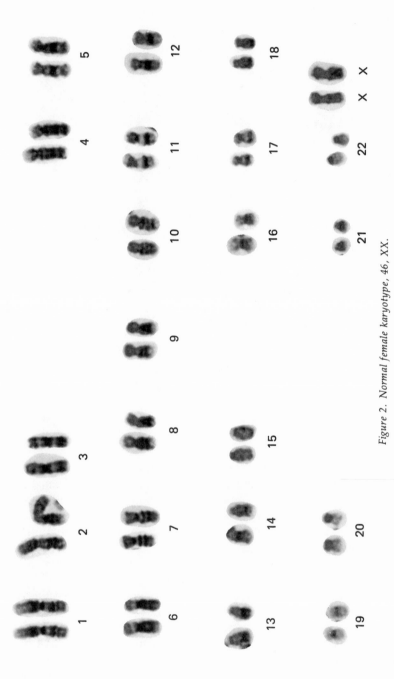

Figure 2. Normal female karyotype, 46, XX.

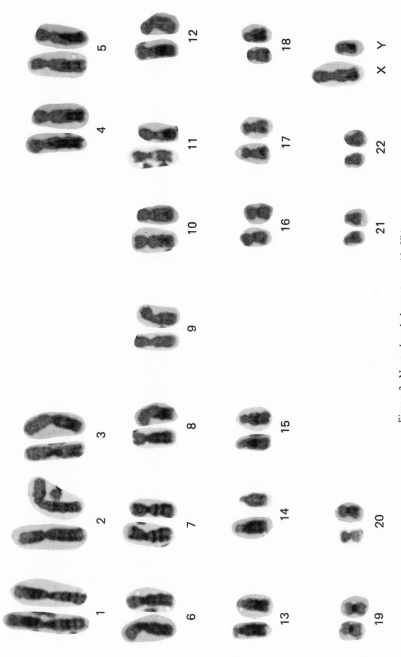

Figure 3. Normal male karyotype, 46, XY.

some disorder is trisomy 21 in Down syndrome, with an overall frequency of 1 in 600 live births.

MENDELIAN (SINGLE-GENE) DISORDERS. More than 2,336 Mendelian (single-gene) disorders have been described, but the frequency of many of these clinical entities is presently unknown.[3] Single-gene disorders follow the classic patterns of inheritance established by Gregor Mendel in 1865.[4] They are classified according to their mode of genetic transmission as autosomal dominant, autosomal recessive, or X-linked recessive.

Mendelian disorders occur because of the presence and action of one or a pair of mutant genes. In order to understand Mendelian patterns of inheritance, it is important to know that genes encoding specific biochemical information occur in pairs and are located at specific chromosomal sites, called loci. Normal individuals receive one member of each gene pair and one member of each chromosome pair from each of their parents. Since human beings possess homologous pairs of autosomal chromosomes, each individual will have a pair of genes each situated at a given locus, one on each chromosomal homologue.

Genes also can occur at the same locus in alternative forms called alleles. Any given individual may have two alleles for a given unique but paired locus.[5] If this occurs, the protein products at such paired loci may not be identical. The term nonallele refers to genes at different loci. For example the hemoglobin molecule is composed of three distinct biochemical subunits, alpha and beta chains and heme. The genes for the alpha chains of globin are nonalleles of the genes coding for the beta chains because there are two sets of gene pairs, each located at different chromosomal sites.

Autosomal Dominant Inheritance. Autosomal dominant disorders arise through mutation and are determined by genes that express themselves in a single dose in the male or female. Affected individuals have a mutant allele on one chromosome and a normal allele on the homologous chromosome at the identical locus. If a given autosomal dominant condition is not lethal and does not interfere with reproduction, the mutant autosomal dominant gene can be passed directly from one generation to the next. It is estimated that affected individuals with known autosomal dominant conditions have a 50 percent chance of transmitting the mutant gene to each of their offspring. There are 1,218 known autosomal dominant disorders.[3] Specific examples include primary hyperlipidemia and Huntington disease.

Five groups of disorders involving elevated plasma lipids have been identified and may affect 1 percent of the general population.[6,7,8] Findings in affected individuals include elevated plasma lipids and a predisposition to premature arteriosclerosis.[9] Evidence of type II disease or familial hyperbetalipoproteinemia can be obtained by testing one or more first-degree relatives. Affected individuals now are treated with appropriate drugs and dietary control of fat intake. At present, there is no mechanism to identify all individuals at risk for this condition. Furthermore, little information exists about the efficacy of the therapeutic regimens in the prevention of vascular disease.[10,11,12]

Huntington disease is a progressive lethal neurologic disorder. Affected individuals usually are diagnosed between thirty and forty years of age.[10] Cardinal features include dementia and rapid writhing of the limbs, trunk, and face. The underlying biochemical defect is not known, and there is no specific diagnostic test available. A positive family history helps determine which individuals might develop Huntington disease but the diagnosis usually can only be made when the clinical manifestations appear. There also is no satisfactory treatment for this disease. The incidence of this disorder in Michigan was reported as 1 in 25,000.[13]

Autosomal Recessive Inheritance. Autosomal recessive disorders occur when both alleles in a particular gene pair are deleterious. Mutation gives rise to gene variants that often are transmitted through successive generations in the benign heterozygous, or carrier, state. However, if two clinically normal carriers of the same harmful gene mate, there is a 25 percent chance that their offspring will receive a double dose of the harmful genes and exhibit the characteristic symptoms of that particular autosomal recessive disorder. Statistically, such a carrier couple has the same 25 percent chance of giving birth to a child with a recessive disorder with each pregnancy.

Investigators have identified 947 autosomal recessive disorders,[3] including many inborn errors of metabolism, such as Tay-Sachs disease. Individuals with Tay-Sachs disease lack a specific enzyme (i.e., hexosaminidase A),[14] which results in the accumulation of a fatty substance (i.e., GM_2 ganglioside) in the cells of the central nervous system, which in turn causes neurological problems. Symptoms first appear in infants of about six months of age and progress, resulting in death at four to six years. There is no treatment for Tay-Sachs disease. It occurs primarily in the offspring of Jews of Eastern European origin, with a frequency of approximately 1 in 3,000 live births.[15] Sensitive, reliable tests can identify the affected homozygote as well as the heterozygote, or carrier.[16]

Phenylketonuria (PKU) is another example of an inborn error of metabolism. Individuals with PKU lack an enzyme that is necessary for the metabolism of phenylalanine, an amino acid. Severe and irreversible neurologic deterioration occurs if an affected individual is not diagnosed and treated shortly after birth.[17] Most states have mandated inexpensive, simple, and accurate tests to screen for PKU in the newborn.[18] A low-phenylalanine diet can be instituted shortly after birth, effectively preventing a substantial amount of the otherwise inevitable mental retardation. There is no carrier test available.

X-Linked Recessive Disorders. The X-linked recessive disorders occur primarily in males and are transmitted by females. Males have a single X chromosome and a single Y chromosome. The Y chromosome bears only the gene or genes necessary for differentiation of the testes. Males have a single copy of the genes on the X chromosome. If a male's X chromosome contains a harmful allele, he will have an X-linked recessive disorder, such as hemophilia A or Duchenne muscular dystrophy. Females are usually heterozygous for X-linked recessive genes and are generally asymptomatic. Females become carriers of X-linked recessive disorders either by inheriting the gene from their mothers or by a fresh mutation.

Recurrence risks can be accurately calculated for X-linked recessive disorders. The sex chromosome makeup of a male is determined by the fact that he inherits an X chromosome from his mother and a Y chromosome from his father. Similarly, a female with an XX chromosome complement receives one X from her mother and one X from her father. Thus, there is a 50 percent chance of having either a girl or a boy with each pregnancy. If the mother's X chromosomes are free of aberrant X-linked recessive alleles, she has a 50 percent chance of having a normal male infant and a 50 percent chance of having a normal female child because she transmits only normal X chromosomes. However, if she is a carrier of an X-linked recessive disorder, she still has a 50 percent chance of having a son, but of her sons, 50 percent are at risk for having an X-linked disorder, and 50 percent will be problem free. Although all of her daughters would be normal, 50 percent run the risk of being carriers of an X-linked recessive allele like their mother, and the remaining 50 percent would not be carriers.

Approximately 150 X-linked recessive disorders have been identified.[3] One of the most common is a deficiency of a red blood cell enzyme, glucose-6-phosphate dehydrogenase (G–6–PD).[19] Many molecular variants of human G–6–PD have been identified. For instance, the A variant associated with G–6–PD deficiency is found in approximately 10 to 14 percent of black males in the United States. Mild hemolysis, or a breakdown of red blood cells, will occur if affected individuals are exposed to drugs such as antimalarials.

Hemophilia A is another X-linked recessive disorder characterized by a coagulation defect caused by a marked reduction of specific plasma factor activity. The frequency of severe hemophilia A is estimated at 1 in 8,600 males.[20] Recent technological advances have made prophylactic therapy possible. Supplies of the necessary concentrate are too limited for a continuing program of prophylactic treatment of a large affected population.[21] Currently, hemorrhagic episodes are managed with concentrates of Factor VIII, fresh frozen plasma, or lyophilized plasma.

MULTIFACTORIAL (POLYGENIC) DISORDERS. Multifactorial problems constitute the third group of genetic disorders. We believe that polygenic disorders result from the interaction of many gene pairs with one another and with environmental factors. This diagnostic category includes many congenital malformations, such as cleft lip, cleft palate, clubfoot, and defects of the developing nervous system. The true incidence of polygenic disorders is unknown. Statistical evidence varies because of differences in the ages of the study sample, diagnostic criteria, methods of ascertainment and skills of the observers. In an Edinburgh study of 8,684 babies, 5.4 percent had congenital malformations, with major abnormalities occurring in 2.1 percent and minor abnormalities in 3.3 percent.[22] A Swedish study of 6,200 infants showed 3.3 percent had major anomalies, and 9.6 percent exhibited minor problems.[23]

The probability of recurrence for most polygenic disorders is low. More accurate recurrence risk figures can be calculated for certain polygenically inherited disorders, such as spina bifida, depending on the exact family history and the number of previously affected offspring.

CLINICAL APPLICATION OF GENETIC THEORY

GENETIC COUNSELING. In the past, genetic counseling was limited to the simple identification of problems that "ran in families." With the acceptance of Mendelian principles, however, physicians soon recognized that a small number of diseases followed specific patterns of inheritance, and they could advise patients about risks of recurrence. Rapid progress in medical genetics in the past two decades led to an expansion of the number of practical applications of genetic information. Initially, the term "genetic counseling" was used to describe the process of collecting genetic data and determining recurrence risks. In 1970, a series of steps in the genetic counseling process was outlined:

1. Establishing the risk of recurrence of disease.
2. Interpreting this risk in meaningful terms.
3. Aiding the counselee to weigh the risk.
4. Reinforcing the risk and estimating its effect on the counselee through follow-up counseling.[24]

More recently, the genetic counseling process has been defined as "the delivery of professional advice concerning the magnitude of, the implication of, and the alternatives for dealing with risk of occurrence of a hereditary disorder within a family."[25] Furthermore, it has been suggested that a ". . . . more comprehensive definition . . . the clear communication of all the medical, social and genetic facts related to the condition under consideration, including the prognosis for the condition as well as the possible consequences of one or another mode of action," is necessary because "counseling is an educational process and should provide emotional support, but should not be directive in the decision-making process of the counselee."[26] This can be extended to consider that ". . . a really effective counselor goes one very important step further in that he continues to support that patient whether he agrees with the decisions arrived at or not."[27:34] Some counselors, however, view genetic counseling as a traditional form of medical practice and give advice, usually directed at decreasing the fertility of carriers of mutant genes and preventing reproduction among couples at risk for having an affected offspring.

People obtain genetic services in different ways. Many are self-referred. Some are seen because a relative has been counseled. Others come at the suggestion of a family physician, medical specialist, clergyman, social worker, or nurse. Some are directed by schools or other community agencies such as adoption services, foster care, or parent groups.

Individuals and families seek genetic services for many reasons. Some have given birth to a child with a genetic disorder or a congenital malformation. Others have clinical evidence of a genetic problem or have an affected family member. Women who are thirty-five and older and are planning to become pregnant should seek genetic information because there is an increased risk that they could give birth to a child with a chromosome anomaly. Some couples wish to discuss problems associated with consanguinity. Many women are worried about the effects of exposure to potential or actual environmental hazards on both the outcome of pregnancy and their own genetic material. Others may have a history of miscarriages. Many individuals come because of problems with growth and with the development of secondary sex characterics. Some come for carrier detection tests.

The number of individuals seeking genetic services increases each year. There also has been an increase in the total number of genetic units so that there are now more than 600 genetic programs in the United States. All of these programs are hospital-based, with associated laboratory services. Some major medical centers have developed satellite clinics to reach out into surrounding communities and into remote geographic areas. Genetic services are delivered by a multidisciplinary team composed of medical geneticists, physicians, nurses, social workers, associates in genetic counseling, laboratory personnel, and office staff.

The genetic counseling process begins with determining the reasons for and the source of referral. If an individual or a family has no knowledge of genetics, time must be spent outlining the scope of the program. Individuals and families should understand that, before they can be advised of their actual risks and options, all aspects of the problem must be fully explored.

The counselor then obtains a complete family history and draws up a detailed pedigree. All past and present medical problems are reviewed systematically. The history includes data about the individual's age, nationality, habits, diet, hobbies, education, and vocation. The patient's possible exposure to infection and environmental hazards, such as X-rays, drugs, and chemicals, is investigated. If pertinent, the counselor reviews the facts concerning conception, spontaneous abortion, stillbirths, and contraception. The counselor will study all available records, including birth, medical, and autopsy reports. Examination of family records and photographs also may prove helpful.

The affected individual and possibly other close relatives then undergo a complete physical examination. If necessary, medical consultation will be obtained from such specialists as neurologists, ophthalmologists, and audiologists. Specific laboratory tests, including biochemical and cytogenetic studies, may be performed. When the information is all gathered, the genetic counselor reviews the assembled data, including the results of any laboratory tests, and arrives at as precise a diagnosis as possible. The counselor first decides whether the problem is genetic or is caused by a known environmental factor. If environmental factors are ruled out, the counselor next attempts to pinpoint the mode of inheritance.

The counselor outlines the conclusions to the concerned individual or family at an informing interview. At this time, the counselor reviews the reasons for referral and the history, the pertinent findings on physical examination, and the laboratory data. Discussion focuses on the diagnosis and the prognosis. The mode of inheritance and the recurrence risks are fully explained. Finally, all possible options are considered, such as appropriate therapeutic and rehabilitation measures or amniocentesis.

Genetic counseling is time consuming. Counselors and their patients need time to exchange information and to absorb facts. Additional follow-up sessions may be necessary in order to answer questions and to more thoroughly communicate genetic concepts. Many counselors send detailed letters to their patients summarizing the results of the genetic workup.

IMPACT OF GENETIC COUNSELING. What happens to individuals who have gone through genetic counseling or even group screening? Do they avoid conception? Do they accept low risks of conceiving children with genetic problems? Are their sex lives disrupted? Unfortunately, genetic counselors have barely begun to ask these questions, and the answers are far from definitive.

One group of investigators studied the responses of 455 couples to a variety of genetic disorders and to counseling. They showed that parents of patients with major medical problems, high mortality, and a high risk of repetition were generally deterred from further reproduction.[28] Parents of patients with less severe handicaps and a high or low risk of recurrence did not curtail reproduction. A follow-up study also revealed that most parents understood the nature of the disorder and their risks. Less optimistic results were reported in a study designed to understand the attitudes of parents toward genetic counseling and the reasons for its success or failure.[29] Reactions of parents with children with known genetic diseases who had received genetic counseling as well as of parents of children with severe nongenetic disorders who had not received counseling were reported. Evidence given by families suggested that reproductive attitudes are determined more by the sense of burden imparted by the disease than by knowledge of its precise risk figures. The term "burden" refers to the medical problems of the disease, including early mortality as well as the parents' perceptions of the physical, emotional, and financial factors involved. Of the families counseled, 50 percent had a good grasp of the information, 25 percent gained some knowledge, and 25 percent learned very little. The authors found that the obstacles to effective genetic counseling include lack of public awareness; limited knowledge of human biology and genetics; differences in the contexts in which the counseling was provided; and the personal qualities, ability to communicate, and knowledge of the physicians providing the counseling. More information is needed about the techniques and results of genetic counseling and about the effect of genetic counseling on larger populations and for a variety of medical disorders. The complexity of the role that genetic counseling plays in decision making for common multifactorial problems remains untouched. More data are needed on the factors that motivate persons to seek or avoid genetic counseling.

CARRIERS OF GENETIC DISORDERS. One possible deterrent to seeking genetic information may be the fear of being labeled a carrier.

Negative attitudes toward carrier status derive from superstitious beliefs and also from ideas originating in the late nineteenth century, which was the era of eugenics, a cultural movement of social reform and betterment that emphasized such concepts as racial fitness and planned breeding. Human eugenics can be divided into positive eugenics and negative eugenics. Proponents of positive eugenics urged the preferential breeding of so-called superior individuals. Champions of negative eugenics encouraged legal prohibitions of reproduction by individuals phenotypically afflicted with so-called genetic disorders or suspected of carrying such undesirable traits.

Today, genetic disorders and carrier status are no longer viewed as threats to society's well-being, but rather as individual and family problems. Emphasis has shifted to concepts of genetic health and prevention of genetic disease. Accurate laboratory tests have enabled the identification of carriers, or healthy individuals heterozygous for deleterious genes.

The ability to detect carrier status improves genetic counseling but also results in the detection of individuals or couples at risk for a specific genetic disorder who were previously unaware of their risks. Screening programs with concomitant carrier status disclosure have already been initiated to test populations at risk for such disorders as sickle-cell anemia[30] and Tay-Sachs disease.[31] The experience with screening has led to concern about how to effectively incorporate information about genetic disorders into the health care delivery system.

The personal significance of being labeled carrier also is not well understood. Despite the fact that each person's stores of nuclear DNA are unique catalogues of genetic instructions, few individuals realize that all human beings are heterozygous, or carriers of altered genetic material. With respect to recessive disorders, it has been estimated that we all carry three to eight deleterious genes, which, if paired with the same mutant gene, result in the birth of an afflicted child.

The disclosure of carrier status leads to the acquisition of knowledge about previously hidden aspects of oneself. Such revelations can cause anxiety and threaten an individual's sense of personal worth and integrity. Labeling an individual a carrier also can lead to changes in social relationships. Carrier detection may impose limitations on mate-selection patterns and on parenthood. For example, if carrier detection for a recessive disorder is carried out premaritally and identified carriers are effectively counseled and no major psychological difficulties ensue, such individuals may restrict their choice of mate in order to prevent the birth of an abnormal child.[32] However, if carrier detection occurs at or after the time of marriage, disclosure can lead to discord and even to marital dissolution. For example, a carefully designed screening program for sickle-cell heterozygotes was carried out in the Greek village of Orchomenos. Prior to the study, approximately four carrier–carrier marriages took place annually. Despite intensive genetic counseling and the fact that the villagers were concerned about the fact that approximately 1 in 100 births resulted in a child with sickle-cell anemia, the author found that four carrier–carrier marriages still took place each year. Although some engagements were disrupted and prevented, many carriers lied about their status to prospective mates.[33]

Parents of a child with a genetic disorder are usually devastated, frightened, and grieving.[34] Studies of mothers of hemophiliac children suggest that they experience severe guilt because they perceive themselves as being genetically responsible.[35] Full disclosure of information about the mode of transmission and carrier status can lead to a variety of emotional responses, including denial, anger, and guilt. As a result, married couples may express ambivalence, curtail family size, or change partners unless such options as amniocentesis or artificial insemination are acceptable and available. More information is needed about the effect and possible stigmatization resulting from disclosure of carrier status. Murray's "Soliloquy on Screening" focuses on the problems posed by carrier detection and genetic screening:

> To screen or not to screen
>   That is the question!
> Whether it is nobler to proceed
>   With a test for mutant genes
> Only after the minds of all have been prepared
>   By proper education
> Or to begin to test, anon, because
>   It is the thing to do.
> One should not ask
>   To test
> Without informed consent!
>   Alas, in time
> Ignorance and confusion
>   In the minds of parents and screenees
> May cause pain, suffering, and stigmatization
>   To those innocents who ask not
> For the genes they are heir to.
>   And, may at some distant day
> Defame those who screen.
>   For whether one should test a pound of flesh,
> A single cell or a drop of blood
>   It is that person tested who must
> Live with and adjust to
>   The label "carrier"
> And therein lies the rub!![36]

AMNIOCENTESIS. The use of amniocentesis has expanded the clinical application of genetic knowledge in medical practice. Amniocentesis is a technique used to obtain samples of amniotic fluid and fetal cells for the prenatal detection of fetal disorders. It was first employed as a diagnostic aid in 1930. During the last decade, it has been a useful tool in the management of problems arising from Rh incompatibility.[37] Since 1968, this technique has been utilized for prenatal diagnoses of chromosome abnormalities, certain biochemical disorders,[38,39] and one type of birth defect, namely, open defects of the fetus's developing nervous system.[40] Prenatal diagnosis usually provides reassuring news since 95 percent of all such studies produce favorable genetic results.[41] When amniocentesis has unfavorable results, couples have the option of therapeutic abortion.

Amniocentesis for antenatal diagnosis is performed by experienced obstetricians as an out-patient procedure between sixteen and twenty weeks' gestation. Local anesthesia is applied to minimize discomfort. The procedure entails the passage of a needle through the abdominal wall into the uterine cavity and the subsequent withdrawal of a small amount of amniotic fluid, which surrounds the developing fetus in utero. The amniotic fluid is placed in sterile containers and should reach the laboratory within twenty-four hours.

ULTRASONOGRAPHY. Ultrasonography usually is performed just prior to or simultaneously with amniocentesis. Ultrasonography is a technique that employs pulsed sound waves[42] to visualize the placenta and the fetus. Sound wave pictures enable physicians to localize the placenta, to diagnose twin pregnancies, and to determine the exact stage of pregnancy. Fetal growth and head circumference also can be measured at appropriate intervals.[43]

The overall risk of amniocentesis performed in early pregnancy for antenatal diagnosis is 0.5 percent. Possible risks include spontaneous abortion, vaginal bleeding, laboratory error, and fetal injury. This overall risk figure was derived from data obtained from a collaborative study sponsored by the National Institutes of Child Health and Human Development.[44] The study involved 1,040 pregnant women who had amniocentesis and 992 who did not. The key issue in the four-year study was whether or not the procedure adversely affected the outcome of the pregnancy. The project investigated the safety, accuracy, and reliability of the procedure; the indications for amniocentesis; and the outcomes of all pregnancies. Data also were obtained on the growth and development of the children born following such pregnancy monitoring. The study determined that amniocentesis was a useful, safe, and accurate procedure: there was no statistical difference in the rate of fetal loss through spontaneous abortion and stillbirth between the women who underwent amniocentesis and the control group. The children born to the women who had amniocentesis exhibited normal growth and development. Reassurance about the positive outcome of pregnancy occurred in 95 percent of the cases.

Specific prenatal diagnosis is still not possible for many congenital anomalies or for all Mendelian disorders. For example, amniocentesis for such X-linked disorders as hemophilia A can only determine fetal sex. Of 115 pregnant women undergoing amniocentesis to determine fetal sex for a variety of X-linked conditions, fifty-four women were found to be carrying male fetuses.[41:59-61] Of these, forty women underwent therapeutic abortions while fourteen decided not to terminate the pregnancy because of the fact that 50 percent of these male fetuses would be unaffected or only mildly or moderately affected and because of theologic reasons or inadequate genetic counseling.

With the increased acceptance and utilization of amniocentesis, more and more prenatal diagnoses will be performed each year. Many observers believe that amniocentesis eventually will become a routine part of antenatal care. At present, obstetricians at major centers offer amniocentesis to all pregnant women past the age of thirty-five because they have an increased risk of bearing a child with a chromosome abnormality, particularly Trisomy 21.[45] A fetal chromosome screening program will be implemented in 1978 in New York City to provide all pregnant women at risk with this option.[46]

All women should have access to information about antenatal diagnosis and the kinds of information amniocentesis can and cannot provide. It is expected that, as public and professional knowledge about genetic disorders and amniocentesis increases, demands for services will soar. The anticipated proliferation of heterozygote detection tests as well as the development of other prenatal diagnostic procedures, such as fetal visualization, will add to the workload of centers providing such genetic services as amniocentesis. Concerned medical personnel are now attempting to devise ways to meet the already growing need for appropriate genetic services for all at-risk pregnancies.

Efforts also are under way to set up guidelines for amniocentesis. Prenatal diagnosis is available for a variety of genetic disorders, which vary in degree of severity and burden. Terminations of pregnancy may not be warranted in all cases. The dilemma becomes more apparent when a treatable genetic disorder, such as phenylketonuria, or a condition with unknown risks, such as an XYY fetus, is diagnosed prenatally. Physicians also are concerned about whether or not they will be obliged to provide amniocentesis to any patient who requests the procedure, no matter what the reason. Some feel amniocentesis should be used only to diagnose severe and untreatable disorders. At the present time, observers must view prenatal diagnosis as ". . . both a life-giving and life-saving procedure. . . ."[27:35]

SEX DIFFERENTIATION DISORDERS. Disorders of sexual differentiation are encountered frequently in the practice of medicine. Many minor anomalies can be easily corrected. Major problems may require the skillful application of surgical procedures, pharmacologic agents, and sex assignment.

Initially, the sex characteristics of humans are determined by the genes of the sex chromosomes. These genes affect sexually bipotential gonads during the later stages of morphogenesis. If a Y chromosome is present, the sexually uncommitted gonad is transformed into a testis. The fetal testis elaborates masculinizing steroid hormones, which in turn act on the ductal system and external genitalia to form the male reproductive organs.[47] The testis also produces a hormone that inhibits the development of certain embryonic structures that have the potential of developing into portions of the female reproductive tract.[48] If the Y chromosome is not present, the fetal gonad undergoes ovarian differentiation, and the reproductive tract is female.

Sex chromosome disorders, hereditary defects of the enzymatic synthesis of testosterone, inborn errors of steroid metabolism of the adrenal gland, peripheral androgen insensitivity that is transmitted as an X-linked disorder, and the treatment of pregnant women with steroids can all result in problems of sexual differentiation. A variety of syndromes including autosomal chromosome disorders also may be associated with anomalies of sexual development.

Depending on the clinical findings and the nature of the underlying problem, the diagnosis can be suspected at various chronologic ages. A definitive diagnosis is made following the collection and analysis of data from the medical history, physical examination, such laboratory assays as cytogenetic studies, and appropriate X-rays. In some cases, biopsy of the gonads and surgical exploration are needed.

Ambiguous genitalia may be recognized in the delivery room or newborn nursery. Sex assignment must be deferred until the diagnostic workup is complete and appropriate treatment is planned. Therapy is designed to promote physical and psychologic well-being. Gender identity may contradict chromosomal, hormonal, or gonadal sex. It more generally agrees with the morphology of a person's external genitalia and assigned sex.

The child's family must be involved in all aspects of case management. Health care personnel working with the family are urged to be humane and diplomatic to

> avoid the freak-show implications of indeterminate sex and use instead the
> explanation that the baby was born with its *sex organs unfinished* or *in-
> completely differentiated*. The medical and surgical implication which fol-
> lows is that they can be finished and the situation is not hopeless.[49:611]

Diagrams and drawings are used to provide the necessary medical information that parents need in order to arrive at an appropriate decision about sex assignment or reassignment. The fact that parents must ". . . feel a sense of conviction that the decision to be made for their baby is the only possible correct one" has been stressed.[49:612] Parents must understand that at birth and up until the age of early language acquisition, psychosexual differentiation depends on the sex of assignment, on family attitudes and rearing practices, and on experience. The critical period is passed in the preschool years, when psychosexual identity is fixed. If the parents feel uncomfortable, negativistic, or doubtful about their decision, these attitudes eventually will be transmitted to the child and interfere with normal maturation.

Parents also must be helped to deal directly with other family members, such as siblings and grandparents. They need to be able to speak comfortably with friends and neighbors in order to avoid fear and embarrassment. It is particularly important to tell parents faced with this problem that such children do not grow up as bisexual or homosexual. Typically, they differentiate according to the assigned sex, developing a monosexual gender identity. Counseling for patients and their families as well as appropriate medical and endocrinologic follow-up should continue as the child grows older. The preadolescent child needs some explanation about his/her condition. Diagnostic and prognostic information can and should be shared in a constructive, open fashion. Teenagers require information about parenthood. Patients who are sterile must be informed of the possibility of parenthood by adoption or by donor insemination. Fertile patients must be informed about possible genetic transmission of their problem. Individuals need guidance in how and when to explain their situation to prospective mates.

Problems of sexual differentiation in older children are far more complicated. Gender identity usually is fixed and irreversible in the older child. Ordinarily, a reassignment of sex would be psychologically disastrous. In a few instances, such as ambiguous or incongruous gender identity, sex reassignment resolves a dilemma and can be assimilated. Careful assessment of each individual's needs and psychiatric preparation is needed prior to treatment. Long-term psychiatric follow-up is essential. Some sex chromosome disorders have been diagnosed on the basis of a constellation of specific clinical findings. Examples of these include Turner and Klinefelter syndromes. Individ-

uals with Turner syndrome are short, infertile females who are missing one X chromosome (45, XO). Persons with Klinefelter syndrome
are eunuchoid males who have an extra X chromosome (47,XXY). Hormonal treatment permits the development of secondary Y characteristics but does not restore fertility.

Some males have been found to have an extra Y chromosome.[50:160]
The discovery of the extra sex chromosome in a male presents many
problems for the counselor. Early reports about the condition indicated that adult XYY males exhibited antisocial behavior. Subsequently, many investigators questioned whether the "discovery of
an extra sex chromosome (i.e., Y chromosome) in a male predicts antisocial behavior with the confidence, for instance, that the observation of trisomy 21 predicts mental retardation."[50:139] A synthesis of all
current information led one investigator to conclude that

> telling the parents of the diagnosis and possible prognosis is likely to in-
> duce more difficulties for both child and family than not informing them,
> particularly since the precise behavioral risks are uncertain and there are
> no therapeutic preventive measures known at present that are specific for
> an individual with the XYY genotype.[51]

Clearly, more data are needed about the prognosis for this condition.

ETHICAL CONSIDERATIONS. In most scientific communities, genetic
principles are considered morally neutral, like arithmetic: there are no
imperatives dictated by this body of knowledge. But the use to which
a society puts this knowledge may well indicate its level of civilization. If genetic principles are neutral, facts that propel patients to particular kinds of actions (such as abortion) must be tinged with the
norms of the society rather than any imperative inherent in genetics.
Current genetic practice includes counseling, screening for carriers of
deleterious genetic traits, and intrauterine diagnosis. The benefits of
these innovations include the reduction of human suffering and the
increase of human joy through the birth of a healthy child.

The benefits gained from the use of genetic technology must be
carefully weighed. Where does genetic responsibility lie? What are the
rights and obligations of the individual, the family, the genetic counselor, and the society? Do parents have the right to determine the
genetic quality of their children? Do individuals at risk have a duty to
undergo genetic counseling? Should the use of genetic innovations be
voluntary or mandatory? It is beyond the scope of this chapter to offer
conclusions or to answer the numerous ethical conundrums facing us.
It is perhaps sufficient for a practitioner to note that the potential
benefits to humankind from genetic knowledge are worth the necessary engagement in the social and moral issues arising out of the discipline.

References

1. Hamerton JL, Jacobs PA, Klinger HP: *Paris conference (1971): standardization in human cytogenetics, Birth defects: Original article series.* Vol VIII, no 7. Edited by Bergsma, D. White Plains, The National Foundation-March of Dimes, 1972.
2. Lejeune J, Gautier M, Turpin R: Les chromosomes humains en culture de tissus. *Comptes Rendus Hebdomadaires des Seances de l'Academie des Sciences 248*: 602, 1959.
3. McKusick VA: *Mendelian inheritance in man: catalogs of autosomal dominant, autosomal recessive and x-linked phenotypes.* Fourth edition. Baltimore, The Johns Hopkins University Press, 1975, pp lviii–lxviii.
4. Mendel G.: Experiments in plant hybridization, in *Classic papers in genetics.* Edited by Peters, JA. Englewood Cliffs, N.J.: Prentice-Hall, pp. 1–20, 1959.
5. Harris H: *The principles of human biochemical genetics.* Second edition. New York: American Elsevier, 1975, pp 278–367.
6. Frederickson DS, Lees RS: A system for phenotyping hyperlipoproteinemia *Circulation 31*:321, 1965.
7. Glueck CJ, Heckman F, Schoenfeld M et al: Neonatal familial type II hyperlipoproteinemia: cord blood cholesterol in 1800 births. *Metabolism 6*:597, 1971.
8. Goldstein, JL, Hazzard WR, Schrott HG et al.: Hyperlipidemia in coronary heart disease. I. Lipid levels in 500 survivors of myocardial infarction. II. Genetic analysis of lipid levels in 176 families and delineation of a new inherited disorder, combined hyperlipidemia. III. Evaluation of lipoprotein phenotypes of 156 genetically defined survivors of myocardial infarction. *Journal of Clinical Investigation 52*:1533, 1544, 1569, 1973.
9. Kennel WB, Castelli WP, Gordon T, McNamara PM: Serum cholesterol, lipoproteins and the risk of coronary heart disease. *Annals of Internal Medicine 74*:1, 1971.
10. *Arteriosclerosis,* report by Task Force on Arteriosclerosis, National Heart and Lung Institute, June 1971.
11. Glueck CJ, Tsang RC: Pediatric familial type II hyperlipoproteinemia: effects of diet on plasma cholesterol in the first year of life. *American Journal of Clinical Nutrition 25*:224, 1972.
12. Kennel WB, Dawber TR: Arteriosclerosis as a pediatric problem. *Journal of Pediatrics 80*:544, 1972.
13. Chandler JH, Reed TE, Dejong RN: Huntington's chorea in Michigan. *Neurology 10*:148–53, 1960
14. Okada S, O'Brien JS: Tay-Sachs disease: generalized absence of a beta-d-n-acetylhexosaminidase component. *Science 165*:698–700, 1969.
15. Aronson SM: Epidemiology, in *Tay-Sachs disease.* Edited by Volk BW. New York, Grune & Stratton, 1964.
16. Brady RO, Johnson WG, Uhlendorf BW: Identification of heterozygous carriers of lipid storage diseases. *American Journal of Medicine 51*:423, 1971.
17. Knox WE: Phenylketonuria, in *The metabolic basis of inherited disease.* Third edition. Edited by Stanbury JB, Wyngaarden JB, and Fredrickson DS. New York, McGraw-Hill, 1972, pp 266–295.
18. Guthrie R, Susi A: A simple phenylalanine method for detecting phenylketonuria in large populations of newborn infants. *Pediatrics 32*:338, 1963.
19. Beutler E: Glucose-6-phosphate dehydrogenase deficiency, in *The metabolic basis of inherited disease.* Edited by Stanbury JB, Wyngaarden JB, Fredrickson DS. New York, McGraw-Hill, 1972, p 1358.
20. *Summary report:* NHLI's Blood Resource Studies, publication no. (NIH) 73–416. Department of Health, Education and Welfare, Public Health Service, National Institutes of Health, 1972, p 101.

21. Meyers RD, Adams W, Dardick K et al: The social and economic impact of hemophilia—a survey of 70 cases in Vermont and New Hampshire. *American Journal of Public Health* 62:530, 1972.
22. Nelson MM, Forfar JO: Congenital abnormalities at birth: their association in the same patient. *Developmental Medicine and Child Neurology* 11:3, 1969.
23. Ekelund H, Kullander S, Kallen B: Major and minor malformations in newborns and infants up to one year of age. *Acta Paediatrica Scandinavica* 59:297, 1970.
24. Fraser FC: Counseling in genetics: the intent and scope, in *Genetic counseling. Birth defects: original article series*, vol. VI, no. 1. Edited by Bergsma D. Baltimore, Williams & Wilkins, for The National Foundation-March of Dimes, 1970, p 7.
25. Sly WS: What is genetic counseling? in *Contemporary genetic counseling, birth defects: original article series*. Vol IX, no 4. Edited by Bergsma D. White Plains, The National Foundation-March of Dimes, 1973, p 5.
26. Murray RF: The practitioner's view of the values involved in genetic screening and counseling, individual vs. societal imperatives, in *Ethical, social and legal dimensions of screening for human genetic disease. Birth defects: original article series*. Vol X, no 6. Edited by Bergsma D. New York, The National Foundation-March of Dimes, 1974, p 189.
27. Macintyre MN: Professional responsibility in prenatal genetic evaluation, in *Advances in human genetics and their impact on society. Birth defects: original article series*. Vol VIII, no 4. Edited by Bergsma D. White Plains, The National Foundation-March of Dimes, 1972, pp 34, 35.
28. Carter CO, Fraser Roberts JA, Evans KA et al: Genetic clinic: a follow-up. *Lancet* 1:281, 1971.
29. Leonard CO, Chase GA, Childs B: Genetic counseling: a consumer's view. *New England Journal of Medicine* 287:433–439, 1972.
30. Bowman JE: Mass screening programs for sickle hemoglobin: a sickle cell crisis. *Journal of the American Medical Association* 222:1650, 1972.
31. Kaback MM, Zeiger RS: Heterozygote detection in Tay-Sachs disease: a prototype community screening program for the prevention of recessive genetic disorders, in *Advances in experimental medicine and biology*. Vol. 19. Edited by Volk BW, Aronson SM. New York, Plenum Press, 1972, p 613.
32. Kaback MM, Becker MH, Ruth MV: Sociologic studies in human genetics, I. Compliance factors in a voluntary heterozygote screening program, in *Ethical, social and legal dimension of screening for human genetic disease. Birth defects: original article series*. Vol X, no 6. Edited by Bergsma D. New York, The National Foundation-March of Dimes, 1974, p 147.
33. Stamatoyannopoulos G: Problems of screening and counseling in the hemoglobinopathies. Read at the Fourth International Conference on Birth Defects, Vienna, Austria, September 2–8, 1973.
34. Golden DA, Davis JG: Counseling parents after the birth of an infant with Down's syndrome. *Children Today* 3:7, 1974.
35. Agle DP: Psychiatric studies of patients with hemophilia and related states. *Archives of Internal Medicine* 114:76, 1964.
36. Murray RF: Soliloquy on screening. *New England Journal of Medicine* 291:803, 1974.
37. Freda VJ: The Rh problem in obstetrics and a new concept of its management using amniocentesis and spectrophotometric scanning of amniotic fluid. *American Journal of Obstetrics and Gynecology* 92:341, 1965.
38. Nadler HL: Prenatal detection of genetic defects. *Journal of Pediatrics* 74:132, 1969.
39. Nadler HL, Gerbie AB: Role of amniocentesis in the intrauterine detection of genetic disorders. *New England Journal of Medicine* 282:596, 1970.
40. U. K. collaborative study on alpha-fetoprotein in relation to neural-tube defects. *Lancet* 1:1323, 1977.

41. Milunsky A: *The prenatal diagnosis of hereditary disorders.* Springfield, Ill., Charles C Thomas, 1973, pp 150, 159–161.
42. Hellman LM, Duffis GM, Donald I, Sunden B: Safety of diagnostic ultrasound in obstetrics. *Lancet* 1:1133, 1970.
43. Campbell S: The prediction of fetal maturity by ultrasonic measurement of the biparietal diameter. *Journal of Obstetrics and Gynaecology of the British Commonwealth* 76:603, 1969.
44. Cooper T: Implications of findings from the amniocentesis registry for public policy. *Public Health Reports* 91(2):116.
45. Harper PS: The prenatal diagnosis of metabolic disorders. *Journal of the Royal College of Physicians of London,* 7:251, 1973.
46. Stein Z, Susser M, Guterman AV: Screening programs for prevention of Down's syndrome. *Lancet* 1:305, 1973.
47. Jost A: Embryonic sexual differentiation, in *Hermaphroditism, genital anomalies and related endocrine disorders.* Second edition. Edited by Jones, HW, Scott WW. Baltimore, Williams & Wilkins, 1971.
48. Josso N: In vitro synthesis of mullerian-inhibiting hormone by seminiferous tubules isolated from the cell fetal testis. *Endocrinology* 93:829, 1973.
49. Money J: Psychologic counseling: hermaphroditism, in *Endocrine and genetic diseases of childhood and adolescence.* Second edition. Edited by Gardner LI. Philadelphia, WB Saunders, 1975, pp 611, 612.
50. Smith PG, Jacobs PA: Incidence studies of constitutional chromosome abnormalities in the post-natal population. *Pfizer Medical Monographs* 5:160, 1970.
51. Hook, EB: Behavioral implications of the human XYY genotype. *Science* 179:139, 1973.

Chapter 5

The Physiological Aspects of Pregnancy

EMANUEL A. FRIEDMAN

PSYCHOLOGY OF THE PREGNANT WOMAN

From a psychological point of view, pregnancy is a "maturational crisis" because it is a critical phase leading to motherhood with all its attendant responsibilities and obligations. The woman is transformed from a state in which she is her own mother's child to one in which she becomes her child's mother. This process involves an interval during which she may find that she must confront and resolve any earlier psychic conflicts in her own developmental phases.[1] Without such adaptive mechanisms, psychological growth and maturation cannot evolve.

The emotional upheaval is potentially great. Moreover, the situation is compounded by a regressive psychologic process in some pregnant women. The normal regression that occurs during pregnancy has been emphasized as one of the keys to understanding many of the psychopathologic symptoms.[2] Awareness of this mechanism aids attendant personnel to comprehend and deal with some of the childlike fears that exist. In addition, awareness that the pregnant woman may be particularly suggestible is of great benefit in terms of the reassurance and security that can be provided.

The commonly encountered admixture of ambivalent feelings toward pregnancy is often unwittingly enhanced by well-meaning but ill-advised attendant personnel. On the one hand, they repeatedly and

EMANUEL A. FRIEDMAN, M.D., Med. Sc. D. • Professor of Obstetrics and Gynecology, Harvard Medical School; Obstetrician-Gynecologist-in-Chief, Beth Israel Hospital, Boston, Massachusetts 02215.

appropriately reassure the patient that childbirth is a normal physiologic experience; on the other hand, they negate these reassurances by warning her about potential hazards and activities that may endanger her and her fetus. It is obvious that pregnant women must be approached on an individualized basis. Most require, and should be given, full assurance regarding specific and general matters that are of concern to them.[3] Wide experience holds that most phobias can be easily managed with simple, confident statements of assurance. And since most fears are not based on realistic concerns, such authoritative assurances usually aid the patient greatly.

Some fears are not expressed; most of these are probably based on deep-rooted fears of childhood or, more prevalently, fears of the unknown. Most women are readily relieved of such worries once they are thoroughly informed, making the situation considerably less stressful and more interesting to them. The effect of removing the fear response to stress as it relates to pain perception is the underlying basis of the psychoprophylactic approach to childbearing, which will be discussed in more detail later.

Unspoken fears, especially among professionals who may have delayed childbearing, stem from the very commonly held view that pregnancy is especially hazardous after, say, thirty years of age. This is based on unsubstantiated, albeit widely accepted, cultural taboos, and it is often reinforced by poorly informed authorities. While it is true that older pregnant women do not fare so well as their younger counterparts, the statistical data are too readily misinterpreted; they refer to rates of complications in the population at large. Even a cursory examination of such data quickly demonstrates that the older women who have difficulties in pregnancy are those with underlying or preexisting medical problems, particularly hypertension, kidney disorders, or diabetes, conditions that tend to appear later in life. The healthy gravida does not need to worry in this regard. Moreover, much of the remaining hazard of pregnancy in older women can be directly ascribed to frequent, closely spaced pregnancies, which take their toll without regard to age, although women who have many babies are perforce older than those who do not. Also, such women are more likely to manifest anemia, malnutrition, and debilitation, thereby compounding whatever obstetrical problem may arise. Although it is frequently stated that labor is longer and more difficult in older gravidas, careful study has failed to substantiate this. As to the fetus, the incidence of twinning increases with advancing age, especially with double ovum, or nonidentical, twins, but the increase in frequency is relatively small. Worth serious consideration, however, are the chromosomal anomalies encountered in about 1 percent of infants born to women over age forty (as contrasted with 0.1 percent under age thirty); fortunately, today they can be diagnosed during pregnancy by amniocentesis, a technique that examines the chromosome makeup of cells shed by the fetus into the amniotic fluid. This information permits such pregnancies to be terminated, if so desired by the gravida. The negative test obtained in most instances (99 percent) is very reassuring indeed and does much to relieve anxiety.

Emotional upheavals during pregnancy may assume many manifestations ranging from somaticized symptoms, such as ptyalism (excessive salivation) and hyperemesis (persistent vomiting), to palpitations, sleeplessness, confusion, or general malaise. More extreme manifestations range from depression to mania. Some may even express suicidal thoughts or the urge to destroy the fetus. When reassurance and symptomatic treatment are ineffective, psychiatric evaluation should be sought.

A growing body of evidence suggests that poor mother–child relationships are detrimental to the child's optimal development. Such serious pathologic processes can have their origins in pregnancy if the mother has a negative reaction to the fetus. The patient who takes a positive attitude will most likely relate well to the fetus both in utero and after it is born. Attendant personnel, by allaying fears, providing emotional support, and inspiring confidence, make it easier for the patient to experience and work through the difficult adjustments to pregnancy and its problems and responsibilities. Pregnancy can thus become a fulfilling and highly rewarding experience for her.

PHYSICAL ASPECTS OF PREGNANCY

The pregnant woman is a species apart. The physical changes that she undergoes are truly phenomenal and are associated with concomitant alterations in the subtle functioning of organ systems, tissues, and cells throughout her body. In general, such changes occur because of the altered hormonal milieu brought about by the pregnancy itself. Regulatory control is thus exerted by that portion of the developing conceptus that surrounds the embryo and that will later form the placenta. This structure, composed of numerous fingerlike projections of fetal tissue, serves not only as the lifeline for the developing embryo but also as an active biochemical laboratory to produce endocrine substances and enzymes that regulate the activities of the reproductive organs, including the adrenal and mammary glands, prepare the uterus for its later essential reproductive role (labor and delivery), and maintain the pregnancy. Under the influence of hormones elaborated by the placenta, uterine muscle undergoes enormous growth and increased production of complex biochemical compounds that will be needed in order for the uterus to generate sufficient contractility to effect delivery by expelling its contents at or near term. Simultaneously, it acts to prepare accessory organs, such as the breasts, so that they will function properly in lactation after delivery. Pregnancy is maintained by independent regulation of the hormonal environment, inhibition of uterine contractility, prevention of the expulsion of the conceptus, interference with the mechanisms of heterograft rejection, and suppression of cyclic pituitary–ovarian function.

The catalogue of physical manifestations of pregnancy extends to every organ system. Fortunately, none is of serious consequence to the healthy female. Aside from the obvious increase in abdominal girth and breast contour, pregnancy may temporarily affect skin pigmentation, producing the "mask of pregnancy" across the forehead, cheeks, and nose; circulation, by increasing heart rate, metabolic demands in terms of oxygen consumption, and blood volume, while simultaneously decreasing blood pressure and often producing relative degrees of anemia; gastrointestinal function, distorting the senses of taste and smell, evoking heartburn, nausea, and vomiting, diminishing appetite, increasing salivary secretion, and commonly yielding constipation. However, nearly all symptoms tend to be negligible or, at most, minor annoyances for most women during the course of pregnancy.

PLACENTAL FUNCTION

As mentioned, the placenta supports oxygenation, nutrition, and growth of the fetus and serves as a pathway for waste disposal. At the same time, it provides the fetus with a barrier against certain agents and organisms present in the mother. Whereas the maternal and fetal blood systems are completely separate and independent, most substances, including gases, ions, sugars, amino acids, and drugs of low molecular weight, cross from the maternal bloodstream to the fetal by way of the placenta. Certain disease states, such as diabetes and hypertension, alter the placental architecture and interfere with the mechanisms of transport of vital substances to and from the fetus. Should this occur, the fetus may be in jeopardy.

FETAL MONITORING

Techniques are currently available to monitor fetal well-being throughout the course of pregnancy and to detect if the intrauterine environment becomes sufficiently hostile to warrant concluding the pregnancy in the interests of the fetus. The surveillance techniques include periodic observations of fetal growth (by means of ultrasonic imaging), analysis of placental endocrine function (determined by maternal urinary excretion of estriol, a steroid hormone elaborated by the placenta from a fetal precursor substance), and monitoring fetal response to the stress of uterine contractions (as demonstrated by changes in fetal heart rate when the uterus is gently stimulated to contract by pharmacologic means). These and other recently developed methods have significantly improved fetal salvage in pregnancies occurring among women afflicted with medical conditions that place the fetus at special risk.

RISKS TO FETUS

In terms of developmental problems, the fetus is in greatest hazard during its early intrauterine life, when it is undergoing rapid organ formation and maturation. This period of organogenesis primarily spans the first eight to ten weeks following fertilization. Malformations discovered at or following birth are not necessarily genetic but may result from abnormal environmental conditions within the womb acting on an otherwise normal embryo, or they may result from the interaction between genetic and environmental factors. Among recognized environmental teratogens (factors causing malformations) are ionizing radiation, certain maternal infections, and specific drugs. Actually, known causes account for only a very small proportion of all fetal anomalies. Our knowledge about their cause and prevention is exceedingly limited.

Since the effects on the fetus of most drugs taken by the mother are at best poorly defined, it is a good working principle to stress that pregnant women avoid any medication that is not clearly necessary: the therapeutic benefits must far outweigh any potential risks. Whenever it is necessary to treat a pregnant woman, the relative safety of alternative measures should be considered carefully. Because this area is so clouded, too often women, when they have delivered anomalous infants, develop great guilt feelings concerning their activities, habits, and exposures during the course of pregnancy, combing their memories in search of some clear-cut causative event or agent. They can be readily reassured and assuaged by the knowledge that the fetus is extremely well protected within the womb and, except for the aforementioned items, is unlikely to have been affected deleteriously by any other intrauterine exposure.

Pregnant women should be encouraged by the knowledge that nature usually does not permit a defective pregnancy to continue for very long. Spontaneous miscarriages occur commonly and probably account for the termination of at least one in every five pregnancies. Most involve a "blighted ovum" in which the embryo has failed to develop properly, if at all. These probably arise primarily from intrinsic defects in the particular ovum or spermatozoon that combined to form the fertilized zygote. A spontaneous abortion does rarely result from other causes, such as inadequate hormonal milieu to support early implantation and development or acute severe local (uterine) or general infection. In the absence of some form of uterine disorder (such as fibroids, anomalies, or incompetent cervix), the woman who has had a spontaneous miscarriage is at no greater risk of repeating this event than anyone else.

IMPORTANCE OF PRENATAL CARE

The principles of preventive medicine are perhaps more important in obstetrics than in any other field. The primary objective of antepartum care is to examine and supervise the woman so that she will experience pregnancy and labor without detriment to herself or to her baby. The great value of such care is well established: the incidence of complications has been reduced because physicians can now detect and treat various medical disorders. Ideally, every woman should be completely examined well before she plans to become pregnant. If carried out routinely, this can uncover any abnormal or potentially serious condition in order to correct it before pregnancy is undertaken. If such prepregnancy examination reveals a medical disorder serious enough to jeopardize the woman's life or health in the event a pregnancy should occur, such information becomes important in her decision to conceive. The same applies for serious conditions uncovered during the course of pregnancy regarding decisions to continue the pregnancy. Aside from screening for maternal disease, antepartum evaluation and care are directed toward optimizing pregnancy potential. This is accomplished by ensuring good nutrition and hygiene.

Most advice given to pregnant women, by both lay and professional people, is based on a heritage of customary practice. Very few stringent restrictions can be supported by substantive evidence. As a general rule, it is probably safe to say that most healthy pregnant women may do just about everything they did before they became pregnant without any risk to themselves or to their fetuses. Nevertheless, fad diets are probably best avoided, and exhausting activities or potentially perilous sports are not advisable. Common sense should apply in all things, such as clothing, exercise, work, travel, rest, and recreation. As long as the woman feels well and does not exhaust herself, no activity has to be curtailed.

LABOR AND DELIVERY

As stated earlier, the anxiety and discomfort of labor may be augmented by stress and fear and relieved by removing the fear response to stress. Psychologic preparation of women for childbearing has gained much attention in recent decades; yet its history has been marked by both exaggerated enthusiasm and vehement skepticism. There can be little doubt, however, that the approach is quite effective. It is the theoretical basis that remains unclear and controversial. All psychoprophylactic techniques are based on essentially the same Pavlovian concept of conditioned reflex training. Painful sensations seem to be blocked by counterstimuli. Various technical approaches are used, and their differences tend to be minimal. All contain elements of didactic, physiotherapeutic, and psychotherapeutic aspects. Since there are no objective criteria for evaluating pain, the results of these approaches have not been subjected to scientific scrutiny. Nevertheless, the many women who have had good experiences and their physicians have expressed great enthusiasm for the techniques.

Psychoprophylactic preparation includes educating women in anatomy and physiology as they relate to childbirth, training them to relax physically and mentally, and concentrating on respiratory exercises to distract from pain. Pain appears to be diminished by familiarizing pregnant women with the process of childbearing and by creating an atmosphere of confidence. The increased suggestibility of pregnant women can be used to establish the confidence necessary for success. Indeed, the methods work best when there are faith, dedication, and trust, both in the method and in an authoritative person, whether monitrice, midwife, or physician. Childbirth can be a rewarding and beautiful experience for the woman, her partner, and all personnel involved.

However, psychoprophylactic preparation is not without its drawbacks, one of the most severe and probably justifiable of which is that patients are accepted without preliminary screening. Results may be disastrous for psychiatrically disturbed individuals, although their experiences could be just as disastrous, if not more so, without the education and preparation. Another drawback is the misguided enthusiasm of some proponents of this approach, who might willingly or inadvertently convince patients that labor is of necessity painless and that the use of analgesia or anesthesia, if it should become necessary, amounts to a failure on the part of the patient. This cultist attitude places some women in serious jeopardy of developing great feelings of anxiety and guilt. Moreover, such feelings will be magnified to pathologic levels if the infant is not completely normal. The essential mother–child relationship may be adversely affected by such feelings, and severe depression may occur.

It is imperative, therefore, that the psychoprophylactic programs be tempered with logic and reason. Extremism must be avoided. The woman who understands what is happening to her and who is emotionally prepared for childbirth undoubtedly will do better than the one who is not. Problems arise when women insist, to the point of fanaticism, on "natural chirdbirth" in spite of a clear-cut need for analgesic or anesthetic intervention, thereby focusing on "natural" (meaning unanesthetized) rather than on "prepared."

The depersonalization encountered so frequently in hospital settings has spurred a movement advocating home delivery. While the sterile atmosphere of the hospital is to be decried, the proposed alternative is clearly retrogressive and anachronistic. The technologic advances of recent decades make it possible for every fetus to be monitored, thereby demonstrating if its intrauterine environment has become so hostile that continued survival without harm is unlikely. The advances are just not available outside of well-equipped hospital obstetrical units.

Whereas many so-called high-risk pregnant women can be identified by documented diseases, such as diabetes or hypertension, many develop serious problems without any forewarning. At least one in five women whose pregnancies have gone smoothly get into some difficulty during labor. At least half the fetuses that develop intrauterine hypoxia are of women who had perfectly normal pregnancies and uncomplicated labors; one-third of all infants requiring immediate, intensive neonatal care are delivered of healthy mothers. Not only is it unfeasible to provide continuous objective surveillance of the fetus in the home setting but facilities for immediate intervention by obstetrician or pediatrician cannot be offered there when such intervention becomes mandatory.

There is little disagreement that a more natural approach to delivery is needed, dispelling the impersonal care common in hospitals. However, the well-meaning advocates of home delivery are unaware of the risks to which this would expose both mother and infant. There is a paradoxical incongruity among those who, on the one hand, are incensed at the prospects of a 1–in–100,000 chance of death or illness from, say, water pollution but who, on the other hand, can blithely accept a greater than 1-in-100 chance of disaster associated with an unattended delivery. A far better solution to this dilemma would be to make the hospital more homelike rather than to reverse the half-century drive to make safe hospital delivery available to everyone.

Much effort is now being exerted to make the hospital environment more homelike. While maintaining standards of safety that cannot be matched in the home setting, one can do a great deal to make the birth process in the hospital an emotionally satisfying experience for the family. Aside from considerations of architecture and decor, attitudes of warmth, personal attention, and caring must be improved.

The presence of the baby's father, once unthinkable, has become more routine both during labor and at delivery. There is a growing movement toward permitting him to be present in order to support the mother emotionally, even during cesarean sections. Needless to say, such partners need to be prepared so that they may contribute to and share in the experience. There must be some agreement that, should problems arise, they will leave when asked. The father undoubtedly can be of considerable psychological assistance to the mother; moreover, his presence may produce closer marital ties, consolidate the family unit, and provide for a warm and intensely meaningful childbirth experience.

On the negative side, unless properly prepared for, the experience can be emotionally upsetting, especially if the woman insists that her partner attend in order to share in her "suffering." Such exceptional circumstances, however, should not be interpreted as a general deprecation of the practice. Most partners are very helpful in this psychologically trying situation. Buxton has put it well:

> The ideal joy, love and togetherness described as existing when the young father and mother achieve the actuality of those first moments with their newborn together is of course a beautiful and sublime aspect of parenthood.[4]

Recently introduced Leboyer principles, while heterodox, have much in their support. Based on the theory that the infant at birth may suffer both physically and psychologically from the shock of the birth process and from the sudden, startling exposure to the light, noise, and cold of the environment, this approach accomplishes delivery in a warm, quiet, and darkened room in an atmosphere of calm and tranquility. The baby is placed on the mother's abdomen and gently stroked until the cord has stopped pulsating. Subsequently, the baby is given a warm bath, and measures are taken to expose him/her slowly to the world.

Babies delivered under such circumstances certainly appear comfortable and content, but there is still some concern that the lack of stimulus may somehow inhibit the lusty respirations and crying that seem to be so effective in clearing mucus and amniotic fluid from the newborn's lungs. Moreover, it is difficult to observe the baby's condition in a darkened room, hampering observations of such conditions as inadequate oxygenation (manifested by a characteristic bluish skin discoloration). The same, of course, applies to the parturient as well, especially regarding vaginal bleeding and repairing injuries to the birth canal. These are not insurmountable obstacles, however, and can be overcome with improvised focal lighting. The benefits of this method to the baby may be difficult to prove objectively for many years, but its seemingly innocuous nature coupled with its indubitable positive psychological impact on the parents suggest that it is an attractive adjunct to the delivery process.

The ability to monitor the fetus continuously throughout the course of labor is a recent major development. Before it was perfected, there was no way to determine with any degree of precision when the fetus was in jeopardy. Today, with the availability of sophisticated electronic instruments, every fetus is ensured that it will be born with its full potential intact and unaffected by unrecognized hypoxic insults.

Uterine contractions, obviously necessary for the labor process, produce progressive dilatation of the cervix and descent of the fetus through the birth canal. Simultaneously, when the uterus contracts, the muscle cells that make up the uterine wall transiently occlude the blood vessels that supply vital oxygen to the placenta, thereby reducing the oxygen available to the fetus. Ordinarily, this causes no problem; it is analogous to holding one's breath. If the contractions are excessively prolonged, however, or if the fetal oxygen reserve has been chronically diminished because the placental exchange has long been reduced (this in turn due to some ongoing maternal disorder), the additional transient reduction in oxygen supply by uterine contraction may affect the fetus adversely. This will be reflected in a characteristic change in the fetal heart rate, designated as a "late deceleration" or "uteroplacental insufficiency pattern." Other varieties of fetal heart rate pattern changes have been identified, but these tend to be less ominous.

Of critical importance is the fact that the various patterns cannot be distinguished by listening with a stethoscope or by periodically counting the fetal heart rate. Only continuously recording instantaneous beat-to-beat rates and simultaneously measuring intrauterine pressure changes for purposes of correlation will indicate fetal jeopardy. There is every reason for women in labor to develop anxiety when first confronted by the equipment involved in fetal monitoring, particularly if they have not been fully advised and familiarized with it. The reassurance it provides to the informed woman, however, should far outweigh this negative aspect.

In the past, cesarean sections often were undertaken whenever an acute fall in the fetal heart rate was detected by stethoscope. It is now recognized that many such instances of "fetal distress" were innocuous episodes. Fetal monitoring now provides the information to make the distinction between such changes and the more serious life-threatening late decelerations associated with fetal hypoxia. It has been said that more cesarean sections are being done as a result of fetal monitoring, and this is undoubtedly true. But the cesarean sections now are being done for different and probably more cogent reasons. Currently, the need to perform a cesarean is much more clear-cut and well defined when the characteristic pattern of persistent late deceleration is encountered. Moreover, whenever doubt exists, the fetal condition can be double-checked by a newly developed technique in which a small sample of scalp blood is obtained from the fetus by way of the vagina and analyzed to determine the fetal acid-base condition, an indirect measure of its level of oxygenation. The combination of fetal heart rate monitoring and scalp blood sampling has raised fetal surveillance in labor to a new level of confidence and reliability without adding any substantive risk to the delivery process.

PUERPERIUM

The most recent outgrowths of natural childbirth programs are the concepts of rooming-in and family-centered care. Growing numbers of hospitals have arrangements whereby the baby may room-in with the mother. While this requires special physical and nursing facilities, its advantages are many. The mother can learn to care for her infant and to acquaint herself with its habits before returning home. It allows for the development of natural mother and baby relationships.

Psychologically, the usual separation of mother from baby as practiced in hospitals may have real disadvantages, particularly as it interferes with certain essential needs for both mother and child. Imposing rigid visiting and feeding schedules does not properly consider the newborn's needs and developmental changes or the mother's stresses in her adjustment to her new role. In the rooming-in system, the infant is on a demand feeding schedule so that the mother tends to get less rest in the hospital than otherwise, but this disadvantage is generally outweighed by its benefits in terms of fostering mother–child relationships.

The constant presence of the baby in the mother's room or in the adjoining nursery is reassuring. When the mother goes home, she will not be caring for a delicate stranger; she will have developed some sense of togetherness. If the mother feels anxious when she first handles her infant, it is much better to uncover such problems in the hospital, where support may be obtained, rather than to wait for their development at home, where supervision, support, and instruction are not available. Rooming-in also may establish an earlier and easier father–child relationship. Parental relations are clearly better if both parents learn to know and to care for the infant during the first weeks of life. This is probably the optimal time to teach parents how to give the infant the love and security it will need during its formative years.

Family-centered care, another new modification, includes the father in the puerperal unit. He is not a visitor but is integrated into postpartum care. In this way, the close father–mother relationships established and fostered during labor and delivery are maintained and further augmented. The father participates in changing and feeding the baby (if it is bottle fed), thus developing some insight into his essential role in the family unit.

Family-centered care is a natural extension of allowing and, hopefully, encouraging the father's participation in labor and delivery. The family-centered care programs ensure that the mother has the best possible experience during pregnancy, labor, and puerperium, enabling her to share this experience with the baby's father, and both return home confident in their ability to care for the baby. The approach treats childbearing as a normal and healthy process and as a major family experience for all concerned. It provides the wherewithal for parents to get to know the new baby and to begin to function as a family unit under guidance and in the security of the hospital environment. Each mother may have her baby with her for as much or as little time as she desires (with some constraints imposed during general hospital visiting hours). Fathers may be present at all times throughout the day to participate in baby care activities. They are afforded hospital courtesies, congeniality, and sound teaching. Thus, when they leave the hospital, they have had the opportunity to gain confidence, security, and a positive attitude toward parenthood.

The postpartum patient is subject to many stresses. Depression during the immediate puerperium is common, taking the manifestation of so-called blues. This occurs when the new mother must adjust to her physical separation from the fetus, analogous to the loss of a love object, and establish a new relationship with her newborn child. Puerperal depression constitutes an anticlimactic letdown. The woman tends to be irritable and unreasonable; she may burst into tears without provocation; she may be moody and unresponsive. Generally, these episodes are mild and self-limiting, lasting no more than a few days. There is cause for concern only if they persist and are associated with unremitting lack of interest in the infant. They may readily be minimized or even averted if the physician forewarns the woman about the benign nature and common occurrence of this particular problem. The severely affected woman may feel weakness, apathy, insomnia, and loss of appetite and libido. Rare instances of psychotic decompensation occur, but they tend to be entirely confined to women with underlying, preexisting psychiatric illnesses, whether or not recognized. The prognosis for the usual minor case of blues is excellent.

BREAST-FEEDING

The controversy surrounding breast-feeding seems to represent an acculturational paradox. By some strange mechanism, latter-day civilization has stigmatized a very natural phenomenon, necessitating discursive polemics to justify it. Breast-feeding is a perfectly normal biological function providing many recognized advantages to both mother and infant. It constitutes the natural extension of the close, harmonious involvement of the pregnant woman with her fetus to the infant. As an act of direct and continued communication, it serves to enhance the mother–infant relationship.

One of our societal disgraces is the exploitation of the female mammary gland as a symbol of erotic sexuality. This in turn generates a cultural repugnance toward breast-feeding as unattractive and animalistic. This is compounded by misinformation about the process, the demands it places on the nursing mother, and its long-term effects on her. The advantages of breast-feeding are well documented and include the obvious facts that it is very convenient, requires essentially no preparation, and is inexpensive. A growing body of scientific evidence shows that it results in healthier babies with less tendency to develop obesity, fewer respiratory infections, and less diarrhea. Breast milk is hypoallergenic and provides the infant with an ideal form of nourishment that cannot be duplicated by any other means (although admittedly reasonably good approximations can be created in formulas for bottle feeding).

Needless to say, breast-feeding does have some drawbacks, but these tend to be minimal and are outweighed by its advantages. It does tie the mother down, although supplemental bottles can be instituted once the milk supply is well established, thereby giving her periodic relief. There is no truth to the oft-stated concerns about loss of figure or damage to breast supports. Occasional discomfort (uterine cramps and breast engorgement) does occur but is counterbalanced by the pleasure derived from the physical stimulation of suckling. The properly initiated and well-motivated mother can overcome both the minor physical annoyances and the possible resistance of attendant personnel and nurse her baby successfully and pleasurably. Nipple fissures or mastitis rarely will develop to interfere. A more commonly encountered disadvantage has to do with depriving the marital partner (and older children) of sharing in this intimate relationship. The husband may need reassurance in this regard. His participation should be encouraged, especially by feeding supplemental bottles to ensure that he does not feel completely left out. A mature relationship recognizes the rewards to be accrued from the joy of sharing this intense experience.

THE UNWANTED PREGNANCY AND ABORTION

Pregnancy undoubtedly constitutes one of life's major stresses because of the complex emotions that are involved. Although it clearly represents the fulfillment of the biological reproductive function, this does not reflect the nature of the associated psychological makeup. Pregnancy may exacerbate or reactivate a preexisting mental illness; moreover, it may be stressful even for women who functioned quite normally and who appeared to be in very good emotional health prior to conception. Thus, all pregnancies, probably without exception, are associated with some emotional upheaval.

Many patients, regardless of whether or not the pregnancy was planned, develop intense feelings of resentment, fear, or anger. Ambivalence is very common,[3] and it often takes the form of outward acceptance conflicting with inward rejection. Feelings of guilt and shame are not unusual, especially among unmarried women, even in today's society. Such feelings, based on real or imagined stigmata, may even be present where social pressures do not exist. Some women look forward to their "ordeal" with great dread because they think that pregnancy, labor, and delivery are terrifying prospects. Many expressed and unexpressed phobias arise relating to pain, mutilation, and death. Similarly, there are anxieties about the fetus, particularly with regard to the possibility of its being defective. Even the most stable women may be concerned over what the pregnancy means to them in terms of increased economic burdens, especially if they give up their own wage-earning capabilities, and the new or increased personal responsibilities it will entail.

MOTIVATION

Some women seem to be motivated, in a complex and seemingly paradoxical fashion, to conceive although there are readily available effective contraception and safe abortion.

The sources of anxiety are manifold. Fears may be overtly expressed or hidden. Ambivalence may take the form of hostility against the fetus because it has caused the patient to become unsightly and uncomfortable and because it is threatening her sexuality and security. Anxieties may arise over the possibility that activity or diet or medication may adversely affect the growing fetus.

ABORTION

In a sense, all pregnancies stir up ambivalent feelings. The situation for the ambivalent woman is not made much easier either by the prevailing and conflicting societal attitudes or even by the readily available facilities for procuring abortion. It is unfortunate that the subject of abortion prior to the viability of the fetus is so clouded by legal, emotional, moral, ethical, and theological overtones. These add to the difficulties that women face in arriving at rational decisions about whether or not to continue an unwanted pregnancy. The Supreme Court in a landmark decision[5] struck down almost all constraining abortion control laws as unconstitutional, acknowledging that it would be inappropriate for the judiciary to speculate about when life may be considered to begin since a consensus on this issue cannot be reached by physicians, philosophers, and theologians. The Court asserted that the decision to abort in the first trimester was strictly a matter of medical judgment between the woman and her physician.[6]

In theory, this should have resolved any legal issues, and indeed, to a large measure, it has. The proliferation of free-standing abortion clinics throughout the country testifies to the great demand for these services. Clandestine abortions, often done under very hazardous conditions, were replaced by safe procedures done in more favorable surroundings. Nonetheless, even under such ideal circumstances, abortion was found to be not totally innocuous.

Although complications tend to be far less serious than in former times and tend to occur far less frequently, it is now clear that abortion cannot be approached as if it were a routine contraceptive measure. The incidence of serious complications ranges from 1 to 20 percent, with fewest occurring in early pregnancy terminated by suction or curettage. Later midpregnancy abortion, done by means of intrau-

terine injection of an abortifacient agent, increases the rate of complications threefold, and a further threefold if the major surgical procedure of hysterotomy is required.

TECHNIQUE OF ABORTION

The most prevalent approach to terminating pregnancies of less
than twelve weeks' duration, namely, dilatation of the cervix followed
by evacuation of the uterus either by suction or less preferably by
curettage, carries with it the least risk. It can be performed under local
anesthesia, making it applicable in nonhospital settings. After about
the twelfth week of gestation, the uterus is generally too large for this
procedure to be undertaken safely. Termination of pregnancy after
twelve weeks, therefore, becomes a major undertaking, requiring hospitalization with its attendant additional anxiety-provoking milieu
and its expense. By means of a needle inserted through the abdominal
wall into the uterine cavity, a drug such as prostaglandin can be injected into the amniotic sac to induce a diminutive labor that will
cause the uterus to contract vigorously, dilating the cervix and evacuating the fetus and placenta vaginally.

The recent introduction of intraamniotic prostaglandin injection
has almost entirely replaced the former use of hypertonic saline, considerably reducing the risks associated with saline, most particularly
the devasting blood-clotting defects that sometimes followed its use.
Whereas this major hazard has thus been eliminated, other problems
with midtrimester abortions persist, including hemorrhage and infection in small but substantive numbers.

When the intrauterine injection fails to effect the abortion, it may
become necessary to undertake the major surgical procedure of hysterotomy, essentially a miniature cesarean section. Seldom is this actually necessary, however, because of prostaglandin's high degree of effectiveness.

It should be clear that an early decision on an unwanted pregnancy will reduce the woman's risks of pregnancy termination. If her
decision is made prior to the twelfth week, her pregnancy can be
aborted by the least hazardous means. If, by virtue of her ambivalence, ignorance, unawareness, denial, or misadvice (the latter too
often based on a misdiagnosis of an early pregnancy), she should opt
for pregnancy termination after the twelfth week, she will be exposed
to considerably greater risk.

Patients who fall into this category tend to be very young, poorly
educated, unsophisticated, and indigent. The woman with good ego
strengths and resources generally recognizes her pregnancy early and

makes her decision in sufficient time to allow her to take full advantage of easily available abortion facilities at minimal hazard. Paradoxically, women who most need the abortion because of physical, medical, psychological, and financial reasons have the greatest difficulty obtaining it. Midtrimester in-hospital abortion facilities are far less available than those free-standing units catering to women needing first-trimester abortions. And both the cost and the risk of the midtrimester procedure are greater.

There has been a most gratifying reduction in unplanned births in the United States in recent years.[7] This is largely attributable to the widespread dissemination of birth control information, coupled with the availability of abortion. It would be most unfortunate if the latter were to be heavily relied on as a primary method of contraception since the new birth control technology has provided a level of effectiveness and safety that cannot be matched by current or foreseeable abortion methods. It is imperative, therefore, that efforts be intensified to provide early education, counseling, support, and facilities for any woman in need of such services.

REFERENCES

1. Bibring G: Some considerations of the psychological processes in pregnancy. *Psychoanalytical Study of the Child 14*:113, 1959.
2. Heiman M: A psychoanalytic view of pregnancy, in *Medical, surgical and gynecological complications of pregnancy.* Second edition. Edited by Rovinsky JJ, Guttmacher AF. Baltimore, Williams & Wilkins, 1965.
3. Nadelson C: Normal and special aspects of pregnancy. *Obstetrics and Gynecology 41*:611, 1973.
4. Buxton, CL: *A study of psychophysical methods for relief of childbirth pain.* Philadelphia, WB Saunders, 1962.
5. Roe v. Wade: U.S. Supreme Court 93:705, 1973.
6. Curran WJ: The abortion decisions: The Supreme Court as moralist, scientist, historian and legislator. *New England Journal of Medicine 288*:950, 1973.
7. Westoff CF: The decline of unplanned births in the United States. *Science 191*:38, 1976.

Chapter 6

"Normal" and "Special" Aspects of Pregnancy: A Psychological Approach*

CAROL C. NADELSON

Pregnancy has been called the fulfillment of the deepest and most powerful wish of a woman, an expression of fulfillment and self-realization, a creative act,[1] which affords many women the opportunity to explore new directions in their lives. However, it may also be a stressful time, requiring adaptation to enable growth and maturation to occur.[2] It may be stressful for a woman who must, for the first time, meet the challenges of pregnancy and the subsequent experience of "mothering."[3] Pregnancy can be compared to other critical life periods which Erikson calls developmental crises.[2] A primary aspect of crisis in pregnancy is that it revives psychic conflicts of previous developmental phases, often enabling new solutions to be found and psychologic growth to occur.

In addition, pregnancy represents a clear turning point in the life of a woman. Bibring et al.[4] point out that pregnancy involves both physical and psychologic changes that are immutable; once a mother, a woman cannot be a single unit again. In addition they feel that the issues involved in resolving this stage are similar to those occurring at other critical life stages—i.e., once an adolescent, one cannot be a

---

*Reprinted from *Obstetrics and Gynecology* 41 (4), April 1973. Published by Harper and Row. Copyright © 1973 by American College of Obstetricians and Gynecologists.

CAROL C. NADELSON, M.D. • Psychiatrist, Beth Israel Hospital; Associate Professor of Psychiatry, Harvard Medical School; Director, Medical Student Education, Department of Psychiatry, Beth Israel Hospital, Boston, Massachusetts 02215.

child again, and once the menopause has passed one cannot bear children.

A physician may perform well in the specific obstetric care of his pregnant patient without understanding the intrapsychic aspects of her experience, but his ability to help with more complex situations occurring during pregnancy may be limited.

For most patients, routine care, including physical attention, factual information and support, are sufficient. For many women, however, the obstetrician may be the only person in a position to observe failing psychologic defenses which might result in decompensation during this stressful time.[5] Psychotic reactions are rare, but many emotional difficulties, with repercussions, may occur after the pregnancy.

On the basis of her work as a consultant for obstetricians in the community and as liaison psychiatrist to the Department of Obstetrics and Gynecology at the Beth Israel Hospital, the author has outlined the *normal* psychologic processes of pregnancy and summarized the kinds of information which, when obtained, can alert the obstetrician to consider psychiatric consultation and referral. Illustrative clinical histories are presented to clarify problem areas.

PREGNANCY, CONFLICT, AND RESOLUTION OF CONFLICT

Under the impact of the early changes that occur during pregnancy, a woman's preoccupation with herself often increases. The beginning of the integration of the fetus, at this point a *foreign object*, as part of the self is enhanced by quickening, which enables the fetus to be perceived as human and real. The next goal is to perceive the baby as a separate entity. This is a dual process, since it requires that a new relationship be established with the baby and that the woman's identity change permanently; she now must learn to see herself as a mother.[4]

The feelings and fears experienced during pregnancy are intense and varied. Women often express concern about the degree of ambivalence they experience in areas that had previously been conflict-free, such as future role and responsibility, marriage and career plans. They become anxious about sexual relations and physical attractiveness during the pregnancy and after delivery.[1,6] Women speak of embarrassment over the exhibition of sexuality, which is definitely and overtly demonstrated with pregnancy. Many kinds of sexual and even homosexual fantasies occur. Other conflicts, basic to the experience of pregnancy, are those concerning the woman's early relationships with her mother and the experience of having been mothered.[7] There is a change in the relationship of the new mother to her mother, as she becomes a mother and her mother becomes a grand-mother. Past conflicts may cause feelings of guilt, anger, ambivalence and remorse. As the new grandmother changes her self-perception, she may see her daughter as a co-equal and no longer as a child.[4] She may become competitive in an attempt to prove that she is a better mother, or she may experience difficulty in accepting the aspects of aging implied in her new role and she may become angry and jealous of her daughter.

When pregnancy is diagnosed, fear and ambivalence are frequently experienced[8] in the same way as with any new and major life change. The initiation is simple, but implications are lifelong and changes are permanent, immutable, and progressive. The experience of pregnancy and of bearing a child become part of the individual's physical and psychic reality. If an abortion, spontaneous or induced, had occurred in the past, the woman often wonders if she can bear a child; she may fear that she is damaged. If a child has been born previously and given up, there is often a revival of the feelings surrounding that child. The woman may feel that this present child will also be lost to her or she may feel guilty for the past rejection of her child and view herself as a *bad* mother.

For the future father, pregnancy confirms his virility, but it is not generally further defined or realized until later in the pregnancy. Sometimes the man experiences ambivalent feelings because of the threat of distance from the woman, or competition with the child for her attention and love, and the potential threat that his needs will not be gratified.[9]

Pregnancy has multiple meanings for both parents together, as well as for each individually. The child's sex or its position in the family may have particular meaning. In addition, sexual problems are often manifested for the first time, because of feelings toward the current pregnancy or future pregnancies, or because of the physical changes occurring during the pre- and postpartum periods. Bearing a child may also represent a hastening toward adulthood.

MOTIVATION FOR PREGNANCY

The motivations for pregnancy are complex and multiple and are not limited to feelings about a specific relationship or to bearing and caring for children.

Concerns about the ability to love or be loved may be motivating factors. Women at times express fear that they cannot be loved by another person; they feel that only by having a child can they be guaranteed love—that of the child. A pregnancy often occurs to resolve questions about the reality or endurance of a love relationship.[1,10]

Another motivating factor for pregnancy is concern about sexual identity,[1] especially in adolescent and younger women. Pregnancy certainly provides the physical evidence of gender, although the psychologic aspects of the dilemma may not be resolved. In the adolescent, one frequently finds a pregnancy which occurs to enable the girl to separate from her parents and to attempt to resolve long-standing conflicts in parental relationships.[11]

A woman may want a child because she wants a mother[10] and needs to resolve an early life experience of deprivation. The pregnancy provides, in the woman's fantasy, a means of having a child and being a child, simultaneously. Many people see a child as an extension and continuation of themselves. These concerns often prevent the parents from being able to see the child as a person.

There are women who, in an unconscious attempt to seek a resolution of oedipal or related conflicts, have a child who is, in fantasy, their father's or mother's child. Often, they attempt to restitute and alleviate the guilt they have toward their mother, about whom they are ambivalent, by giving her the child to care for or even to keep.[1]

Another aspect of the motivation for pregnancy is seen in the passive, masochistic woman who deprives the man of his child as an aggressive act, but whose underlying motive of self-punishment forces her to deprive herself of the relationship.[1]

Freud[12] hypothesized that the frustration caused by the lack of a penis was central to a woman's desire to become pregnant, and that bearing a child was the fulfillment of the wish to have a penis. Deutsch[1] added that when pregnancy occurs, the drive toward aggressiveness and masculinity in the healthy woman is given up. This implies that aggressive feminine drives are associated with masculinity and the healthier woman becomes more passive. These views have both been questioned by others.[13,14]

When an unwanted pregnancy occurs for reasons other than accidental, it is crucial to understand the motivating factors. Once understood, it is then possible to intervene and attempt to help the woman deal with those problems which were instrumental in motivating her to become pregnant.

PHYSIOLOGIC CHANGES AND PSYCHOLOGIC CONCOMITANTS OF PREGNANCY

Early in pregnancy, changes are apparent. These result both from the recognition of and the implications of pregnancy, as well as from the physiologic changes taking place. Fatigue, nausea, and vomiting are almost universal[15]; in excess, however, they *may* represent ambivalence toward the pregnancy. Emotional lability is frequent and depressive feelings are not uncommon, especially in the first trimester. These feelings may occur normally; however, they also occur at times when feelings of guilt or ambivalence are present.[10]

Early nausea, vomiting, and fatigue are often accompanied by a sense of disappointment, since the expected sense of excitement and well-being is absent. The effect of quickening is to usher in this sense of well-being, and it is related to the visibility of pregnancy and the perception of its reality, as well as to the relief at the disappearance of the unpleasant symptoms of the first trimester.

Late in the second trimester, women begin to report an increased feeling of dependency, passivity, and a desire to be alone. These feelings peak in the third trimester and do not disappear until sometime during the postpartum period.[16] They may, in part, occur for physiologic reasons; they also involve the relationship of the mother to an unseen baby and the development of new identifications. Regressive fantasies may also occur as part of the experience of pregnancy, particularly in the last trimester.

As the pregnancy nears term, women have reported many increased anxieties and fears.[10] They are concerned about the realities of becoming a mother and the changes in marital and family relationships which necessarily occur. They are concerned about the process of labor and the difficulties they may experience with delivery, especially if they have had a previous experience or fantasy about the process. The sex and health of the infant and possibilities of death or injury to mother and/or child preoccupy a woman during an often sleepless and restless period in the last trimester.[17]

Labor and Delivery

The process of labor is always a new experience, even for a multipara, since each pregnancy is different and a woman never knows exactly what can be expected. Women report feeling supported and encouraged more often by the presence of another woman, such as a nurse, because of a sense of sharing and familiarity with a maternal figure.[18] Extreme anxiety can interfere with labor, delivery, and the care of the child. Often this anxiety is related to fear of giving up a sense of unity with the child or to real concerns about not having the capacity to love and care for the infant. The sex of the baby, the sibling order, and the special meanings of the particular baby to the parents also affect these processes.

It is possible that effect of heavy medication during labor, and the consequent failure of the mother to experience the delivery, may interfere with early mothering. Many women report feelings of unreality and disbelief that they have borne a child, and uncertainty that the child presented to them is actually their child.[18]

Instruction for natural childbirth is aimed at reducing fear and tension, which theoretically leads not only to pain reduction[19] but also enhances the experience of birth and facilitates the development of the relationship between mother and child. There are multiple and often interconnected reasons, however, for difficult childbirth, which may be physiologically and/or psychologically determined. Understanding the individual woman helps those involved in care during labor to be prepared to use analgesia and anaesthesia when suitable, and to avoid making uniform rules or having unrealistic expectations for the rate of progress or the degree of discomfort. When either natural childbirth or heavy sedation is presented as mandatory, without fully appreciating individual needs and abilities, a woman may feel inadequate and/or guilty about not being a good enough woman or mother, and may experience greater anxiety.[10] Such an experience, at delivery, may leave its residues in terms of continued self-doubt and interfere with a successful resolution of the *crisis* of pregnancy.

THE POSTPARTUM PERIOD

In our society the breakup of large, extended family groups and the prevalence of small, isolated nuclear families have changed pregnancy from an experience of family involvement, concern, and attention to an experience of isolation, wherein a woman may be alone and unsupported by those who care and have shared the experience.[17] Because of technical advances, delivery may occur in a foreign environment, and the normal early postpartum dependency and expected feelings of depression may be accentuated by the isolation and lack of familiarity.

In the early postpartum period, concerns about breastfeeding are prominent and may be accentuated if a woman feels that performance is a major factor in determining her adequacy as a mother or as a woman. There frequently are social pressures brought upon her either to continue breastfeeding or to give it up which may intensify the pressure and increase the conflicts.

Depressive feelings, often related to the *loss* of the pregnant state and the sense of *oneness* with the infant, are very common in this period. The state of ego depletion, experienced at this time, involves a feeling of inability to tolerate any additional burdens or stresses, however minor they may seem. The early postpartum period can be seen as part of the total crisis of adaptation during pregnancy.[20] Most commonly, symptoms begin within a few days. The woman may weep without apparent reason, feel that she is *falling apart* and sense that she is unable to cope with any more than the most immediate details of living and caring for her child.[17] Minor inconveniences may be viewed as major traumas. Many new, intense feelings and impulses are experienced by the mother. She often is in conflict about being able to meet tasks and responsibilities and to integrate the new experience which can seem monumental.

The process of adaptation is gradual; the course is generally several weeks. The sleep-wake cycle of the infant and its feeding habits play a large part in the evaluation of the postpartum depressive period. Sleep deprivation may, in fact, be a major factor in the emotional distress of new parents.

Severe emotional disorders or postpartum psychoses occur at approximately the rate of 1 to 2 per 1000 live births.[21] They are more often associated with obstetric abnormalities, such as toxemia of pregnancy, malpresentations, hydramnios, and placental defects. There does not seem to be any relationship between pre- and postpartum emotional disorders. In fact, it is unusual to find them both occurring during the same pregnancy.[22] Physical stresses increase the emotional strain of this period. Symptoms of psychoses usually appear between the first and fourth postpartum weeks. One-third of the women who experience puerperal psychosis develop similar difficulties during subsequent pregnancies.[21] Other important etiologic factors in postpartum psychosis are the possibility of organic (biochemical, endocrinologic)[21] causes, as well as the psychologic which include unresolved conflicts about pregnancy, child rearing, and the relationship with the child's father.[4,23] Patients with postpartum psychosis present with delirium, restlessness, and confusion. Depression usually occurs later.[24] The physician and family must be alert to potential destructive acts toward the self or the infant and psychiatric consultation should be sought immediately. Treatment consists of support, reinforcement of the patient's ability to function as a mother; at times, medication and hospitalization may be necessary.

MOTHERHOOD

Mothering has long been seen as an instinctual process. However, Erikson[3] pointed to the need for social experience in achieving satisfactory motherhood. His thesis is that to be a good mother, a woman must have: (a) the past experience of being mothered, which provides a model for this new experience; (b) a conception of mothering shared with a husband and/or people in the environment; and (c) a world image linking past, present, and future.

Harlow[24] demonstrated that monkeys reared in isolation do not react as *natural* monkey mothers, but show rage at their infants. Robson and Moss[25] reported a study of 54 primiparous mothers in which the data indicate that the infant's behavior, particularly visual fixation and smiling, intensify maternal feelings, and that attachment is not an immediate phenomenon, but grows with the interaction between mother and infant during the first months.

The evidence seems to indicate that a part of mothering behavior may be learned, in much the same way fatherhood has been considered to be learned by fathers. Feedback and personal interaction are crucial in the experience of motherhood and fatherhood.

Whiting[26] reported on mothering patterns in other cultures. She finds a general belief in the need for mothers and grandmothers to teach their children directly how to respond to and care for infants, and not to rely on innate knowledge or ability.

THE UNMARRIED MOTHER

A discussion of mothering and parenthood leads inevitably to the person who may have no outside support but, in fact, experiences negative feedback at each phase during her pregnancy and afterward—the unmarried mother. In addition to the problems of sociocultural factors, the pregnancy may have had its origin in psychologic problems which then add to the woman's burdens as she attempts to master the *crisis* and adjust to this phase in her life. She may have struggled initially to decide if she should have an abortion or if she should bear the child and then perhaps have to give it up. The implications in the decision to abort are intrapsychic, moral, and legal.[27] The problems involved in giving up a child include, among others, loving and separating from the child with a resultant negative self-image as a rejecting, bad mother.[28] The solution to this kind of dilemma, which recurs repeatedly, is not settled in one decisive act, but must be resolved repeatedly, rarely unambivalently.

As we observe the complex process of pregnancy, we must be aware that each woman comes to terms with the multiple changes in relationships and roles of pregnancy in her own way. It is necessary for those caring for her to respect her way of coping. Frequently, it is the family physician or obstetrician-gynecologist who carries this responsibility during the pregnancy, labor, and/or delivery. As discussed earlier, pregnancy is an opportunity for mastery and maturation; it is also a time of major stress with which most women cope admirably. However, for some it appears as an almost insurmountable obstacle.

Such a person can be helped to confront and resolve conflicts at this time if clues to this problem are observed early in the pregnancy.

There are some elements of the patient's history which the obstetrician can be alert to, to enable him to modify his approach or technic, or to request consultation with a psychiatrist, in order to help the woman resolve some of the conflicts she is experiencing. A complete initial history is a primary requisite in the treatment of any patient; this is also true for the obstetric patient. The following are some suggested signal areas for the obstetrician to attend to:

1. Previous history of psychiatric treatment or hospitalization
2. A past history of difficulties at other critical maturational stages, such as puberty
3. A history of early maternal deprivation or loss
4. Conflicts involving separation from parents
5. Conflicts about sexual identity
6. Conficts about role as a mother, concerns about adequacy as a mother or ability to care for a child
7. Marital or other family difficulties
8. Past difficulties with pregnancy, delivery, or postpartum depression
9. Major individual or family medical problems or deaths
10. Familial or congenital diseases
11. Unmarried status
12. History of pseudocyesis, infertility, habitual abortion, premature births, stillbirths, hyperemesis, or prolonged or difficult labor
13. Previous birth of a defective child and/or possibility of defective birth with this pregnancy
14. Extremes in age range (under 17, over 40)
15. Previous poor relationships with physicians (delineation of this aspect may be an important guide to approach)

The following case histories illustrate some of the special difficulties discussed.

CLINICAL MATERIAL

Case 1

Mrs. L was a 23-year-old, recently married secretary when she was first seen. The referral was made by her gynecologist after she told him of her wish to have a child and her intense fears of pregnancy.

She had grown up in a very chaotic home, with an impulsive mother who was sexually active with many men, and a passive, compliant father to whom she could not relate. A sister, 10 years older, provided some warmth and stability during her early childhood. Upon reaching adolescence she was ostracized by her peers because of her mother's reputation. She felt that the implication of this action was that she too was "bad." When she was 20, she married a man 10 years her senior, with a cardiac problem that was minimally limiting but not seriously life threatening. He tended to deny his disease and project his underlying feelings of defectiveness onto her. She readily accepted the position of the defective member of the family.

Mrs. L appeared to be a warm, attractive woman who tearfully unfolded her story, concluding with the statement that she was convinced that she could never be an adequate mother. She started psychotherapy and responded well to support, reassurance, and a gradual exploration of the past and current depressive feelings. The early focus of therapy was on her relationship with her mother, her inability to separate and her inability to express any negative feelings because she was fearful of being rejected. As her anger emerged and she became able to tolerate it, her depression diminished.

Mrs. L became pregnant after approximately 6 months of therapy. She was seen regularly throughout the pregnancy. Her anxieties and fears about her own and the child's health were similar to those feelings expressed by most women, but her focus on her fears of inadequacy progressively intensified and became overwhelming as she approached term. She was also fearful that her mother would not accept being a grandmother and would reject her and/or the child.

When her child was born with a minor congenital foot defect she became extremely upset. She felt that this occurrence proved that she was the *bad* person she had seen herself to be, and she stated: "God is punishing me." She was seen daily during the first 2 postpartum weeks, and frequently for the next 3 months. She did remarkably well, integrating her own feelings of guilt with emerging feelings of anger toward her husband. She was able to begin to accept that fault or blame could not be assigned, and that her overreaction related to her own sense of herself as defective.

She continued to do well at home and was seen irregularly, most often at times of increased stress, for the next 2 years.

It is possible that Mrs. L could have been an obstetric *casualty* without appropriate referral and treatment. Her difficulty, conceptualizing herself as a mother, had implications in her ability to conceive, adjust to a pregnancy, and develop an image of herself as a mother. Her own experience of inadequate mothering made her fearful that she would also be inadequate; her anger at her mother could potentially have been directed toward her husband or child; her difficulty separating from the ambivalent relationship with her mother may have made separation from her child impossible for her; and her child's birth defect could have overwhelmed her with guilt and prevented her from functioning.

Mrs. L's pregnancy was a maturation step for her largely because of the intervention. She was able to report, in subsequent visits, that her therapy continued to help her cope with a periodic upsurging of fears of rejection by her mother and her friends. She regarded the therapist as a *giving mother*, who could tolerate negative feelings and allow her to grow. In the course of treatment, Mrs. L was able to give up much of her depressive, dependent position.

Case 2

Mrs. A is a 40-year-old housewife, the mother of two children aged 15 and 10. She was being seen in couples therapy with her husband because of marital difficulties stemming from her almost total absence of sexual interest which intensified after the birth of her second child.

Mrs. A had grown up in a rigid Catholic home, the second of five children. Her father was an alcoholic, and her mother had periodic hospitalizations for mental disorders. Mr. and Mrs. A were married when both were 24, after a year of courtship. Shortly thereafter they moved to a distant city where Mr. A planned to attend graduate school. Mrs. A had never been away from home before and was quite apprehensive about the move.

When Mrs. A discovered she was pregnant she was delighted at first but became increasingly more anxious. She developed severe nausea and vomiting, fatigue, and insomnia. Her husband expressed considerable anger toward her since he expected her to be better able to cope with pregnancy, as the women in his family had always been.

Her fantasies were terrifying: she was fearful of the birth of an abnormal child and of her own death. She was lonely, unable to make friends, and she pressed her husband to be with her constantly. The pregnancy ended at term with toxemia and a prolonged difficult labor and delivery.

After the birth of a daughter, Mrs. A developed a severe postpartum depression. As a result, it became necessary for the couple to return to the home of Mr. A's parents where Mr. A's mother was able to care for the new mother and child. Mrs. A gradually improved but she retained a fear of another pregnancy and was reluctant to have sexual relations.

Her desire for a family, despite the difficulty, led to a subsequent pregnancy with a similar course. After the birth of her son, another postpartum depression occurred and she was referred for psychiatric treatment. Her depression cleared but the sexual difficulty intensified. It was not until the A's daughter reached puberty and began to show her own sexual interests that they sought consultation, ostensibly for their daughter. The etiology of the difficulties in their relationship became increasingly clear during the evaluation and the A's started psychiatric treatment.

The early history of family difficulties that is evident here is important since it can serve to alert the physician to the possibility of problems with pregnancy. Despite her background, Mrs. A had done well until the pregnancy occurred, simultaneously with separation from home. These stresses triggered internal conflicts which had previously been well defended. Mrs. A's experience with her own mother made it impossible for her to master these two concurrent crises. It is possible that earlier active intervention might have helped to avoid the subsequent marital disruption. In the current therapy, Mrs. A is attempting to move from her dependent, asexual position with her husband to a more mature, self-sufficient, and sexually interested position where she feels that she is not necessarily doomed to repeat her mother's experience, and where they are both able to communicate with each other more openly.

Case 3

Mrs. M is a 25-year-old married mother of a 2-year-old daughter and was first seen when she was 21. She presented with a history of a symbiotic early relationship with her mother followed by a stormy adolescence with sexual acting out, including two illegal abortions by the time she was 20. She had failed out of school and was taking drugs indiscriminately when she decided to start psychiatric treatment because she recognized the self-destructive course she was taking.

After about a year of treatment she married a rather disorganized, dependent man and became pregnant shortly after the marriage. She was referred to an obstetrician who was aware of her difficulties and with whom her psychiatrist could work closely.

Mrs. M had a difficult pregnancy with considerable anxiety, marked by daily telephone calls to her obstetrician. She was fearful that *something terrible* would happen, that she would abort or give birth to a *monster*. She was unable to control her appetite and gained 60 pounds. She was preoccupied with the *ugliness* of her pregnant body and intolerant of her husband's sexual interest. She was angry with him for any demands he made on her.

Her labor and delivery were unremarkable. However, her early postpartum period was marked by concerns about the weight, health, and body functions of her baby, as well as by feelings of depression and inadequacy. She received psychiatric treatment throughout this time and was able to make a good adjustment and function in her maternal role.

In her psychotherapy, Mrs. M primarily dealt with the differentiation of herself as a person and as a mother, separate from her mother. She gradually came to see herself as a person who could perform capably, and who could control impulses. She had the gift of humor and enough ability to be self-observing to make it possible for her to work effectively with each new, daily crisis. Her daily telephone calls with questions and demands for more care were responded to patiently and firmly. The result of the coordinated effort of psychiatrist and obstetrician was that Mrs. M mastered a developmental crisis and successfully entered a new life phase. While Mrs. M is not totally well, the crisis intervention technics offered her models for the future, and the motivation to continue to work on her problem.

Case 4

Miss V was a 35-year-old, single, computer programmer when she was referred by her gynecologist because of a severe intermittently recurring depression.

She was the oldest in a large family. Her father was a rigid, authoritarian man and her mother a weak, passive woman. She had few peer relationships during childhood or adolescence. Generally, she mistrusted people, and for that reason she also dated infrequently. When she was 25, she met a married man at work. Shortly thereafter, she began to see him frequently. After 3 years she pressed him, by becoming pregnant, to divorce his wife and marry her. When he did not accede to her demands she made a serious suicide attempt, but continued her relationship with him. After the birth of her son, she attempted to keep the child for 6 months but finally succumbed to family pressure to give him up. Again she made a suicide attempt but refused her obstetrician's referral for psychiatric treatment.

Miss V entertained the fantasy that some day her boyfriend would marry her. However, there was little change in their relationship. She had depressive episodes almost yearly on the anniversary of the child's birth. During these times she would take massive indiscriminate doses of medication and then inform her boyfriend and family, who would rescue her. It was not until the boyfriend threatened to leave her if she did not seek psychiatric treatment, that she called her obstetrician–gynecologist and requested a referral.

Early in psychotherapy Miss V began to deal with the reality of the relationship with her boyfriend, and she confronted the fact that part of its unchanging character had to do with her desire to maintain distance from him.

Within the first weeks of psychiatric treatment she discovered that she was pregnant again, an event which was apparently motivated by the 10-year anniversary of their relationship. She decided that she wanted an abortion after considering the trauma of her previous separation from her child. She felt that she could not subject herself to *that pain again*. She also felt that she was unable to care for the child alone. The pregnancy mobilized considerable feeling; she was able to talk about her anger, sadness, and loneliness. She obtained a therapeutic abortion and continued her psychiatric treatment.

The working out of the previous loss of a child in this patient's life was crucial to her ability to develop a realistic view of her goals. It is important to emphasize that, although major character changes did not occur, she did master the crisis and she matured. Miss V was able to settle an issue that had been active as a cause of her depressive symptomatology and acting out. She accepted the reality of the relationship with her boyfriend, as a result of her needs as well as his, and decided to continue this relationship.

These four case histories illustrate different aspects of the problem of working with some pregnant women. They underline the need to be familiar with the past experiences and personalities of each woman, and the benefits of appropriate consultation and referral. The end of a pregnancy cannot be regarded only in terms of the birth of a child but should be seen also as a time for growth and maturation even in the face of previous failures to master life crises.

References

1. Deutsch H: *The psychology of women. Motherhood.* Vol 2. New York, Grune & Stratton, 1945.

2. Bibring G: Some consideration of the psychological processes in pregnancy. *Psychoanalytic Study of the Child* 14:113, 1959.
3. Erikson E: *Childhood and society*. New York, WW Norton, 1950.
4. Bibring G, Dwyer T, Huntington D et al: A study of the earliest mother-child relationship. *Psychoanalytic Study of the Child* 16:9, 1961.
5. Parks J: Emotional reactions to pregnancy. *American Journal of Obstetrics and Gynecology* 62:2,339, 1951.
6. Pleshette N, Asch S, Chase J: A study of anxieties during pregnancy, labor, the early and later puerperium. *Bulletin of the New York Academy of Medicine* 32:436, 1956.
7. Depres MA: Favorable and unfavorable attitudes toward pregnancy in primiparae. *Journal of General Psychology* 51:2,241, 1937.
8. Menninger WC: The emotional factor in pregnancy. *Bulletin of the Menninger Clinic* 7:15, 1943.
9. Daniels PS, Lessow H: Severe postpartum reactions: an interpersonal view. *Psychosomatics* 5:21, 1964.
10. Benedek T: Sexual function in women, chap 37. *American handbook of psychiatry*. Vol 1. New York, Basic Books, 1959.
11. Bernard V: Psychodynamics of unmarried motherhood in early adolescence. *Nervous Child* 4:26, 1944.
12. Freud S: Some psychological consequences of the anatomical distinction between the sexes. 1925 *Collected Papers*. Vol 5. New York, Basic Books, 1959, p 185.
13. Thompson CM: Penis envy in women. *Psychiatry* 6:123, 1943.
14. Horney K: Flight from womanhood. *International Journal of Psycho-Analysis* 7:324, 1926.
15. Schaefer ES, Manheimer H: Dimensions of perinatal adjustment. Presented at the Eastern Psychological Association Meeting, New York, April 1960.
16. Caplan G: Psychological aspects of maternity care. *American Journal of Public Health* 47:25, 1957.
17. Shainess N: Psychological problems associated with motherhood, chap 4. *American Handbook of Psychiatry*. Vol 3. New York, Basic Books, 1966.
18. Nadelson C: Unpublished data.
19. Dick-Read G: *Childbirth without fear*. New York, Harper, 1953.
20. Winnicott DW: Pediatrics and psychiatry. *Collected Papers*. New York, Basic Books, 1958.
21. Paffenberger RS: Epidemiological aspects of parapartum mental illness. *British Journal of Preventive and Social Medicine* 18:189, 1964.
22. Pugh TF, Jerath BK, Schmidt WM et al: Rates of mental disease related to childbearing. *New England Journal of Medicine* 268:1224, 1963.
23. Arieti S: Introductory notes on the psychoanalytic therapy of schizophrenics, in *Psychotherapy of the psychoses*. Edited by Burten. New York, Basic Books, 1960.
24. Harlow HF, Harlow MK, Hansen EW: The maternal affection system of rhesus monkeys, in *Maternal behavior in mammals*. Edited by Rheingold HL. New York, John Wiley & Sons, 1966.
25. Robson K, Moss H: Patterns and determinants of maternal attachment. *Journal of Pediatrics* 77:6,976, 1970.
26. Whiting B: Fold wisdom and child rearing. Presented at the American Association for the Advancement of Science, 1971.
27. Nadelson C: Psychological issues in therapeutic abortion. *Woman Physician* 27:12, 1972.
28. Notman M: Personal communication, 1972.

Chapter 7

The Sense of Mastery in the Childbirth Experience*

ANNE M. SEIDEN

INTRODUCTION

There are three basic goals in attempts to assist the process of labor: (1) enhancing safety for mother and child; (2) allowing freedom from undue pain without the loss of positive and indeed ecstatic aspects of the experience; and (3) setting or maintaining the best foundation for a solid, exuberant relationship between mother and child (and the rest of the family).

Modern obstetrics has concentrated on attempts to enhance safety and to decrease pain, using both pharmacologic analgesia and "prepared childbirth" in its various varieties. The third goal, favorably beginning the mother–child relationship, has been more problematic and less systematically studied until recently, but is of obvious importance to the family and society as a whole.[1]

In lower mammals, the normal healthy neonate will predictably elicit nurturant care from the normal mother. If the mother is removed or damaged, other adolescent or adult females or males may take over, sometimes quite adequately, other times not.[2] Thus, "foster mothering" is possible, but not inevitable, in many species. Similarly, if the infant is abnormal or damaged, the mother may or may not provide adequate nurturing.

---

* An earlier version of this paper was presented at the Third Annual Conference on Psychosomatic Obstetrics and Gynecology, Sugar Loaf Conference Center, Temple University, Philadelphia, Pennsylvania, February 2, 1975.

ANNE M. SEIDEN, M.D. ● Director of Research, Institute for Juvenile Research, Department of Mental Health and Developmental Disabilities, Chicago, Illinois 60612.

In many ways, human mothering in present-day America often resembles the responses of other mammalian adults—"foster mothers"—more closely than it resembles the predictable and dependable response of the mammalian "natural mother." Some mothers and children establish strong and effective bonds with one another, but many do not. Severe neglect and gross physical abuse of infants occur with alarming frequency.[3] And in turn, young married couples with children tend to report less happiness than those without children.[4,5,6]

While these social problems have many other determinants, there is reason to believe that often they are caused or compounded by *impaired initial establishment of the mother–infant bond*. We do not know to what extent this occurs because human mothers and infants lack dependable "instinctual" bonding repertoires, or to what extent social learning and current obstetric/pediatric practice interfere with otherwise adequate repertoires. But we do know: (1) Even in lower primates, so-called instinctive nurturant behavior is heavily dependent on the mother's prior life experience.[7] (2) Mammalian mothering behavior is obliterated by decortication of the mother and, in some instances, of the child.[8] (3) Drugs habitually used in labor either cause varying degress of cortical depression (e.g., barbiturates, scopolamine, analgesics) or suppression of activity in those subcortical circuits most likely to be involved in "instinctive" behaviors (e.g., phenothiazines, which affect the limbic system).[7] These effects last longer in the infant than in the mother and have been shown in the human infant to alter EEGs and depress the sucking reflex up to a week or more after birth, thus potentially interfering with the baby's initial response to its mother.[9] (4) Medication-induced sucking depression, especially when combined with mother–child separation during the early hours of life, can delay adequate sucking until after the breasts have become engorged. Thus, the infant may fail to receive colostrum, and initiation of adequate lactation can be complicated or even prevented.[10,11] (5) Maternal response to infants is very highly dependent on infants' response to mothers, and there is evidence to suggest a very important critical period during the first postpartum hour and days.[12,13,14] Eye contact with the infant may be a critical releaser during the first hour.[15]

Thus, there is reason to scrutinize practices that produce a sedated infant or mother immediately postpartum or that separate the pair or impair eye contact during the first postpartum hours. These procedures entail a risk of impairing initial attachment and of producing a variable rather than a dependable beginning of the mother–child relationship.

The need for procedures that sedate and separate mothers and infants can potentially be reduced by effective preparation for childbirth. All three major approaches to "prepared" or "natural" childbirth claim to reduce or eliminate the need for analgesic medication during normal birth.[16,17,18] Controlled studies indicate that this result can be achieved and that it is in fact related to the preparation itself, not merely to the selection of women or their general education about pregnancy and birth.[19,20] Of course, a major reason for the usual postpartum separation of mother and infant, in this country, is the fear that the sedated mother might not be able to provide ordinary infant care and that the sedated infant might require close expert nursery observation.

In recent years, organizations promoting prepared childbirth and breast-feeding have assumed many of the characteristics of a social movement.[21] However, the impact of these groups on general obstetric and pediatric practice has been somewhat fragmentary, in part because of the demographic characteristics of the people that they have reached. Just as medically sound obstetric care has been more available to advantaged segments of the population, childbirth preparation also has been unequally distributed and tends to reach first a population that is educated, informed, and articulate. This population has been predominantly married and under relatively advantaged circumstances at the time of giving birth. Childbirth preparation may therefore not reach the disadvantaged populations, which need it most.

Thus, while many advances in safety and comfort are now theoretically available through modern, prepared obstetrics, there remain major problems in the broad achievement of good childbirth experiences in the United States. These problems appear to occur mainly in two areas: (1) there is a great need for a wider and more rational distribution of available knowledge and skills and (2) there is a great need for relevant professional and consumer groups to recognize that advances in the pursuit of safety and comfort have sometimes endangered mother–infant attachment while not necessarily achieving safety and comfort.

In conceptualizing possible remedial action, this paper will use three models: First, a psychological model emphasizing as an organizing principle the mother's sense of mastery, in all of its aggressive and libidinal implications. Second, a medical model based on *primum non nocere*. Third, a community health model involving clear delineation of first-, second-, and third-line services (i.e., primary care for normal situations with several levels of expert backup as needed). These will be further explained below. All three work together. A woman cannot achieve a sense of mastery if she is either at high risk of severe pain or death or, on the other hand, if she is treated as an ill or incompetent patient when, in fact, she is not.

PROBLEMS IN ACHIEVING SAFETY, DECREASING PAIN, EXPERIENCING MASTERY

Some very real questions are raised about the extent to which the three goals of freedom from danger, freedom from pain, and freedom from intrusion on normal birth and bonding are mutually compatible or conflictual. Quite often an action taken to avoid one hazard introduces another. Thus, anesthetic medication to avoid pain may increase danger, impair the mother's sense of participation and mastery, and produce sedation, thereby necessitating the separation noted above. A hospital environment chosen to promote safety by permitting quick intervention when needed may inherently increase risks of cross-infection. It also may enhance the need for medication when unfamiliar surroundings exaggerate the cycle of anxiety leading to muscle tension and to increased pain. But avoiding all intrusions prevents using those that might be needed to increase safety to mother and child. Thus, to a certain extent, the attempt to achieve all three goals simultaneously has elements of wanting to have one's cake and eat it too.

Haire's thoughtful review of American birth practices [10] discloses a number of paradoxes. Our expensive and heavily interventionist system of delivering obstetric care has yielded disappointing outcomes when measured by the usual parameter of infant mortality: fourteen industrialized nations surpass us with more favorable statistics. [22] This has been attributed by some to our economic and ethnic diversity, but actually, black women, who are more often poor and tend to receive less modern obstetrical care, had a lower incidence of brain-damaged children than white women in the major national study of this point. [23]

In one recent survey, hospitals having fewer than 2,000 deliveries per year showed less favorable standards of anesthetic care for mothers and children than those with larger services. [24] In another survey, hospitals not having specialized facilities for high-risk infants or rapid transport to such facilities showed much higher risks for infants. [25] Yet the National Study of Maternity Care found rates of neonatal death, maternal deaths, and stillbirths to be lower in small community hospitals than in larger teaching centers: the larger the hospital and the closer the tie to a medical school, the more neonatal deaths occurred. It is still unclear what proportion of this variance is accounted for by a higher loading of higher risk patients at the teaching centers and what proportion by the fact that large, impersonal centers may enhance the fear-pain-medication syndrome; moreover, teaching needs may lead to interventions that increase risks more than they lower them.

CULTURE, PERSONALITY, AND CHILDBIRTH PREPARATION

The question "How intrinsic is pain to childbirth?" is often referred to observations of primitive societies. The answer appears to vary somewhat, depending on which primitive group is studied.[26] A woman physician drawing on her own obstetric experience and on Dutch methods of preparing women for birth drew a vivid analogy: yes, there is pain in childbirth, but its impact varies—like the difference between suturing a 3-centimeter chin laceration on an eighteen-year-old football player and repairing a similar wound on a confused and frightened four-year-old.[27] Similarly, pain in the chest when one is running a winning race is associated with pride and mastery rather than humiliating dependency. In a somewhat different vein, Bradley[18] has observed that women may be made more vulnerable to obstetric pain by socialization that discourages them from being sufficiently insistent on their own comfort or by overly rigid toilet training that conditions tension and shame to bodily exposure or "making a mess." Birth, he observes, is not "ladylike."

Indeed, Newton found that "cultural femininity," as measured by conventional psychological masculinity–femininity tests, correlates negatively with what she calls "biological femininity," or interest in and success at the tasks of animal mothering: confident delivery, successful breast-feeding, and related attitudes and behaviors.[28] More recently, she has noted that in the female reproductive triad of coitus, birth, and lactation there is a tendency in our society to place special emphasis on the first, presumably because of its special pertinence to the adult heterosexual relationship, and to ignore the sexual aspects of the latter two.[29]

The point is that childbearing, like childrearing, is an aggressive and libidinal task—tough and demanding, sometimes exciting, often exhausting. Parents must confront the world to protect the child's survival needs, set firm limits at times to the child's behavior, cuddle the child for fun or for soothing, and in general have a strong sense of confidence that they know what they are doing or can find out. This aggressive mastery is such characteristic behavior for female mammals during parenting that folklore has generated the old saying, "The female of the species is deadlier than the male."

These parenting tasks are greater, not fewer in the human mammal because of the longer duration of childhood dependence (extended in modern society even beyond biological adolescence[30]) and because of the plasticity of human responses, which makes them more subject to the influence of learning or social expectations. Thus, we cannot assume that "maternal instinct" will make all women assertive enough to be good mothers. Furthermore, our culture has generally discouraged female assertiveness, aggressiveness, and sexuality. This has been specifically extended into the childbearing situation, where it has been regarded as normal and even intrinsic.

Thus, for example, the psychiatric chapter of an obstetrics text widely used only a decade ago reads as follows:

> The *nature of childbearing* [italics added] is such that . . . for nearly twelve months the obstetrician takes over the guidance of an adult woman, supervises her food intake, regulates her activities, answers her questions, clarifies her puzzlements, advises her about the handling of her baby when it comes, and generally charts her conduct during the twenty-four hours of the day.[31]

Obviously, this psychology has led to many problems. It does not seem surprising, after being told by her society that she needs this kind of infantilization, that when the baby comes a mother might have questions about how to handle it and become or remain addicted to "experts." Tough, effective, confidently warm human parenting is not encouraged by beginning with twelve months—or many years—of treating the mother like a puzzled, fragile, dependent creature. On the contrary, everything that is done with or for a pregnant woman should be done to increase rather than decrease her sense of mastery. And this should begin long before the actual pregnancy.

Childbirth education, if provided during the prenatal period, can help women achieve mastery, but it has some limitations. First, it tends to reach the middle-class married population predominantly; both theory and practice have recently tended to emphasize the place of the husband.[18] Second, like so much remedial education, for example, sex education courses in high school, it comes too little and too late, and often not at all to those who need it most. Women whose sense of mastery might be most vulnerable would likely be lower-class, adolescent, unmarried mothers, who are a large group (current estimates are that 10 percent of American women will become pregnant during their high school years: the majority will not marry at this time, but will keep their babies[32]).

The mothers of one out of three firstborn children are unmarried at the time of conception, although over half of these marry before the birth, and in a high proportion of cases, the marital bond is unstable. One-fifth of all births occur to mothers below age twenty.[33] We ignore these facts when we rely on the role of the husband and on a few prenatal classes late in pregnancy to set the stage for confident child-bearing and childrearing. Such confused thinking is common and is contaminated by exaggerated or inconsistent concepts of what is normal or optimal. For example, in a recent paper[34] the Queen of England's gynecologist deplores the facts that (1) so many children are born outside of optimum maternal age, which he defines as eighteen to twenty-five; (2) children are often born into unstable marriages; and (3) many people marry at a young age, less than twenty, which predicts more unstable marriages. Obviously, one cannot have it both ways! These expectations for the social maturity required to establish a stable home for children and the biological maturity for optimal childbirth are grossly incompatible.

If such a high proportion of pregnant women are by definition considered less than suitable subjects for even the kind of late and abbreviated childbirth education we now offer, it is not surprising that there is widespread pessimism about psychoprophylaxis as a predominant approach to pain control. For example, a prototypic paper on safe anesthetic management indicates that the "vast majority" of women want and need anesthesia (despite the author's own figures that show a threefold increase over the last decade in the number of women not receiving it in his own hospital).[35]

Even our language reveals our attitudes. The physician is the one who "delivers the child"; he does not attend the mother, who delivers the child. One recent textbook states, "The obstetrician of today and tomorrow must be more than a physician who 'follows' a woman through pregnancy, labor, and delivery. He [sic] must be able to 'lead' the mother and fetus through these periods. . . ."[36]

There is a widely held belief that the only women who object to this philosophy are unusual, middle-class, educated, or "liberated" women who embrace an "ideology," implying that those who want to experience and manage their own births are deviants. Yet lower-class black adolescent women, when seen in supportive groups during prenatal care, frequently ask about delivery, "Will they tie my hands down?"[32] While this may be a concrete expression, the message appears to be the same. A healthy adult does not wish to be rendered helpless and immobile during a significant life event, unless there are enormous compelling reasons.

Cross-cultural research reveals a great diversity of rules about who may attend a laboring woman, from cultures in which birth is a tribal community event, to others in which strict taboos limit the number and kinds of persons who may be present. Our society frequently allows or requires a woman to pass significant portions of labor alone and excludes all familiar persons, while admitting strangers.[26] Our taboos against allowing birth to be witnessed, other than by professionals and perhaps now by the husband, seem to be related to taboos against witnessing coitus or breast-feeding. As Newton suggests, there may be biological reasons for some of these taboos. Any of the three acts, coitus, birth, and lactation, place the participants in a poor position for fight or flight. Observations of animals also support the belief that the presence of frightening strangers or unfamiliar surroundings can inhibit all three activities.[29] Thus, it seems important not to exclude familiar persons, whose company the mother values. Rather we should scrutinize the practice of including a bewildering array of professional strangers, some of whom are there for the mother's benefit, but not subject to her control, others for a diversity of staffing or training needs.

Birth has been ambivalently perceived and, curiously, both underplayed and overplayed in its importance in contemporary American culture. On the one hand, the parturient is in a sense the "invisible woman." Boy Scout manuals and first-aid books tell how to stop arterial bleeding but not how to assist in childbirth. Movies and television depict death and violence, but childbirth is seen rarely, if at all, despite the fact that birth plays as significant a part in the human drama as death.

On the other hand, too much emphasis can be placed on the few hours surrounding birth. Many factors determine the quality of mother–child relationships, and focusing on, or romanticizing, these few hours might well lead to neglect of other major factors. Women and men who have never experienced parenthood establish excellent nurturant bonds with children they adopt. Many parents establish excellent attachments to premature infants even though they are separated from them for weeks after birth, although the incidence of bonding failure is much greater here.[15]

There are two peculiar trends in Western society, particularly in North America, that tend to be carried over into education for prepared childbirth. First, pregnancy is regarded as something very special and unusual in a woman's life. Western society is unusual because the average woman wears special garments, maternity clothes, during half of her pregnancy, and later finds both these and her ordinary clothes inconvenient for breast-feeding. We segregate maternity education—like maternity clothes—into the few months of pregnancy.

Second, our culture avoids the education that is inherent in daily life experience, isolates children from life experiences that teach, and develops a curriculum that artificially provides structured remedial education to fill in knowledge gaps that would not have existed had children been permitted to use their own eyes and ears.[37] Birth education in this regard is like sex education: we go to great trouble to set up separate bedrooms, thick walls, careful time schedules, and the like—all to make sure that children will not observe sexual behavior. Then, at what we regard as an appropriate time, we show them carefully produced films and books to provide the knowledge we now recognize they need.

There is a difference between daily life learning, where one has the option of growing up and teaching one's own children, and the teaching done by professionals. A woman receiving childbirth knowledge and labor encouragement from more experienced women can look forward to identifying with and later passing her experience on to other women. But a woman who is encouraged to regard her mother's and friends' life experiences as "old wives' tales" can well anticipate that her own experience will be similarly depreciated.

To summarize, we see many trends in North American culture in general, obstetrics in particular, that impair both the safety of and the mother's sense of mastery in birth. In recent years, professional and consumer awareness of this has increased, and there is a growing interest in what might be called a birth reform movement, which is often explicitly critical of obstetric practices. However, obstetricians may be unfairly criticized for what is in part the result of general cultural attitudes, and there may be real risks in denying the need for expert obstetric care.

THE BIRTH REFORM MOVEMENTS: STRENGTHS AND LIMITATIONS

Rossi[38] noted that the contemporary women's movement had placed more emphasis on women's economic and sexual equality with men than on those rights that support women's unique needs when bearing and raising children. There has been, however, a significant feminist push to assert women's rights in the maternal area. The Boston Feminist Health Book Collective's best-selling book, *Our Bodies, Ourselves,*[39] emphasizes knowledge about childbearing, and the Chicago Women's Liberation Union has provided courses in prepared childbirth, as well as in abortion and contraceptive services.

The theme of controlling or mastering the childbearing experience has a long history, as does the opposite theme of questioning the woman's right to do so. In fact, the Biblical account that equates pain in birth with the human condition assigns the cause to Eve's eating the fruit of the tree of knowledge of good and evil, and therefore knowing too much. The introduction of obstetrical forceps by the

Chamberlens allowed mastery over some otherwise intractable situations, and the introduction of general anesthesia during the Victorian era provided one approach to mastery over pain. While theological authorities at the time questioned the morality of relieving pain in labor, neither forceps nor anesthesia placed the mastery in the woman's hands. It has been pointed out that the celibacy of many early Victorian feminists was not necessarily mere prudery and resistance to male domination, but a rather positive means of asserting mastery over the otherwise considerable danger and pain that were then associated with birth.[40]

Along with the increased use of anesthesia after Queen Victoria herself used it and the more frequent use of forceps that anesthesia permitted came the increased medicalization of what had formerly been midwifery. Once Semmelweis developed aseptic technique, obstetricians could perform autopsies without carrying infection to laboring women. Obstetricians then began to approach the more favorable safety record for normal births that midwives had hitherto enjoyed, and the stage was set for discrediting midwives.[41] Control over the birth process then passed rather rapidly out of the hands of women wherever advanced medical technology was available.

Alternative approaches to modifying labor pain were explored in the 1930s by Dick-Read in England[42] and by a number of Russian workers in the Pavlovian tradition,[43] whose methods were brought to Western attention with modifications by Lamaze,[44] Vellay,[45] and others.

The first formally structured consumer organization directed at helping women with birth-related problems was the La Leche League, started in 1956 in Franklin Park, Illinois, by a group of nursing mothers. They were alarmed at the lack of assistance from hospital personnel and even positive interferences that were experienced by women who wanted to nurse their infants.[46] Their book says that ". . . you may need to be prepared to assert yourself, in a nice way . . . you can't win . . . smile and smile, and get out of there as fast as your doctor will let you." Indeed, many of the original members of the group attributed part of their success in nursing their later children to returning to the home to give birth.[47]

More recently, a number of other organizations have been formed to promote collaboration between consumers and professionals.[48-53] To varying degrees, some of these organizations or their members have tended to place birth within the context of nineteenth- and early twentieth-century assumptions about woman's role, to support large families and relatively undifferentiated pronatalism, and to oppose abortion. Literature published or endorsed by these groups tend to emphasize husband dominance, question whether a hospital that performs abortions can be sensitive enough to the emotional needs of infants and mothers, and the like.[54]

However, the desire to exercise sexual equality, freedom from unwanted pregnancy, and the right to control one's own birth and lactation experience are in no way intrinsically opposed. Sherfey[55] has discussed ways in which civilization has required, or thought it required, the inhibition of women's "inordinate sexuality." This is as true of the libidinal aspects of a woman's relationship with her child as it is of her sexual demands from a mate. Newton[29] has discussed how desexualizing the maternal experience tends to inhibit its spontaneous enjoyment and contributes to difficult births and lactation. Women who sleep with their infants are more likely to breast-feed successfully. Women also may experience orgasm with breast-feeding.

Thus, in both standard obstetric practice and the more formally organized birth-reform movements, there is a paradox. On the one hand, medical and surgical obstetrics tend to present birth as an illness, an abnormal event that is medically risky and sexually taboo. On the other hand, attempts to balance this attitude through prepared childbirth tend to emphasize excessively the nuclear family as the "normal" social situation, organizing support around the presence of the husband and even his dominance.

The battle to help the husband regain access to the birth of his own children, and to the side of his laboring wife, has been necessary and is by no means fully won, particularly for cesarean births. However, as noted above, not all mothers are married and not all marriages are stable or supportive. The husband may be "allowed" to be present and then be as intimidated as the wife by hospital rules and personnel. Or he may be coopted into sharing an authoritarian role with the hospital staff.[56] Some women might prefer other companions, such as their own mothers, sisters, a friend who has successfully given birth, or their own older children. What remains is a profound ambivalence about "letting" the woman in normal labor control the situation, using companions of her choice, including medical personnel, as sources of support, consultation, and technical expertise on an informed consent basis. This becomes a more serious problem as families get smaller; the woman who bears only one or two children cannot as readily draw on prior childbearing experiences.

While the earlier phases of the birth reform movements have been obstetrically based and/or quite respectful of the authority of the "right" physician, the past several years have seen a veritable flood of publications taking a different tone.[39,54,57–64] These books share a number of similarities: critiques of our disappointing obstetric outcomes, careful documentations of data, searching examinations of the

extent to which current poor outcomes may be at least in part iatrogenic (via excessive intrusions on normal births, perhaps made necessary by lack of preparation or unfavorable psychosocial settings for
normal births). Unlike the earlier birth reform literature, they tend to
be profoundly pessimistic about achieving medically safe and psycho-
socially optimal conditions for normal births within present hospital
settings. They differ somewhat in philosophical base, but they are
mostly directed at the committed, heterosexual couple. Most of these
books include accounts of couples' earlier experiences with hospital
births, which were characterized by iatrogenic complications, psychological trauma, or both; a common theme is the unsuccessful and ultimately abandoned search for a physician who could assure a couple
that he would help them achieve a more satisfactory experience. Many
of these books provide directions or advice on how to conduct a
home birth without any professional attendants! They differ in the extent to which they caution realistically against risks that may be involved in doing so.

In summary, a variety of birth reforms have been proposed over
the past decades; some have been associated with organized movements, others have not. A majority fall short of truly comprehensive
plans for a system of maternity care delivery, because they apply more
specifically to the complicated birth only (medical reforms), to the uncomplicated birth only (home birth movement), or to the needs of relatively mature and committed heterosexual couples only. Thus, ex-
panding any one of these approaches to cover the whole spectrum of
maternity care would deny some important aspects. Hence, a comprehensive blending of medical, psychosocial, and public health models,
outlined in the introduction above, would permit us to use available
expertise without impairing the mother's sense of mastery.

RECOMMENDATIONS: PHILOSOPHY AND SERVICE DELIVERY SYSTEMS

Philosophically, the broad achievement of good birth experience
in this country is delayed when planning is hampered by adherence to
the following:

1. *The myth of the so-called traditional feminine personality.* Passivity, dependence, ineptness, emotional lability, and sexual inhibition are so exactly opposite to the requirements of good birth experience and good motherhood that one suspects that they are desired
because of a poorly worked-through fear of mature women.[65] Excessive dependence on the obstetrician or surrogate (including the ob-
stetrician-trained husband as birth coach) could be a temporary substitute for active mastery in childbirth. But one wonders about the
longer range implications for childrearing: to infantilize women, after
all, is to rear children by infants.

2. *The myth of the nuclear family as the only or optimal context for birth or for childrearing.* As noted above, many pregnancies do not occur in marriage, and others only appear to because the marriage is transient. But even if the marriage lasts, birth can be made unduly conflictual in this country because there is far less sharing of child care responsibilities than is characteristic of other cultures.[66] Birth is the beginning of what is perceived as an oppressive trap by many women.[67,68] Women in other cultures count on relatives (older children as well as adults) to help in child care; in other industrial nations, the women count on group day care that is near enough to the workplace to permit nursing.[69]

In our society, childbirth often means loss of employment (therefore, loss of income, status, achievement, and independence), loss of mobility, and virtual isolation from society with the child. Fear of entering this trap is dysphoric in itself and may contribute to psychological hazards of pregnancy or the puerperium.[68]

3. *The myth of maternal maturity and competence.* Despite its conflict with the first myth and its relation to the second myth, we expect even the primipara to have a degree of solo responsibility and childbearing competence that is unlikely to be achieved before the age of menopause, if then. Much of human childrearing involves learned responses, and the sources of learning are relatively few. The memory of one's own childhood is subject to retrospective distortion and is only a sample of one. Care of younger siblings is increasingly a rare experience, as families become smaller. Doll play is very poor preparation: live children do not act like dolls. The experience of older and wiser humans who have seen a number of children come and grow up is inevitably necessary. The myth of maternal maturity contributes to the difficulty in accepting advice from mothers and mothers-in-law. Seeking an alleged "expert" seems somehow more consistent with maturity. Like the general public, "experts" in childbearing and childrearing have incomplete knowledge and controversial issues are subject to "scientific" fads and fashions. "Old doc's tales" often are about as scientifically based, and less experiential, than "old wives' tales." Not too long ago both the public and the experts believed that masturbation caused insanity; more recently, rigid feeding and toilet schedules were considered essential; even now many physicians advocate unfounded restrictions of prenatal diet or postpartum body contact with children. Mothers often learn from their own experience to disregard this kind of advice, but only after the first or second child. For a high percentage of mothers, however, childbearing will be over by then.

4. *The myth of the one best solution.* Many mothers have complained of having to fight for the privilege of seeing their babies born or of rooming-in; yet a few years later, every mother in the same hos-

pital will be pressed to participate regardless of her preference. Abortions were seen as damaging and were difficult to obtain just a few years ago. Married women, inadvertently pregnant, would often be pressured into keeping the child by obstetricians. Today, many women going in for prenatal care for a third or fourth pregnancy report that they are asked to explain to the obstetrician why they do not want abortion or sterilization. The one constant issue is that the woman's own choice is ambivalently respected. We know, however, that the best outcomes are obtained by following women's preferences. Women who are denied requested abortions raise less healthy children.[70] Women who are persuaded to nurse against their impulses have lower percentages of successful nursing.[71] Women who are employed out of necessity rather than choice or who are persuaded to give up jobs they want to keep produce less well-adjusted children than women who are able to exercise their own choice in the matter.[72] Women who desire active participation in childbirth or who come into the hospital wanting "a rest" or "to get away" usually have sound reasons for their preferences, which need to be respected. Doing whatever is necessary to enhance the beginning of good mother–child relationships would appear to be a good investment of professional time in an era when the prevalence of child abuse, delinquency, reactive behavior problems, and other miscarriages of the childrearing process are matters of national concern.

How then, in health planning, is it possible to provide good systems of obstetric services, which save life and promote comfort, maternal joy, and mastery, all within some reasonable cost–benefit calculation?

1. We need a clear delineation of when the illness model applies—that is, to the birth with complications, some of which can be predicted and some of which cannot. There is no need to base maternal confidence on a false assumption that complications never occur—they do. The issue is similar to driver education: there is a sense of great power from being at the wheel with two hundred horses under one's foot. That sense of mastery does not have to be impaired by knowing that there is a distinct possibility of accidents: some things can be done to prevent them (like enhancing your own skill, not driving under the influence of drugs, keeping your car in good repair), to minimize their consequences (like wearing seat belts), or to assure prompt effective treatment if they do occur (like having a well-organized system of trauma centers, with fast transportation to them).

2. We need a commitment of professional energy and expertise to the really adequate provision of emergency obstetric care. This includes both the concentration and the organization of highly skilled personnel and the needed equipment. It includes good prenatal

screening for high-risk situations, mobile units for prompt response to unexpected emergencies (if we can do this for heart attacks, we can do it for obstetric emergencies), and provision for rapid transfer of high-risk infants and their mothers to centers able to provide for their special needs.

3. At the same time, for the normal delivery we need to restore the mother's choice and control. A continuum of services is currently being explored, ranging from home births, to extramural hospital-affiliated maternity centers,[73] to intramural homelike labor-delivery rooms in hospitals.[74] These gradations may be appropriate for varying degrees of anticipated risk or for availability of backup services: for those who live too far from the hospital for adequate emergency response and for those who, for practical or psychological reasons, need to get out of their home environment in order to give birth. Such facilities should look homelike and be familiar, part of or coordinated with the space in which prenatal care occurs. Unless the woman has some psychiatric disorder impairing her competence for decision making, she should be treated as a guest in a facility that employs medical personnel as consultants and assistants, not as dictators; she should have, as nearly as possible, the same degree of control over her activities and companions as she has in her own home. The assumption is that she is in the birth center rather than in the hospital because she is not ill.

4. If she does require hospital delivery, only those intrusions that are absolutely necessary should be imposed. Watchful waiting does not require an environment more restrictive than the labor-delivery room. Even major interventions such as cesarean section need not require general anesthesia or separation from the father or other chosen companion. The baby, if healthy, can then be put to breast immediately after birth.

5. All of this ideally implies a model of lifelong childbirth education, predominantly in natural contexts. Prenatal education should be a review of learned knowledge and a provision of special support, if needed, rather than a source of new and secret knowledge. Some of the breathing and relaxation exercises that minimize the need for medication during birth could be taught earlier in gym classes and used to control other kinds of pain and tension without medication. Birth itself needs to be reviewed against the background of a renewed recognition of women's personalities and potential. In the education of girls, we need to support toughness as well as tenderness, assertiveness as well as empathy, proud endurance of some pain in the service of desired goals (as in contact and endurance sports). We need, and are achieving, some decrease in body taboos. Nursing, in public and on films, should be common enough not to be particularly

noteworthy. It is important to see some births, either in real life or on film, at a time when the issue is not especially emotionally loaded: that is, not just at adolescence or during prenatal classes, not just one's own or one's mother's birthings. If it is true that being able to insist on one's physical comfort during labor is an important prerequisite for labor to go well, then we need to raise women who know how to insist on their needs in other situations before and after childbirth. In short, we need to loosen the apparent and artificial conflict between our "human" and "animal" selves that contributes so much to making an existential crisis out of birth.

These broad cultural and educational changes cannot be the responsibility of obstetricians alone. Today's major technical advances are new enough to be novel. One can confidently predict that further research will narrow the indications for their use, and mature clinical judgment will supplant some of the eagerness to use new "toys." Appropriate interventions, replacing "overkill," should improve our outcome statistics. The same process of improving service delivery that is needed to restore the mother's sense of mastery may well be expected to enhance the professional competence and confidence of the appropriately used high-risk obstetrician.

References

1. Sugarman M: Paranatal influences on maternal–infant attachment. *American Journal of Orthopsychiatry* 47:407–421, 1977.
2. Lehrman DS: Hormonal regulation of parental behavior in birds and infrahuman mammals, in *Sex and Internal Secretion*, Vol. 2. Third edition. Edited by Young WC. Baltimore, Williams & Wilkins, 1961.
3. Gil D: *Violence against children: physical child abuse in the United States*. Cambridge, Harvard University Press, 1970.
4. Campbell A, Converse PE, Rogers WL: *The quality of American life: Perceptions, evaluation, and satisfactions*. New York, Russell Sage, 1976.
5. Feldman H, Rogoff M: Correlates of changes in marital satisfaction with the birth of the first child. Paper presented at the 76th Annual Conference of the American Psychological Association as part of the symposium on Variation in Contemporary Marriage Patterns, Aug. 10-Sept. 3, 1968, San Francisco, Calif.
6. Falicov CJ: Interpersonal perceptions during pregnancy and motherhood. Doctoral Dissertation—Committee on Human Development, University of Chicago, 1971.
7. Harlow HF, Harlow MK, Hansen EW: The natural affectional system in rhesus monkeys, in *Maternal behavior in mammals*. Edited by Rheingold H. New York, John Wiley & Sons, 1966.
8. Ford CS, Beach FA: *Patterns of sexual behavior*. New York, Harper & Row, 1951.
9. Brazelton TB: Effects of prenatal drugs on the behavior of the neonate. *American Journal of Psychiatry* 126:1261–1266, 1970.
10. Haire D: The cultural warping of childbirth. Seattle, Wash., *International Childbirth Education Association Special Report*, 1972, 1976. Also reprinted in *Environmental Child Health* 19:171–191, June (Special Issue), 1973.

11. Applebaum RM: The obstetrician's approach to the breasts and breast-feeding. *Journal of Reproductive Medicine* 14:98–116, March 1975.
12. Klaus M, Jer Auld R, Kreger N, McAlpine W, Steffa M, Kennell J: Maternal attachment: importance of the first post-partum days. *New England Journal of Medicine* 286:460–463, 1972.
13. Salk L: The critical nature of the post-partum period in the human for the establishment of the mother–infant bond: a controlled study. *Diseases of the Nervous System* 31:(Suppl.)110–116, November 1970.
14. Robson KS, Moss HA: Patterns and determinants of maternal attachment. *Pediatrics* 77:976–985, 1970.
15. Klaus MH, Kennell J: *Maternal-infant bonding: the impact of early separation or loss on family development*. St. Louis, CV Mosby, 1976.
16. Dick-Read G: *Childbirth without fear*. Fourth edition. Revised and edited by Wessel H, Ellis HF. New York, Harper and Row.
17. Vellay P: *Childbirth without pain*. Translated by Lloyd D. New York, EP Dutton, 1960.
18. Bradley RA: *Husband-coached childbirth*. New York, Harper & Row, 1965.
19. Enkin M. et al: An adequately controlled study of the effectiveness of P.O.M. training, in *Psychosomatic medicine in obstetrics and gynecology: proceedings of the 3rd International Congress of Psychosomatic Medicine in Obstetrics and Gynecology, London, March 29–April 2, 1971*. Basel, S. Karger, 1972.
20. Doering SG, Entwisle DR: Preparation during pregnancy and ability to cope with labor and delivery. *American Journal of Orthopsychiatry* 45:825–837, 1975.
21. Langman L, Black R, Black R: Prepared childbirth as a social movement. Paper presented at Conference on Psychosomatic Obstetrics and Gynecology, 1973.
22. *United Nations statistical yearbook: 1972*. New York, 1973. Table 21, pp 89–94. Cited in Galog J: A new look at our infant mortality. *Birth and the Family Journal*, 3:15–23, 1976.
23. Niswander KR, Gordon M: *The collaborative perinatal study: the women and their pregnancies*. First edition. National Institute of Neurological Diseases and Stroke. Philadelphia, WB Saunders, April 1972.
24. Phillips OC: Preferable methods of pain relief in labor, delivery, and late pregnancy complications, in *Controversy in obstetrics & gynecology II*. Edited by Reid D, Christian C. Philadelphia, WB Saunders, 1974.
25. Quilligan EJ: Introduction, in *Risks in the practice of modern obstetrics*. Edited by Aladjem S. St. Louis, CV Mosby, 1972.
26. Mead M, Newton N: Cultural patterning of perinatal behavior, in *Childbearing—its social and psychological aspects*. Edited by Richardson SA, Guttmacher A. New York, Williams & Wilkins, 1967, pp 142–244.
27. Shaffer IB: Naturally it hurts—but not that much. *Medical World News*, October 3, 1969.
28. Newton N: *Maternal emotions: a study of women's feelings toward menstruation, pregnancy, childbirth, breastfeeding, infant care, and other aspects of their femininity*. New York, Hoeber, 1965.
29. Newton N: Interrelationships between sexual responsiveness, birth, and breastfeeding, in *Contemporary sexual behavior: critical issues in the 1970's*. Edited by Zubin J, Money J. Baltimore, Johns Hopkins University Press, 1974, pp 77–98.
30. Seiden A: Sex roles, sexuality, and the adolescent peer group, in *Adolescent Psychiatry*. Vol. IV. Edited by Feinstein S, Giovacchini P. New York, Jason Aronson, 1975, pp 211–255.
31. Kanner L: Psychiatric aspects of pregnancy and childbirth, in *Williams' obstetrics*. Twelfth edition. Edited by Nicholson, Eastman et al. New York, Appleton-Century-Crofts, pp. 354–372, 1961.

104   ANNE M. SEIDEN

32. Halsted L: The use of group process in prenatal counseling. Thesis submitted in partial fulfillment of requirements of master's degree in psychiatric nursing, University of Illinois, Chicago, 1973.
33. Williams TM: Childrearing practices of young mothers: what we know, how it matters, why it's so little. *American Journal of Orthopsychiatry* 44:70–78, 1974.
34. Peel J: Maternal health, in *Quality of life: the early years*. Edited by the American Medical Association. Acton, Mass., Publishing Sciences Group, 1974, pp 237–243.
35. Weiss LB: Preferable methods of pain relief in labor, delivery and late pregnancy complications, in *Controversy in obstetrics and gynecology II*. Edited by Reid D, Christian C. Philadelphia, WB Saunders, 1974.
36. Quilligan EJ: Introduction, in *Risks in the practice of modern obstetrics*. Edited by Aladjem S. St. Louis, Mosby, 1972, pp xi–xii.
37. Illich I: *Deschooling society*. New York, Harper & Row, 1971.
38. Rossi AS: Maternalism, sexuality, and the new femininism, in *Contemporary sexual behavior: critical issues in the 1970's*. Edited by Zubin J and Money J. Baltimore, Johns Hopkins University Press, 1974, pp 145–173.
39. Boston Feminist Health Book Collective: *Our bodies, ourselves*. New York, Simon & Schuster, 1973, 2nd ed, 1976.
40. Haller J, Robin M: *The physician and sexuality in Victorian America*. Urbana, University of Illinois Press, 1974.
41. Ehrenreich B, English D: *Witches, midwives and nurses: a history of women healers*. Old Westbury, N.Y., The Feminist Press, 1973.
42. Dick-Read G: *Childbirth without fear*. Fourth edition. Revised and edited by Wessel H, Ellis HF. New York, Harper & Row, 1972.
43. Chertok L: *Motherhood and personality*. London, Tavistock, 1969.
44. Lamaze F: *Painless childbirth: the Lamaze method*. New York, Regnery, 1970, Pocket Books, 1972.
45. Vellay P: *Childbirth without pain*. Translated by Lloyd D. New York, EP Dutton, 1960.
46. La Leche League International: *The womanly art of breastfeeding*. Franklin Park, Ill. La Leche League, 1963.
47. Tompson M: Why do responsible, informed parents choose homebirths? Presented at conference of National Association of Parents and Professionals for Safe Alternatives in Childbirth, Arlington, Va., May 15, 1976.
48. International Childbirth Education Association.
49. American Society for Psychoprophylaxis in Obstetrics.
50. American Academy of Husband-Coached Childbirth.
51. National Association of Parents and Professionals for Safe Alternatives in Childbirth.
52. Association for Childbirth at Home (called Home Oriented Maternity Experience in some states).
53. American College of Home Obstetrics.
54. Sousa M: *Childbirth at home*. Englewood Cliffs, NJ, Prentice-Hall, 1976.
55. Sherfey MJ: *The nature and evolution of female sexuality*. New York, Vintage, 1972.
56. Scully D: Unpublished data for Ph.D. thesis, Department of Sociology, University of Illinois, Chicago Circle Campus, 1975.
57. Arms S: *Immaculate deception: a new look at women and childbirth in America*. Boston, Houghton Mifflin, 1975.
58. Lang R: *Birth book*. Cupertino, Calif., Genesis Press, 1972.
59. Shaw NS: *Forced labor: maternity care in the United States*. Elmsford, NY, Pergamon Press, 1974.
60. Wessel H: *Natural childbirth and the family*. New York, Harper & Row, 1973.

61. Milinaire C: *Birth: facts and legends.* New York, Harmony Books, 1974.
62. Seaman B: *Free and female.* New York, Coward, McCann & Geoghegan, 1972.
63. Ward C, Ward F et al: *The home birth book.* Washington, D.C., Inscape Publishers, 1976.
64. Hazell LD: *Commonsense childbirth.* New York, Berkeley, 1969. Revised edition, 1976.
65. Lerner HE: Parental mislabeling of female genitals as a determinant of penis envy and learning inhibitions in women, in *Female psychology: contemporary psychoanalytic views.* Edited by Blum HP. New York, International Universities Press, 1977, pp 269–283.
66. Minturn L, Lambert W: *Mothers in six cultures: antecedents of childrearing.* New York, John Wiley, 1964.
67. Peck E: *The baby trap.* New York, Phoenix, 1971.
68. Parlee MB: Psychological aspects of menstruation, childbirth, and the menopause: an overview with suggestions for further research. Paper presented at Conference on New Directions for Research on Women. Madison, Wis., May 31–June 2, 1975.
69. Sidel R: *Women and childcare in China.* Baltimore, Penguin, 1975.
70. Forseman H, Thuwe I: One hundred and twenty children born after application for therapeutic abortion refused: their mental, social adjustment, and educational level up to the age of 21. *Acta Psychiatrica Scandinavica* 42:17, 1966.
71. Newton N: Interrelationships between sexual responsiveness, birth, and breastfeeding, in *Contemporary sexual behavior: critical issues in the 1970's.* Edited by Zubin J, Money J. Baltimore, Johns Hopkins University Press, 1974, pp 77–98.
72. Howell M: Employed mothers and their families. *Pediatrics* 52:252–263, 327–343, 1973.
73. Wilf R: Childbearing and maternity centers: alternatives to home births and to hospitals. Presented at conference of National Association of Parents and Professionals for Safe Alternatives in Childbirth. Arlington, Va., May 15, 1976.
74. Summer P, Wheeler JP, Smith S: The labor-delivery bed simplified obstetrics. *Journal of Reproductive Medicine* 13:158–161, 1974.

Chapter 8

The COPE Story: A Service to Pregnant and Postpartum Women

Maureen Finnerty Turner and Martha H. Izzi

The questions of motherhood, its place in a woman's life, and the strains that an increasing population is placing on shrinking resources are issues that have been addressed in recent years by feminists and ecologists alike. In many cases, the weight of these questions has provoked anxiety and isolation among women who find themselves pregnant—by accident or by design.

Ecological and feminist concerns, together with the acknowledged decline of the extended family, have isolated the pregnant woman/couple, who are often without the traditional support systems essential to family strength.

An additional consideration for the pregnant woman/couple has been the emergence of birth and parent technologists, with all eyes focused on the baby. The mother wanders in a maze of obstetrical and pediatric faces and probes, and often has little encouragement to deal with the new emotional and life patterns facing her.

Sandwiched between blood pressures, weigh-ins, childbirth classes, fetal monitors, breast-feeding and childrearing theories is the woman. The pervasive cultural assumption is that in an age of contraception, legal abortion, and wider options for women, she has made a conscious decision to plan her family and "knows what she is getting into."

But indeed, none of us knows what we are getting into. Intrinsic to pregnancy and infant parenting adjustment are major physical, hormonal, emotional, and life-style changes that span more than a two-

Maureen Finnerty Turner, R. N. and Martha H. Izzi, B. S. • COPE (Coping with the Overall Pregnancy Parenting Experience), Boston, Massachusetts 02215.

year period. Ambivalence about having children is a common reaction even among those who have planned their pregnancies. At the same time, a range of emotional turbulence can be triggered internally by physical and hormonal changes and externally by the cultural image that at least some "craziness" is inherent in the pregnancy experience.

COPE

Coping with the Overall Pregnancy/Parenting Experience (COPE) support groups exist to bridge these conflicts and enable a woman to focus on her needs, motivations, and questions surrounding her experience. They draw pregnant women and new mothers together in small groups to share their mutual experiences and knowledge under the guidance of a group leader, herself a parent trained by COPE in perinatal psychology. Other groups include pregnant teenagers, single parents, fathers, couples, mothers of toddlers, all of whom share and learn under the direction of a new specialist *who has been there*. The COPE model also encompasses groups for postabortion women.

Founded in 1972 by psychiatric nurse group therapist Maureen F. Turner, COPE's birth coincided with that of her second child and her realization that, despite months spent in the intimacy of a consciousness-raising group, she and others ignored her pregnancy, impending birth, and postpartum issues. Sisterhood at that time did not necessarily include motherhood. An important psychological preparation had been eclipsed in favor of more militant concerns. And for her, new motherhood rested on its traditional foundations. "One was alone, tired, and isolated."

COPE groups evolved with enthusiastic media attention and support that, in turn, generated the first of (to date) over 12,000 phone calls. More than 600 women have participated in peer-led support groups. Presently, COPE groups are operating in sixteen metropolitan Boston communities, and by 1978, that figure will rise to twenty. A COPE in Atlanta, Georgia, is currently being licensed as well.

The COPE Support Group Model

The COPE group format encourages and assists women to focus on and come to terms with what they are experiencing. The atmosphere is supportive and focused on problem solving. In contrast to the encounter group model, the immediate goal is to reduce rather than to heighten anxiety levels to facilitate easy discussion of problems, joys, conflicts, and the whole network of belief systems that women bring into their pregnancies. The group setting is based on a support model but with a professional peer leader who eschews a lecturing posture in favor of relating personal experiences and insights.

COPE groups, meeting once a week for two hours, are limited to eight members, the optimal number for securing an intimate environment and developing group responsibilities. This is an important difference from other support models, such as Alcoholics Anonymous or Weight Watchers, which attract large, often listening audiences and tend to be leader dominated. A round-robin technique lifted from the consciousness-raising model is employed, allowing each member to develop a sense of "her" time and topic with time allotted at the end of each session for a summation or feedback.

As a normal adjustment reaction to multiple changes, some depression is inherent in the pregnancy and postpartum process. Severe and prolonged depression can be prevented as a postpartum reaction. The support group counteracts severe depression because it cuts through the isolation of pregnant women and new mothers, isolation being both a cause and a symptom of depression.

Variables that affect the group process and the isolation factor include wide spans in maturity levels, socioeconomic positions, age, racial makeup of the group, feminist and nonfeminist ideology, and stages of pregnancy/parenting.

For this reason, when possible, we group persons who have the same frames of reference, and because of the geographical spread of the organization, this often is feasible. For instance, if we cannot put at least two single parents together in a group, we will encourage the single parent to travel a bit farther to where there are other single parents in a neighboring community group. Also, we try not to start a newly pregnant woman with a group who have long since delivered. However, a woman's need for support and sisterhood immediately outweighs the group leader's concept of what might be an "ideal group makeup."

We find the urban groups more often able to tolerate and utilize a wide variety of variables quite well. This supports an axiom in group therapy that the more diversified the group in roles and backgrounds the more growth potential. It is a matter of keeping the group together. The main exception is the immature adolescent. She needs her own peer support and mixes uncomfortably with adult women.

An important COPE innovation was using mixed groups of pregnant women and new mothers. The new mothers often find great pleasure in sharing their new knowledge and experiences, while pregnant women pose poignant questions that new mothers might be reluctant to ask of one another. Many pregnant women also welcome the opportunity to offer the new mother babysitting services, often holding a baby for the first time.

COPE groups, such as pregnant women/new mothers, have been conducted for five years, involving over 600 women. Our experiences contradict an historically strong cultural bias that unveiling emotional issues among pregnant women could lead to serious consequences for the unborn child. Instead, they are a vehicle for positive transition into parenthood. This also is borne out by the fact that attendance at group meetings is characteristically high, with dropout rates extremely low.

The role of the professional peer leader is to maintain group focus, lead discussion, and serve as a technical resource on pregnancy and childrearing issues. She assists in developing decision-making skills for the woman faced with the often conflicting and controversial options open to the pregnant woman and new mother.

Group leaders are encouraged to share personal experiences with group members when such sharing strengthens the connection between them. This provides a role model and allows group members to follow suit. Further, members are not patients in the you-patient–me-therapist tradition, but are women with a mutual sense of purpose who often form friendships external to the group.

THE COPE COUNSELING MODEL

In the beginning, little research on the normal emotions of pregnancy and postpartum was available to Turner. Two important resources were the newly published *Pregnancy: The Psychological Experience*[1] by Libby and Arthur Coleman, which charted normal emotional stages of pregnancy, and *Our Bodies, Ourselves*,[2] which underscored the need for women to reclaim the pregnancy–childbearing experience. Most other available data focused on the pathology of pregnancy and postpartum psychoses. Beyond these limited resources, the field of normal perinatal psychology lay largely barren. In fact, McDonald states in his review of ten years of research on the emotions of pregnancy and the postpartum period, "There is a paucity of research and most of it is poorly done."[3] And yet it was the absence of data and reliable pregnancy models that enabled Turner and subsequent group leaders to listen to and closely examine the myriad emotional issues and experiences of pregnant and postpartum women and, hence, to avoid the pitfalls of incorporating them into existing therapeutic models.

Fundamental to the COPE counseling model is the recognition

that the pregnancy experience is a series of psychological stages identified by the Colemans and modified and expanded by Turner. The
following psychological stages of pregnancy and postpartum are the
theoretical framework within which the group and individual issues
are interpreted.[4]

PREGNANCY EMOTIONAL STAGES OF THE WOMAN

STAGE I—MOTIVATION STAGE. This stage is applicable to all pregnancies except birth control failures (i.e., the pill, IUD, and diaphragm) and rape.

Motivation for pregnancy can be conscious and unconscious.
Conscious planning can range from the pitiful cry of a fourteen-year-
old, "I want a baby for someone to love me," to the mature awareness
of a couple that "It is time" to share their love and understanding of
themselves and each other by creating offspring. Unconscious motives
for pregnancy are multiple.[5] They range from wanting a baby to replace a loved one to getting pregnant to test one's femininity. Most
often the reasons are a mixture of the mature and immature for both
men and women. The baby is seen as helper, curer, playmate, catalyst
for better things to come, or guest to arrive at a convenient time.

A great deal of growth can evolve from identifying one's less mature and self-serving motivations. The maturational level of one's motivations are not considered irrevocable or rigid and are utilized to
improve the context of parent–child relationships.[4:5−6]

STAGE II—INCORPORATING PREGNANCY REALITY (FIRST TRIMESTER).
This stage as identified by Libby and Arthur Coleman[1] is the psychological process of (1) realizing that one has missed a menstrual period;
(2) wondering if it means one is pregnant; (3) "feeling pregnant" in
some way—whether it be breast tenderness, abdominal swelling, nausea, tiredness, crankiness, and so forth; (4) having the initiative to get
a pregnancy test; (5) having pregnancy medically confirmed; (6) psychological acknowledgment of the pregnancy, that is, putting the
pregnancy into the context of one's life. This may or may not mean
making a *decision* about the pregnancy.

This decision phase of the incorporation stage is rapidly becoming the norm rather than the exception. Fewer women are taking the
confirmed pregnancy as something "to accept," and more women are
participating in making a decision to accept or to terminate the pregnancy. In order to make a "decision," the psychological *acknowledgment* (step 6) of the pregnancy has to have occurred. This is where
immature women and adolescents fall prey to denial defenses of the
reality of the pregnancy. This psychological acknowledgment is de-

layed, and preventive action is often put off to a point where intervention is too late.

Women who have planned their pregnancies seem to feel that they have less license to reexamine their decision and often experience guilt when considering an abortion. The "I made my bed and I'm going to lie in it," "The baby didn't ask for this—it was no accident" syndromes are common. Married women seem to follow this pattern even more than single women who have planned their pregnancies because there is no "reason" other than their fear *not* to have a baby.

Once the decision has been made, the pregnancy will be accepted or terminated.[4:17-22] (See section for Decision Making below.)

STAGE III—DIFFERENTIATION—OF THE PREPREGNANT SELF AND ESTABLISHMENT OF A PREGNANCY ROLE (SECOND TRIMESTER). The process of establishing a pregnancy role was described by Reva Rubin.[6] The Colemans identified this stage as beginning in the pregnant woman with an increased fixation with her own relationship to her mother. This is seen as a transitory response marking the end of the incorporation stage and the beginning of differentiation; no matter if it is the woman's first or sixth baby. Other key issues in the differentiation stage include dealing with the relationship to the baby's father, sexual readjustments, and feeling both a loss of control over one's body and an increased need to control and test one's environment. Fear of birth defects and retardation is probably the most universal anxiety variable in the pregnancy experience. The March of Dimes and other birth education groups have significantly raised public awareness about birth defects and retardation. Many women now are aware of the possible hazards of tranquilizers, alcohol, aspirin, and German measles and know about amniocentesis to test for mongolism and other diseases associated with advanced maternal and paternal age.[4:24-25]

STAGE IV—SEPARATION STAGE (THIRD TRIMESTER, LABOR AND DELIVERY). At about the seventh month of pregnancy, the two separate realities—that one is pregnant and that one is going to deliver a baby—begin to merge. The pregnancy role has been realized psychologically, and the impending birth and termination of the role begins to surface. The baby and especially the delivery become paramount concerns.

One of the growing dangers in the psychological process of the separation stage is the "option glut" of delivery choices and the emerging "scorecard" for the "best" kind of delivery to have. Depending on one's background, the "best" kind of delivery can vary from a home birth, with the father delivering, to being "put to sleep." It is important to help the pregnant woman/couple articulate the ideal delivery, making sure that they are informed of the pros and cons of each choice. The growing danger lies in the failure syndrome, which occurs when a complication obstructs the nature of the planned delivery. For example, a cesarean instead of a vaginal delivery may be required (the incidence is rapidly increasing to at least two out of ten deliveries and approaches five out of ten in some hospitals), or perhaps a paracervical block is needed at the last minute. One COPE group scored deliveries and developed a status chart that all eight members easily rattled off with consensus. It is this scorecard mentality that causes problems and is so prevalent. If women feel that they "flunked delivery," what psychological handicap may they take into the next stage? [4:15]

POSTPARTUM EMOTIONAL STAGES OF THE WOMAN

Postpartum stages are beginning to be identified because of research into the infant–mother relationship.

Postpartum technically means after the delivery and medically is considered "over" for the mother at six to eight weeks when her uterus has returned to place. Psychologically, there has been no clear definition as to when one is over the postpartum period. Speculation runs from six months to six years (or when the child begins school). Postpartum has most often been attached to psychosis and depression in the literature; yet there is still wide disagreement as to whether postpartum depression and postpartum psychosis are, in fact, different from other depressions and psychoses.

An important piece of research on postpartum behavior of the *mother* to be published for the general public is the new Klaus–Kennell book entitled *Maternal–Infant Bonding*. [7]

The original mother–infant bond is described as "the well-spring for all the infant's subsequent attachments and is the formative relationship in the course of which the child develops a sense of himself (or herself)". [7:1-2] The importance of the mother to the infant has been acknowledged in the infant-focused research of the past forty years. What is little understood empirically is the importance of the infant to the mother—that is, the development of attachment in the opposite direction, from mother to infant; what stimulates it, how it grows, develops, and matures, and what distorts, disturbs, promotes, or enhances it.

The study of maternal behavior came about as a result of studying infant behavior and is still in primitive stages. Again, most research has focused on pathology or on cross-cultural studies, leaving out American mothering patterns as part of the study.

The normal progression of the emotional stages of maternal development through the first three years of parenting (the postpartum period) has not been charted out. Margaret Mahler and her colleagues have been forerunners in researching in detail the emotional stages of the infant through three years of age.[8] This work and others can be utilized as a guide. Brazelton has identified the "dance" between parent and child and the dependency of each on the other for stimulation, growth, and development.[9] It seems reasonable, then, to look at the infant psychology research for clues as to what "step" the infant's dance partner, the mother, might be in. Along with establishing theory deductively, an inductive approach will be utilized by simply asking the mother.

The outline of postpartum stages that follows is a sketch based on more comprehensive charts.[4:35-37] It attempts to reflect the "hard research data" of maternal psychology and to interweave the "soft research" of watching, asking, and listening to hundreds of mothers in the past five years.

STAGE I—INITIAL BONDING—"THE SENSITIVE PERIOD" (DELIVERY TO 10 DAYS). The first phase of maternal postpartum adjustment was identified by Klaus and Kennell as the "maternal sensitive period."[7:51] This is to be distinguished from the "infant's sensitive period" identified by Yarrow and Bronfenbrenner when the infant is able to establish a stable, affectionate relationship with its mother at two to six months.[10,11]

The maternal sensitive period is described as an "enigmatic period" when "complex interactions between mother and infant help lock them together." The premise is that the events that occur during this time have long-lasting effects.[7:51]

The ability to have eye-to-eye contact and to touch the infant triggers further maternal instinct and emotional responses. The first two hours after delivery are considered pivotal since the infant (who has been delivered without medication) is at its most alert stage (Level 4 out of six stages of consciousness from sleep to crying) and remains alert for the longest consecutive period of time (up to two hours) in the early neonatal period.[12] Extended eye-to-eye contact is possible between both parents and their baby.

The tenuousness of the initial bonding behavior of mother to baby is underscored in the research. A jaundiced baby, an infant needing minor special attention, or early feeding problems can cause the new mother to "switch off" her bonding response or at least turn down the volume of interest as an "anticipatory grief reaction." Maternal-infant bonding research has bolstered the movement for family-centered maternity care and enlightened as well as grieved many of us who had our babies whisked away from us upon the delivery. The guilt of not feeling instant maternal love some twelve hours later when

a sleepy puffy-eyed baby is brought to you now has some interpretation. How different it might have been if you had seen your baby and
had that wide-eyed baby staring at you in the first few hours!

In one investigation[13] involving fourteen first-time mothers of
normal full-term infants, mothers were given their nude babies in bed
for one hour during the first two hours after birth. On each of the next
three days of life, they were given their babies for five extra hours
while a control group of mothers received the routine care still common to many hospitals in the United States: a glimpse of the baby at
birth, a brief contact at six to eight hours, and then visits of twenty to
thirty minutes for feedings every four hours. The infants and mothers
have been observed and tested over a five-year period.

The "extended contact" mothers and infants demonstrated significant differences in interaction at two years with the mothers asking
twice as many questions and giving fewer commands than the control
mothers.[14] The children at five years of age tested out at higher IQ and
language test scores than those who did not receive those extra hours
of contact with their mothers within the first three days of life.[15]

The birth-educated mother, that is, the woman who is seriously
examining traditional obstetrical birth practices and taking other measures, is learning about this research and planning with her doctor or
midwife accordingly, whereas many other women are highly medi-
cated, see the hospital stay as a vacation, and will begin to take care
of the baby only when they get home.

It is important that this sensitive period be used and not abused.
Failure to establish bonding behavior has long been seen as privation
for the infant. Now the question of privation and deprivation of the
mother is being raised. Are the postpartum pathologies of depression,
psychosis, and child abuse manifestations of interruptions of the
mother's bonding mechanism? If so, all the more reason for the *relationship* between the mother and infant, rather than the mother alone,
to be the "patient." At this point very few studies of postpartum emotional pathology in the mother even mention the infant's behavior.

STAGE II—INCORPORATING THE ROLE OF PARENT (10 DAYS TO 6–8
WEEKS). The psychological realization that one is no longer pregnant
but has a baby takes a while to incorporate. A brief grieving period for
the old pregnancy may well occur before the baby can become a reality. Once the initial bonding process has taken hold, the realization
that one *really* has a baby begins to dawn. Part of the incorporation
process appears to be dealing with one's fears of inadequacy as a
parent.

Ambivalence as to whether one really wants to take on the responsibility and self-sacrifice required of a mother to a newborn is

normal. These negative feelings frighten both women who are prepared for them and those who are not. To be able to acknowledge the ambivalence in a supportive setting is often a relief and catalyst to inner growth.

The mother deals with varying degrees of inadequacy and ambivalence depending upon her experience, situation, and support. Concurrently, the newborn is progressing psychologically from a "normal state of autism," which is an almost purely biological organismic dance with the mother, to the beginnings of a "normal symbiotic phase." This latter phase is a period of from one to five months of life where there is a sociological stage of interdependence with the mother, according to Mahler.[8:290]

Meanwhile the mother is still adjusting to the infant while watching, caring for, and recording the infant's activity. Part of this process is a need for "reporting on the baby from numbers of bowel movements a day to identified smiles."[4:32] This appears to be part of the incorporating process of the parenting role, just as counting calendar days, urine testing, and doctor exams are part of incorporating the reality of pregnancy. There is a one-dimensional focus that is important in the incorporation stage for the parenting role to take hold.

The baby stimulates the maternal role and helps the mother weather sleep deprivation, isolation, and the willingness to change some one hundred diapers a week. Developing the sense of history they share via "record-keeping" behavior seems to concretize their relationship. It appears to be disruptive to baby and mother if someone else takes over this role of overseer, as often happens with the help of well-meaning relatives. A common complaint among new mothers is that their mother (or aunt, or mother-in-law) came and took over and when they left the new mother felt more inadequate, abandoned, and "lost" than she would have had she been left by herself. The father can offer a great deal of support at this time and can protect the mother and baby from intrusion. The new mother often wants and needs teaching, not "take-over," at this time.

During the incorporation stage some semblance of a regular schedule is necessary before the next stage of differentiation (the reinstituting of other facets of one's life) becomes possible. A baby that sleeps through the night seems to accelerate this process. Sleep deprivation of the mother is a real danger and mothers and fathers of new infants have to be encouraged to "take it slow" for those first six to eight weeks.[4:36]

STAGE III—DIFFERENTIATION STAGE OF PARENT AND SELF (6–8 WEEKS TO 8–12 MONTHS). Once a loose schedule and plenty of sleep have been established, one can start taking back other familiar activities and interests to a greater degree. There begins to be a flow between the mother and infant in establishing priorities, whereas up to this time infant's needs and schedule have been the focus of attention. Now the mother gradually begins to establish some of her own priorities when possible.

Mahler sees the infant beginning a differentiation stage of its own between four and five months to ten to twelve months.[8:55] This is when total physical dependence on the mother begins to decrease and the development of partial locomotion brings about the first tentative moving away from her.

The realization that one is a parent of a child as opposed to an infant starts to dawn dimly as the baby begins rolling over, sitting up, and crawling.[4:37]

STAGE IV—EARLY SEPARATION STAGE (8–12 MONTHS TO 14–16 MONTHS). The realization that the baby is becoming a child and a separate entity from the mother seems to be clinched when the child begins walking. Sometimes, neither mother nor baby are emotionally ready to begin this separateness. The process for mother and baby of realizing these separations, independence and dependence, is both exciting and painful. Child specialist Margaret Mahler sees the infant progressing through a "Practicing Stage" from nine or ten to fourteen to sixteen months where the world is explored actively with relative lack of concern about the mother's presence.[8:65] This gives many a mother a false sense of autonomy and leaves her unprepared for the "Rapprochement Phase" identified by Mahler.[8:78]

STAGE V—MID-SEPARATION STAGE (14–16 MONTHS TO 24 MONTHS– 3 YEARS). Many a mother thinks that her child has reached the "terrible twos" prematurely when at fourteen to sixteen months, their delightful toddler becomes whiny, demanding, and literally clutches her leg at her first step away. As the toddler's awareness of separateness grows, she(he) wants her(his) mother. Mahler stresses the importance of the optimal emotional availability of the mother during this subphase.[8:77] Often, this is the time when many mothers, fooled by the carefreeness of their young toddler, begin to plan returning to work part-time or have begun making involved plans for time away from home. The "clings" of the sixteen- to twenty-four-month-old hark back to the immobility of the newborn period and fears that the mother has truly "spoiled" the child run rampant. A common complaint is that the only time the mother can get away from the child is while taking a shower. At this stage mother and child literally "dance" to each other's song of ambivalence about being separate people, with "No, no" often being their common refrain. Reassurance from other mothers who have been through it is extremely helpful in developing a more relaxed and playful attitude toward the toddler, which in turn facilitates the child's growth and independence.[4:38]

STAGE VI—LATE SEPARATION STAGE (24 TO 30 MONTHS). This is the final stage of "letting go" of mother–infant interaction. Mahler sees the mother's willingness to let go and give the toddler a gentle push toward independence as crucial.[8:75] Here the mother and child can talk to each other calmly and with dignity. The child has a sense of self and object constancy and does not need to see her (his) mother every minute to be aware of her presence. The mother now is aware that she is indeed the mother of a child and not a baby. The mother's postpartum period is ended.[4:39]

SPECIAL AREAS RELATED TO COUNSELING

DECISION MAKING. Counseling for decision making about pregnancy is difficult due largely to time constrictions and the nature of a major life decision. Most often a woman seeking help is between eight to ten weeks pregnant and has been referred by one of the abortion clinics because of doubts she has expressed to them. She has anywhere from two weeks to a few hours to make her decision about a suction abortion since most clinics will not perform a suction after ten weeks. If she does not make her decision in that time limit, she must wait at least four weeks before a hospital will do a prostaglandin or saline procedure; most prefer sixteen weeks and in Massachusetts will not perform an abortion after twenty weeks.

COPE counselors have found that second trimester abortions cause considerably more psychological complications and repeated unwanted pregnancies than the suction procedure. We therefore try to facilitate a decision at the earlier period if possible.

In the decision-making appointments, we try to help the woman understand her motivations as clearly as possible in as short a period of time as possible. The sessions, held in person (and never by phone), rarely last less than two hours each and will be scheduled as often as the woman and a staff member can manage. We will marshall as many resources as possible. A client can expect a session alone with a counselor who will help her sort the pros and cons of each choice and will try to deal with the various obstacles in the way of each choice. In some cases, she may wish to speak with a woman who has had an abortion and worked it through and/or a successful single parent. The danger of allowing this is that she may like the personality or lifestyle of one over the other and make the choice on this basis. This is discussed beforehand. Within COPE's counseling framework, Turner adapted and modified Gilligan's research on levels of women's moral development: (1) the undifferentiated self; (2) self-centered level; (3) concern for others as the reason for a decision; and (4) the most mature level—integrating the needs of the self and others in the decision-making process.[16]

POSTABORTION COUNSELING. If a woman agreed to an abortion on the demands or wishes of others in her life and/or has received little preabortion counseling, she will often contact COPE depressed, unable to define her needs, fearing that "to talk about it will make things worse."

Ambivalence about engaging in a COPE counseling group is a common characteristic in postabortion women. Her second thoughts and hesitancy about whether she really wants to open up a "can of worms" makes scheduling of postabortion groups very difficult. We have found that many women, perhaps eight out of ten, will come to an individual interview, spend hours recounting their experiences and insights and then not show up or opt for a group. Therefore, the rewards in working with postabortion women are not always as immediate as in working with pregnant women and new mothers who are not as easily able to repress their pregnancy and parenting experiences.

COPE's postabortion program began on an experimental basis. Group formats, time limits, and leadership roles were varied to adjust to the psychic and emotional wounds of women who have made a major life decision, often for the first time.

A workable group format evolved gradually that entailed an hour-and-a-half session each week for six weeks. Five to eight women, either married or single, comprise the group. All group leaders have experienced the abortion process and share in the group.

Topics focused on are:

First week. *The Abortion Experience.* Views on abortion prior to pregnancy. The clinic or hospital experience. Starting with what the women have in common helps solidify the group and gives a feeling of esprit de corps. We try to put the women who have had saline and saline prostaglandin procedures together and have found that women who have just recently had abortions and women who are working through old (one to ten years) abortions are helped by each other—one by experiencing new pain and the other by giving some perspective.

Second week. *Family and Friends/The Decision.* Reactions are sorted out by the women as to where they have received support and can continue to look for support and where they have felt rejected and abandoned.

Third week. The Man/How to Deal with Detachment, *Abandonment and General Male Disinterest.* Anger toward the male involved is a very common reaction along with feelings of being abandoned. "He gets off scot-free, while I go through a pregnancy and abortion and have to put my life back together alone" is a frequent response.

Fourth week. *Anger/Guilt and Outlets*. Here the women explore how they have been dealing with their anger. Many do not even realize that they are very angry. This is an extremely important session since it pulls together the anger and guilt expressed in the first three weeks and puts it in some perspective. Statistics indicate a range from 12–50 percent in abortion repeat rates. The highest risk appears to be among teenage women. We have worked with women having had up to six abortions who have had no repeat abortions in the program's three-year history. We will go through each abortion with them, helping them to get at the motivations for each pregnancy.

Fifth week. *Loss and Grieving*. Whether a woman feels that it is "just a bunch of cells," "potential life," "a growing fetus," or a "miniature baby" that she aborted, she needs to deal with grieving in proportion with what she felt she lost. Most often, we see women who are trying to figure out what it is they feel they lost and why they are feeling so bad or in more severe cases, not feeling anything at all. "I feel numb," "I feel like I'm dead inside" are heard repeatedly. A number of women we have worked with in individual therapy have found that the grief reaction they were having was, in fact, directed more toward a dead relative, most notably a parent, and have come to realize the pregnancy was an attempt to replace this loss.

Sixth week. *Birth Control and Our Future*. This is not a technique demonstration but focuses on why and how the diaphragm stays in the drawer, the pills are forgotten, the foam stays in the can, and most commonly, the condom stays in the wallet.

ADOLESCENT PREGNANCY COUNSELING. Our street level office in Boston is currently realizing a dramatic increase in walk-in, teenage, pregnant clients. They are referred by schools, courts, clients, and friends.

The pregnant adolescent population is growing by 10 percent annually at a time when the national birthrate is declining markedly. Historically, the myth existed that positive support and personal encouragement would induce a young woman to repeat the pregnancy experience and more unwanted social dependents would appear on the scene. The recent studies of Currie, Jekel, Klerman[17] do not support that widely held image. And in fact, they show that the more personalized and competent the pattern of counseling care during pregnancy and postpartum, the less likely they are to repeat a pregnancy.

The needs of the pregnant/parent teenager are great. COPE provides individual counseling, single parent groups, couple counseling, pregnancy decision-making skills, day-care referrals, educational/career counseling, even recycled maternity and infant clothes.

Subsequent family planning and birth control education is offered as well.

While the mature pregnant woman is awhirl with concerns ranging from the myriad birth processes open to her to deeper fears of ability to mother adequately, the pregnant adolescent is quite likely to appear at COPE's door announcing that she is eight months pregnant and "should I be doing something?". Another common reaction is "What's the big deal?" "I've babysat before, I know what's involved." Ninety percent will keep their babies, at least for a while, despite their boyfriends, many of whom favor abortion and often question paternity.

The COPE counseling model is individualized for this population. In fact, the support group process is less successful than a one to one counseling relationship, largely due to the issue of confidentiality and an adolescent inability to share intimate feelings and experience. Teenagers are often very curious about the counselor's behavior and surprised that she will share personal experiences. But this very sharing often serves as a role model to imitate, allowing motives, fears, anxieties, and fantasies to surface.

"Having a baby will make me a woman" is perhaps the most commonly expressed motive for adolescent pregnancy. In fact, a class pretest given by a COPE counselor at a large Boston high school revealed that 90 percent of those tested responded that the ability to have a baby is equated with womanhood.

Inherent in the complex issue of adolescent pregnancy counseling is pre- and postabortion counseling should she make a decision to terminate. A critical variable—the motivations for becoming pregnant—applies as much to the postabortion model as it does to the entire pregnancy counseling framework. In our view the high rate of repeat abortions within 12 months—so common to adolescents—will continue until her motivations are understood. The counselor must recognize the adolescent's loss of innocence and her need for varying degrees of grieving. Utmost skill is required to help her regain a sense of dignity and self-worth.

CONCLUSION

COPE was founded in November 1972 by Maureen Finnerty Turner. At this writing, it is in the final stages of the clinic licensure process and by Summer 1978 will become the nation's first perinatal mental health center. Its contribution to the new field of perinatal psychology—its practice and theory—is being acknowledged. As an organization, its immediate task is to provide for teaching and replication. Seminars, workshops, in-service counselor training, and consultation are an increasing part of COPE's services.

REFERENCES

1. Coleman A, Coleman L: *Pregnancy: the psychological experience*. New York, Herder & Herder, 1972.
2. Boston Women's Health Book Collective: *Our bodies, ourselves*. Revised Edition. New York, Simon & Schuster, 1976.
3. McDonald RL: The role of emotional factors in obstetric complications, a review. *Psychosomatic Medicine 30*:222–237, 1968.
4. Turner M: Psychological stages of pregnancy and postpartum. *Manual in Perinatal Psychology*, second draft (unpublished material) 1977, p 5–40.
5. Notman M, Kravitz, Payne et al: Psychological outcome in patients having therapeutic abortions. *Psychosomatic Medicine in Obstetrics and Gynecology*. Third International Congress. Edited by Morris, N. Basel, Karger, 1972.
6. Rubin, R: Attainment of the maternal role. *Nursing Research 16*:237–245, 342–346, 1967.
7. Klaus M, Kennell J: *Maternal-infant bonding: The impact of early separation or loss of family development*. Saint Louis, CV Mosby, 1976.
8. Mahler M, Pine F, Bergman A: *Human infant*. New York, Basic Books, 1976.
9. Brazelton TB, Tronick E, Adamson L, et al: In *Parent-infant interaction*, Ciba Foundation Symposium 33, Amsterdam. New York, Elsevier, 1975.
10. Yarrow LJ: Maternal deprivation: toward an empirical and conceptual re-evaluation. *Psychological Bulletin 58*:459–590, 1961.
11. Bronfenbrenner V: Early deprivation in mammals: a cross-species analysis. In *Early experience and behavior*. Edited by Newton G, Levine S. Springfield, Ill., Charles C Thomas, 1968.
12. Brazelton TB: The growth and development of parents. Speech delivered at Wheelock College Parenting Conference, Oct. 21, 1977.
13. Klaus MH, Jerauld R, Kreger N et al: Maternal attachment: importance of the first post-partum days. *New England Journal of Medicine 286*:460–463, 1972.
14. Ringler NM, Kennell JH, Jarvella R, et al: Mother-to-child speech at 2 years—effects of early postnatal contact. *Journal of Pediatrics 86*:141–144, 1975.
15. Ringler NM, Trause MA, Klaus MH: Mother's speech to her two-year-old, its effect on speech and language comprehension at 5 years. *Pediatric Research 10*:307, 1976.
16. Gilligan C: In a different voice: women's conceptions of the self and of morality. *Harvard Educational Review 4*:481–516.
17. Currie J, Jekel J, Klerman: Subsequent pregnancies among teenage mothers enrolled in a special program. *American Journal of Public Health 62*:12, Dec. 1972.

Chapter 9

Adolescent Sexuality and Pregnancy

CAROL C. NADELSON, MALKAH T. NOTMAN, AND JEAN GILLON

According to recent estimates, one out of ten American women becomes pregnant during her high school years, and two-fifths of fifteen- to nineteen-year-olds risk unintended pregnancy.[1,2] Despite the decline in the total birth rate in the United States, there has been a dramatic increase in adolescent pregnancy during the past decade.[3] Two-thirds of all pregnancies and one-half of all births to adolescents are unintended.[1] The most consistent findings in this group of teenagers is the failure to use contraceptives by those who are sexually active, and the adolescent's poor understanding of sexuality.[4] Lack of information, however, does not appear to be the major factor in the nonuse of contraception.[5] Most teenagers seeking contraceptive advice from family planning agencies have already been sexually active for several years, frequently without contraceptive use.[6] Psychosocial data on sexually active adolescents reveals that the majority are neither very disturbed nor promiscuous.[7] In fact, a recent study of adolescent sexual behavior reported that sexual affairs were seen as moves toward physical and emotional intimacy, not as casual encounters.[8] Clearly there is a need to improve and develop more appropriate educational and counseling programs that take into account the developmental and familial context of the adolescent.

CAROL C. NADELSON, M.D., MALKAH T. NOTMAN, M.D., AND JEAN GILLON, B.A. • Department of Psychiatry, Harvard Medical School, Beth Israel Hospital, Boston, Massachusetts 02215.

ADOLESCENT DEVELOPMENT

The adolescent developmental process involves a complex series of physical and emotional changes. It is a turning point, in which the implications of physiological change are often difficult to understand or to incorporate into an evolving self-concept. Menarche confronts the adolescent girl with unpredictable changes in feelings and behavior. She is often inadequately prepared or unable to respond to these changes. When menarche occurs early, biological maturation may take place in the framework of a childhood developmental phase. The physical events and attendant emotional changes may be difficult for the youngster to understand or to cope with. Formation of a stable self-image, a sexual identity, and the concept of self as separate from parents are the final goals in the maturational process.[9] This process does not occur in an orderly sequence, and thus the adolescent does not always integrate the perception of herself as a woman capable of procreation at the same time as she becomes physically able to do so. In addition, many adolescents, particularly younger ones, have not yet developed a set of personal values regarding sexual behavior when they begin to be sexually active. The consequences of sexual activity may not be clearly perceived, and often the ramifications of sexual acts are poorly conceptualized.

CONTRACEPTIVE USE

To use contraception effectively one must be oriented toward planning for the future, and one must acknowledge one's sexuality. Impulsiveness, lack of future orientation, and denial of consequences clearly do not provide protection against pregnancy, and these characteristics hallmark the adolescent developmental process. For the young adolescent, denial is a major ego mechanism that is used when confronted with a conflictual issue. Since the use of contraception implies acknowledgment of and responsibility for sexuality, it may not be consistent with the ego development of adolescents. Uncertainty about what is considered appropriate sexual behavior is frequent among adolescents, and parents are often uncertain or insecure and provide no clear guidelines. Nonuse of contraceptives may seem to conceal or deny sexual activity, or it may be a response to fear of being seen as "too" sexual, or guilt about sexual activity itself. The possible consequences of contraceptive nonuse are often difficult for the adolescent to face.

When one considers the complex reasons for the nonuse of contraceptives, the conscious or unconscious motivations to become pregnant must be considered as well as some of the more concrete aspects of availability of contraceptives. The adolescent may feel empty or isolated; she may see a baby as a means of receiving the care she lacks, or of replacing a loss in her life. The urge to mother is often an expression of the need to be mothered.[10] If the adolescent feels guilty about her sexual activity, she may see her pregnancy as a just punishment. Pregnancy may be seen by the adolescent who is unsure of her sexual identity as a statement of her femininity and womanhood. It can also be a vehicle for achieving independence from parents and for asserting adulthood, or it may provide a sense of security and status. At times the family may communicate, overtly or covertly, that a pregnancy is desirable. Often this occurs after the last child has been born to the parents, or when there are family stresses or disruptions.

CONSEQUENCES OF ADOLESCENT PREGNANCY

Teenage pregnancy is a major concern because of the medical, psychological, social, and economic sequelae of early childbearing. Premature birth, perinatal loss, and complications of labor and delivery are more frequent in the young adolescent and appear to be related to poor prenatal care.[11] In addition, the younger adolescent is less likely to develop and realize life plans and goals.[12] Premarital adolescent pregnancy has been shown to increase greatly the probability of eventual marital dissolution.[13] Pregnancy has been cited by one-half to two-thirds of female dropouts as the principal reason for leaving school.[14] The potential unplanned child also has difficulty; maternal ambivalence or rejection has long been acknowledged as a major contributing element in the development of human psychopathology and physical pathology.

THE DILEMMA OF PREGNANCY

When an adolescent becomes pregnant, there is no "good" alternative. She can continue the pregnancy and face the future with a child with whom she is emotionally unprepared to cope; she can give up the child and face the pain of separation and loss; or she can have an abortion and attempt to work through the resulting feelings. For the adolescent, this conflict is of particular developmental significance. It may represent the first time she must make decisions with lifelong implications. Even passive acceptance represents a decision to continue the pregnancy, and the consequences cannot be avoided or permanently denied.[15] Pregnancy itself constitutes a developmental step in the life cycle; however, the adolescent may not be prepared to move from the position of being an individual to seeing herself as part of a combined mother–child unit.[10] This conflict is important and can either be a significant maturational experience in which the adolescent assumes control of and finds direction for her lifelong decision, or can increase her feeling of failure, inadequacy, and inability to cope. A teenager who has not worked through maturational issues or those conflicts related to becoming pregnant initially is more at risk of becoming pregnant again. The high recidivism rates reported in adolescent pregnancy confirm this view.[11]

There is an increasing tendency for young mothers who do not have abortions to want to keep their babies. The young woman thus places herself in the position of combining her own maturation processes with the care of a baby whose needs she is not fully prepared to separate from her own. Pressure for adoption by persons who ignore these needs may result in repetition of the pregnancy.

For the girl who continues her pregnancy, realistic planning is important. The young adolescent who is passive and regressed may turn the responsibility for the baby over to someone else—to parents or an institution. Denial of the real implications of having a baby and sensitivity to social criticism make exploration of these issues difficult. Later, when attachments have developed and the repercussions for both mother and child are more serious, separation is potentially more damaging and older children may be more difficult to place for adoption.

A PILOT STUDY OF ADOLESCENT SEXUALITY AND PREGNANCY

In our own work with pregnant and nonpregnant adolescents, we have explored sexual knowledge and attitudes of a group of predominantly female adolescents. A questionnaire was given to the following groups of girls: those applying for abortions, pregnant girls carrying their pregnancy to term and staying in maternity homes, and a group of nonpregnant girls in a surburban high school. Although the groups varied in age, demographic characteristics, and stage of pregnancy, making rigorous data analysis impossible, there were suggestive results from the 350 responses that are consistent with those of other studies.[16]

KNOWLEDGE AND ATTITUDES. Those adolescents who had had sexual information courses indicated greater knowledge of basic areas of sexual information, including information about homosexuality, venereal disease, masturbation, and abortion. However, these adolescents do not appear to integrate and utilize this knowledge, since sexual education courses did not seem to contribute to the *use* of contraception. Thus, as has been noted above, sexual information alone may not change behavior when there are stronger motivations or conflicts that a pregnancy will resolve.

Use of Contraceptives. The adolescents revealed some knowledge of various forms of contraception. Most had obtained this information predominantly from friends, the mass media, or "the street," rather than from parents or school. Those sexually active adolescents who were seeking abortions and those who were not pregnant were more likely than those in the maternity homes group to have used some form of contraception at some time. A fourth of all the adolescents failed to use contraception because they did not predict or consciously acknowledge the consequences of sexual activity. They felt that pregnancy could never happen to them. Others attributed nonuse to fear of discovery, guilt, or shame. Some were embarrassed, fearful, or reluctant to confront their boyfriends directly with the need for protection during sexual activity; some blamed them for not assuming responsibility. Some expressed explicit conscious motivation or indicated unconscious motivation for pregnancy. The remainder saw birth control methods as "messy or unnatural."

Those young women in the maternity homes group were more likely to respond affirmatively to statements like: "Sometimes I feel so lonely that I'd like to have a baby," and "Deep down I might want to get pregnant." They felt lonely and wished for a pregnancy. The abortion group had the lowest percentage of respondents choosing these as possible motivations. There also appeared to be a relationship between age and contraceptive use. The likelihood of pregnancy decreased with age. The peak incidence of pregnancy was at age sixteen with diminishing incidence occurring at seventeen and eighteen. With increasing age, contraceptive use increased.

Attitudes toward Pregnancy. Those adolescents who were seeking abortions were similar to the nonpregnant high school students in their statements about how the dilemma of pregnancy was to be resolved. They searched for active solutions to the conflict created by the choice between abortion or carrying an unwanted pregnancy. Issues of responsibility and active confrontation with the problem were prominent.

The responses from the abortion group expressed their concern about autonomy and responsibility—"It's up to the girl herself!" "It's her choice and her body, no one else's," "It's better if that's what she wants," "She should make her own decision," and "If she decided on the abortion, not her parents." These statements describe the adolescent's striving for autonomy. In some responses other considerations are also communicated, such as: "She might not be ready to take care of the baby and she should not quit school at such a young age,"

"Having a baby and not being able to provide for it is worse than any other thing for both mother and child," and "Abortion is a good choice because she couldn't give an innocent baby the love and care it deserves."

The nonpregnant high school students gave very similar kinds of responses, for example, "If she didn't want the child, if she couldn't care for it—then I see her point!" "It's up to the person, you can't decide for anybody else," and "It's better than getting married if she doesn't want to."

The responses from the maternity homes group were different. Their responses included statements like, "Her mother and father should have helped her with the baby until she got on her feet," indicating an expectation of parental help. Other responses tended to imply that continuation of the pregnancy was a just punishment because the adolescent was guilty and/or lacked responsibility for her sexual activity. Examples of these are: "I don't think she should because it's wrong to get one even if she don't want it she should still keep it," and "She had the baby, she should have kept it, she was the cause." Many were willing to assume the responsibility and bear the guilt for their actions, dismissing their male partner from any responsibility.

Those girls who chose abortion focused on the importance of finishing school, the practicality of caring for a child, and the need to take responsibility for one's actions.

Those from the maternity homes more often indicated that there was no real choice for them or, at least, that the choice was passively made. Undoubtedly many made their decision to carry to term because of religious or ethical considerations, some out of a desire to have a baby, and some because they were unable to bear the abortion loss. Since becoming pregnant is often a way of replacing a loss, under the circumstances abortion might not have been an alternative that could be considered.

FAMILY ISSUES. The pregnant adolescent's relationship to her family is complex and varied. Adolescents from the maternity homes indicated they never fought with their mothers; however, denial of conflict or fear of confrontation may have contributed to these responses. Their passivity and acceptance may perhaps reflect a defensive attempt to reduce internal conflict. Since adolescents who carry to term either continue to live with their families or leave home and live on welfare, having a baby may also be a means of maintaining or breaking familial relations. Adolescents from the abortion group more frequently indicated that they fought with their mothers and that their mothers were more strict than other people's mothers. Perhaps their drive toward autonomy as reflected by this conflict with authority, resulting in their becoming pregnant, enabled them to make an active choice (in this case abortion) to resolve the unwanted pregnancy.

SUMMARY

Adolescents live in a changing society where values are being questioned, sexual mores are changing, traditions are weakening, and social performance pressure is high. The teenager is often confused as to what is appropriate sexual behavior and has often had to seek guidance outside of the family. Becoming pregnant in adolescence for many teenagers appears to be strongly related to unresolved familial issues and difficulty in making the transition to adulthood. Motivations for the nonuse of contraceptives as well as the messages communicated by an unwanted pregnancy are diverse. Clearly, no single resolution for an unwanted pregnancy is appropriate for all young women. The handling of this stressful period for the unmarried adolescent is critical, as its implications are lifelong and are instrumental in the young woman's development.

REFERENCES

1. Jaffe F, Dryfoos J: Fertility control services for adolescents: access and utilization. *Family Planning Perspectives* 8(4): 167, 1976.
2. National Institute of Child Health and Human Development, Center for Population Research, RFP No. NICHD-BS-75-7, 1974.
3. *New York Times*, September 20, 1977.
4. Goldsmith S, Gabrielson W, Gabrielson I et al: Teenagers, sex and contraception. *Family Planning Perspectives* 4(1):32–38, 1972.
5. Nadelson C, Notman M, Friedman C: Sexual knowledge and attitudes of teenagers. Presented at American Psychiatric Association meetings, Honolulu, Hawaii, May 1973.
6. Akpom A, Akpom K, Davis M: Prior sexual behavior of teenagers attending rap sessions for the first time. *Family Planning Perspectives* 8(4):203, 1976.
7. Bernard V: Psychodynamics of unmarried motherhood in early adolescence. *New Child* 4:26–45, 1944.
8. Chess S, Thomas A, Cameron M: Sexual attitudes and behavior patterns in a middle-class adolescent population. *American Journal of Orthopsychiatry* 45(4):699–700, October 1976.
9. Nadelson C: The pregnant teenager: problems of choice in a developmental framework. *Psychiatric Opinion* 12(2):8–12, 1975.
10. Schaffer C, Pine F: Pregnancy, abortion and the developmental tasks of adolescence. *Journal of Child Psychiatry* 14:511–536, 1975.
11. Mecklenberg F: Pregnancy: an adolescent crisis. *Minnesota Medicine* 56(2):101–104, 1973.
12. Presser H: Social consequences of teenage childbearing. In *Social demography: the state of the art*. Edited by Peterson, Day. Cambridge, Mass., Harvard University Press, 1977.

13. Lowrie S: Early marriage: premarital pregnancy and associated factors. *Journal of Marriage and the Family* 27:49, 1965.
14. Coombs J, Cooley W: Dropouts: in high school and after school. *American Educational Research Journal* 5:343, 1968.
15. Nadelson C: Abortion counselling: focus on adolescent pregnancy. *Pediatrics* 54:6, December, 1974.
16. Sorenson R: *Adolescent sexuality in contemporary America*. New York, World Publishing, 1973.

Chapter 10

Conflicts between Fertility and Infertility

Ruth W. Lidz

Today, a woman can avoid pregnancy by using one of the highly effective methods of contraception available to her, or by having an
abortion when necessary. It has become clear, however, that many
women cannot accept that choice comfortably and that psychological
conflicts often interfere with the planning of a family and motivation
to use contraception. Prior to the availability of effective contraception, a woman could avoid sexual intercourse, use a partially effective
contraceptive method and hope not to get "caught," or depend on her
husband to prevent conception. It was psychologically useful for her
not to have to make a definite decision about pregnancy and to be
willing to accept what happened each month. Maintaining an ambivalent state of mind was a common and highly useful adaptation of
married women that served well in case of an unexpected or even
unwanted pregnancy. Now that a woman can prevent pregnancy herself, she has to come off the fence, reach a decision, and take the responsibility for choosing fertility or infertility.

The sequence from sexual intercourse through conception, pregnancy, childbirth, and the rearing of a child is usually considered as a
continuum, and the assumption is often made that a woman who does
not want a child will be well motivated to use contraception. However, an understanding of women's feelings, fantasies, and behavior
in family planning and abortion clinic settings makes it apparent
that many psychological complexities are involved in the process.
There is, for example, a basic difference between the gratifications a

RUTH W. LIDZ, M.D. • Clinical Professor, Department of Psychiatry, Yale University,
New Haven, Connecticut 06519.

woman gains from sexual intercourse and even from proving that she is fertile by conceiving, in comparison with the gratifications and responsibilities derived from the birth of a child and motherhood. Sexual relations are often sought not only for pleasure and release but also because of the woman's need for closeness and dependency. A less mature woman may seek to become pregnant to prove to herself and others that she is a woman, and has the capacity to create a child—a highly ego-supportive experience. Being a mother, however, requires commitment, self-discipline, and the ability to empathize with the child and to accept the child's needs as equally important, if not more important, than her own. Although many women will gain satisfaction and pleasure from intercourse, being pregnant, and having and rearing a child, some women will be more attracted to having intercourse and becoming pregnant, while others will be more attracted to having and rearing a child. Unconscious factors play an important role. Indeed, we find women who appear to need to have frequent pregnancies and then seek repeated abortions since they do not wish to have a child. Some young women become pregnant simply to show that they are now as grown up as their mothers or sisters. Others wish to have a baby to have someone to love or who will love them, but cannot sustain their investment when the infant makes demands upon them and limits their activities. And a woman may need to prove her fertility much as a man needs to prove his potency.

FAMILY AND CULTURAL PRESSURES

Besides the inner pressures motivating a woman to become pregnant, there may be family and cultural pressures toward fertility before a woman is ready to accept and bring up a child. For example, a young woman's mother—possibly going through menopause herself—may wish for a grandchild and pressure her daughter to produce one before the latter feels settled in her marriage.

Women who already have several children and do not wish or cannot afford another may also feel considerable conflict about using contraception regularly. Men and women from backgrounds in which women traditionally have been primarily mothers and housekeepers can have difficulty separating the sexual act from procreation. Such men may not appreciate or respect women who are not fertile. Thus, a man called his wife a "dud" when she was taking the pill. Some men feel frustrated about the "waste" of their semen and one compared his infertile wife to a broken-down vending machine by saying, "One can get kind of resentful when one keeps putting a dime in a machine and nothing comes out." Men's and women's self-esteem and pride may be tied in with the number of children they produce. Women may feel that sex is unexciting or "does not make sense" when they cannot conceive. A woman complained, "I have to feel fertile to enjoy sex." Many women prefer to expose themselves to the possibility of becoming pregnant for such reasons even when they do not wish to have a child. Spouses may be unable to discuss their feelings about what contraception does to their sexual desire and self-esteem, and major marital conflicts may ensue. The woman may then abandon her contraception to restore harmony. Such difficulties can often be avoided by inviting the husband or partner to participate in family planning from the beginning.

Some women from traditional, particularly religious, backgrounds feel guilty about rejecting motherhood and feel that they would be "selfish" or lazy if unwilling to accept more children. Such women are apt to feel conflicts about doing something against nature or the will of God and may even punish themselves for using contraception by inadvertently having another child. Some feel uneasy about being "aggressive" in controlling their fertility or in denying their husbands the "self-expression" or "right" to father another baby. Many prefer to have their husbands use condoms and adjust to the man's decisions or indecisions, or to blame their husbands for making them pregnant. Perhaps the conflict in these women derives from the need to remain passive in relationship to their husbands' wishes while resenting their husbands' control over their lives. They may feel that their husbands keep them tied to the home by impregnating them over and over again. Nevertheless, they allow themselves to become pregnant, even when they do not want another child. If the husband refuses to accept the responsibility for contraception, the wife who is caught in such conflicts may take her pill irregularly. One woman said she felt sorry for her husband and wanted to give him "a chance" and so did not take her pills on weekends.

In marriages of this type where the woman has habitually adjusted passively or passive-aggressively to her husband's wishes or what she thinks are his wishes, there is little chance for consistent use of contraception unless the husband is brought into the planning process, the couple agrees on using contraception, and the husband reinforces the wife's use of the contraceptive or uses a condom himself.

Simply because a woman smilingly says that she already has "too many" children, one cannot assume that she is well motivated for contraception. A woman can have serious conflicts because she cannot afford another child and yet feels the urge to become pregnant, having found pregnancy the most hopeful, exciting, and creative experience of her life. Such women talk longingly of the desire to be pregnant, to have "something alive inside." Their lives are basically oriented toward having and caring for babies. When an IUD is inserted, they may become depressed, feeling that the future holds nothing for them, that they are "no good any more," or that it is like being post-menopausal.

The loss of a loved or needed person, or a severe blow to a woman's self-esteem can consciously or unconsciously lead her to expose herself to pregnancy. During bereavement, feeling lonely and lost, she seeks closeness to a man. This may lead to pregnancy, particularly when she seeks to reaffirm life through creating a new life in the face of death.[6]

Pregnancy can also serve to reestablish self-esteem or to provide a way out of an intolerable situation. A graduate student who had used contraception successfully for several years became upset and discouraged when her proposal for her Ph.D. thesis was rejected. She decided to spend the next weekend with her boyfriend to "think of something else." The next month, she found herself pregnant but realized only after counting her pills that she had forgotten to take them while with her boyfriend.

Factors in Teenage Pregnancy

At present, there is great concern with the high number of teenage pregnancies, sometimes in twelve- or thirteen-year-old girls, which frequently run counter to the long-term interests of the girls themselves as well as their children and society. Experience has shown that having a child at this age is often the beginning of a destructive cycle of failure to continue education, dependence on the welfare system, day-to-day living without a plan, and further pregnancies arising out of a feeling of desperate emotional need.[1,4] In the 1960s such patterns were observed more frequently in black inner-city ghettos;[2] in the 1970s teenage pregnancy has become a general problem. Lack of family life, hostilities toward parent figures, longings for dependency and love as well as need for prestige often play decisive roles in short-term motivation for pregnancy. Babies are often fervently wanted but with little thought, awareness, or knowledge of the investment needed to care for the baby and growing child.

Statistically, education has been identified as the single most significant variable favoring small or smaller families.[5,7] In clinical work with women of varied backgrounds and ages, we have been impressed by the discovery that it may not be the number of years of education, or sex education in particular, that make the decisive difference but rather, that the woman develops interests and a plan for her life that allows her to postpone having a child and lessens the need to use pregnancy as an ego-supportive experience.[4] Educational and work opportunities for women are therefore of great importance, as are counseling and help with career planning as well as sex education and counseling throughout high school and the early college years.

Gaining pleasure from sexual relations tends to lessen rather than increase the need for procreation. It tends to undermine the old attitude that "a man gets pleasure from sex and a woman a baby," a feeling expressed by many women who were having trouble using contraception consistently. To maintain her contraceptive planning, a woman must be able to separate sex for recreation from sex for procreation, and to enjoy the relationship involved as well as the act—a relationship that needs to be open and cooperative rather than manipulative or sadomasochistic.

From the above, it becomes evident that services in family planning clinics need to include a study of the woman's relationship to her husband or mate and their attitudes to help them carry out their contraceptive plans. To understand the couple's commitment to or difficulties with the use of contraception, one needs to investigate their cultural background and relationship with each other, family and peer influences, as well as their personal attitudes toward infertility, sexuality, pregnancy, childbirth, and parenthood.[3]

SUMMARY

There are many reasons why women fail to use effective contraception or slip up on its usage despite their expressed intention not to have a child, and why many women seek abortion despite the availability of effective contraception. In the simplest terms, there are differences between sex for passion or recreation and sex for procreation, between the desire to be pregnant and the wish for a child, and between the wish for a baby and the desire to rear a child.

We have noted the sources of some conflicts that can arise in the sequence that leads from sexual relations to the rearing of a child. A young woman may become pregnant to prove her femininity or fertility to herself or others or to hold a boyfriend, but she may be too immature to give birth and assume the responsibilities of motherhood. A woman may need the sense of creativity and fulfillment that comes with bearing a child, but may lack a husband or the self-sufficiency needed to raise a child. Despite a conscious decision to pursue an occupation for a time, a young married woman may feel unfulfilled in any role other than that of mother and housewife. She may consider infertility depriving or degrading or may be unable to gain sexual pleasure if she cannot conceive. A wife may seek the attention and tenderness received from her husband and family when she is pregnant despite the limitations, financial and otherwise, that could result from having another child. Some find it more comfortable to adjust in a passive-aggressive manner to whatever their husbands decide or fail to decide, rather than to assert their own needs or preferences about having another child. Others fear that their own reluctance to have a child and their use of contraception will encourage their husbands to demonstrate their virility by making another woman pregnant. Women who may have little or no desire for a baby may consciously or unconsciously utilize pregnancy as an affirmation of life after losing a loved or needed person; and some will become pregnant as an ego-sustaining means of recouping from a defeat, or as a way of escaping from a dilemma. With conception and having a baby, as with many other aspects of life, conflicts and unconscious motivations commonly interfere with intentions and even with resolutions.

REFERENCES

1. Balsam A, Lidz RW: Psychiatric consultation to the Teenage Unwed Mothers Program. *Connecticut Medicine 33*:447–452, 1969.
2. Lewis DO, Klerman L, Jekels J, et al: Experiences with psychiatric services in a program for pregnant school-age girls. *Social Psychiatry 8*:16–25, 1973.
3. Lidz RW: Emotional factors in the success of contraception. *Fertility & Sterility 20*:761–771, 1969.
4. Sarrel PM, Lidz RW: Psychosocial factors: the unwed. In *Manual of family planning and contraceptive practice*. Edited by Calderone M. Baltimore, Williams & Wilkins, 1970.
5. Stycos JM: *Ideology, faith and family planning in Latin America*. New York, McGraw-Hill, 1971.
6. Swigar M, Bowers MB, Fleck S: Grieving and unplanned pregnancy. *Psychiatry 39*:72–80, 1976.
7. Zelnik M, Kantner J: Sexual and contraceptive experience of young unmarried women in the United States, 1976 and 1971. *Family Planning Perspectives 9*(2), March–April 1977.

Chapter 11

The Problem of Infertility

MIRIAM D. MAZOR

> And when Rachel saw that she bore Jacob no children, Rachel envied her
> sister; and she said unto Jacob: "Give me children, or else I die."
>
> GENESIS 30:1

Infertility represents a major life crisis to more than 10 million people in the United States[1]—as individuals, as partners in marriage, and as members of families and society. Few people who have not been personally involved are fully aware of the emotional impact of recognition of the problem, the diagnostic and therapeutic procedures that may be undertaken, and the eventual outcome of such an investigation.

This chapter will first deal briefly with the medical aspects of infertility, in order to provide a better understanding of the emotional issues. It will then describe the psychological and social issues involved in facing the problems of infertility, in reactions to various aspects of the infertility study, and in coming to terms with an acceptable resolution of the problem. Although the focus will be on the problems of the infertile woman, many of the issues are similar for the infertile man, and many issues involve the couple as a unit, regardless of which partner has the infertility problem.*

DEFINITION AND INCIDENCE OF INFERTILITY

Infertility is generally defined as the failure to achieve a successful pregnancy (i.e., leading to live birth) following a year of regular sexual

---

*Throughout this discussion, I am deeply indebted to Barbara Eck Menning, founder and director of Resolve, Inc., a support organization for infertile people, and to the members of Resolve whose candid statements about their problems provided many of the quotations used here.

MIRIAM D. MAZOR, M.D. • Clinical Instructor, Department of Psychiatry, Harvard Medical School; Associate in Psychiatry, Beth Israel Hospital, Boston, Massachusetts 02215.

relations without contraception. Primary infertility means that a pregnancy has never been achieved; secondary infertility refers to situations in which there have previously been one or more living children.
Sterility is defined as absolute infertility—for example, after a hysterectomy, or for the male, total inability to produce sperm.

In the absence of contraception, about 25 percent of all sexually
active couples will conceive in one month, 63 percent in six months,
and about 80 percent in a year. In a second year, another 5 to 10 percent will achieve a pregnancy. The remaining 15 percent or so have a
diminished chance of becoming pregnant in the absence of treatment,
and it is this group of people who are considered to have an infertility
problem.[2]

Some evidence suggests that this group is increasing.[1] In part this
is due to the postponement of marriage and child-bearing, for personal, social, and economic reasons, until the thirties or even forties.
For both males and females, fertility appears to be maximal at about
age 24 to 25.[2] Other factors include the increased prevalence of venereal disease in all sectors of the population, especially among teenagers. An unfortunate sequel in both males and females, if treatment
is not obtained early enough, may be scarring and blockage of the
reproductive tract. Also, certain contraceptive methods may lead to infertility problems. For example, the IUD may cause infection and subsequent scarring of the Fallopian tubes. Oral contraceptives may
present problems in ovulation when their use is discontinued, especially in women with histories of irregular menses prior to the use of
the pill.[1] Therapeutic abortion, even under conditions that minimize
the risk of infection, may, through rapid or over-vigorous dilation of
the cervix, lead to problems in maintaining desired pregnancies later
on.

Still other factors may lead to a rise in the number of people seeking help with infertility problems. People today are less likely to adopt
a fatalistic or reticent attitude. Medical advances offer greater treatment possibilities, and the social climate fosters a direct approach to
problems previously considered shameful or embarrassing. Although
infertility usually is not a problem of sexual dysfunction, its relation to
the reproductive organs causes many people to associate it with sexual
problems. Since it has become more acceptable to discuss sexual matters freely, it has become easier for infertile people to acknowledge
and discuss their problems. Also, as aware consumers of medical services, people demand and expect help in the area of infertility, as in
other health-related matters.

Still another push toward recognition and treatment of infertility
is that adoption no longer represents the easy solution it was once

thought to be. Since 1970, abortions have become more available to women who want them. At the same time, less stigma is attached to unwed motherhood. Healthy infants of all races available for adoption are extremely difficult to find in the United States.

Medical Aspects of Infertility

In about 70 percent of couples who have been thoroughly investigated, an organic problem can be found. Of these, about 50 percent can be helped to achieve a pregnancy and 40 percent a living child. In about 50 percent of couples the infertility problem resides in the female partner; in another 30 percent the problem is with the male, and the remaining 20 percent represent a combined problem.[3]

The old notion that infertility is a predominantly "functional" disorder is not only unsubstantiated, but tends to alienate patients and thus deprive them of the sources of psychological help that may be very important. Psychological factors and stress reactions probably play some role in infertility, but the influence of higher nervous system centers on human reproduction is complex and not well understood. Perhaps the strongest evidence comes from observations of women who stop ovulating in times of stress. Sperm production in the male may also be somewhat sensitive to stress, and some evidence suggests that psychological factors may inhibit sperm transport within the female genital tract.[2] However, current research indicates that these factors are not the critical ones in the majority of infertility patients, and experience tells us that pregnancies can and do occur under even the most trying environmental and psychological conditions.

An excellent discussion of the common causes of infertility, diagnostic procedures, and treatment modalities can be found in Menning's book *Infertility: A Guide for the Childless Couple*.[1] Those readers who want a more comprehensive, detailed account of the medical issues are referred to Behrman and Kistner's *Progress in Infertility*.[2] For this discussion, however, a brief review of the anatomy and physiology of reproduction is given in Figure 1.

Problems in the Female

These can be grouped roughly into (1) mechanical barriers to fertilization, (2) endocrine disorders, and (3) structural disorders of the reproductive tract.

Mechanical Barriers. Mechanical barriers to the union of sperm and ovum probably account for the majority of cases of infertility in

ESSENTIAL FACTORS
FOR REPRODUCTION

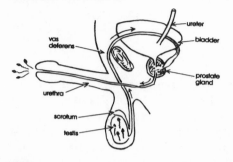

Male — He must be able to produce sufficient numbers of normal, active sperm in his testis which, on ejaculation, can be discharged from the penis.

MALE
Sperm Production
Ejaculation

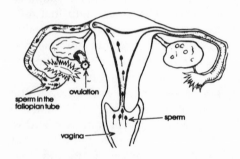

Male and Female — The sperm must be deposited in the female vagina in such a way that they reach and penetrate the cervix (neck of the womb) and ascend through the uterus to the fallopian tube. For pregnancy to occur the sperm must reach (or be present) at the end of the tube within hours of the time that the ovum (egg) has been released from the female ovary.

MALE AND FEMALE
Sperm Deposition in Vagina
Normal Uterus and tubes

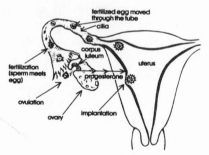

Female — She must produce a normal ovum (usually at monthly intervals) which can enter the fallopian tube and become fertilized (union of the egg and sperm). The resulting conceptus must then move into the uterus, implant itself in the wall and there undergo normal development for nine months.

FEMALE
Ovulation, Fertilization and Implantation

Figure 1. Copyright © Boston Hospital for Women Division Affiliated Hospitals Center, Inc. 1976. All rights reserved. Reprinted with permission.

women. Problems in tubal patency may account for 30 to 35 percent of all infertility cases.[2] Some of the more common causes are:

1. Infection of pelvic organs. The uterus, tubes, ovaries, or their ligaments may become infected and inflamed. Following the acute inflammation, stringy scar tissue called adhesions may form and interfere with the normal functioning of the reproductive tract. Infections may be introduced from the vagina (as in venereal disease), from outside the body (as in septic abortions), or from a leaking or ruptured portion of the digestive tract (as in appendicitis).

2. Endometriosis. In this condition, endometrial tissue grows in areas other than the uterus—usually in the tubes, ovaries, and around the uterine ligaments. This tissue bleeds at each menstruation. Irritation of the surrounding tissue causes scarring and adhesion formation. Although its cause is not fully known, endometriosis is most commonly diagnosed in women over thirty who have not been pregnant.

3. Cervical problems. Sperm may be impeded or destroyed by components in the cervical mucus.

ENDOCRINE DISORDERS. These represent the second greatest cause of female infertility. Because of the delicate hormonal balance required for normal function, dysfunction of the pituitary, thyroid, adrenals, or ovaries can affect fertility. Some women are unable to ovulate at all; others do so irregularly. In Turner's syndrome there is a congenital absence of functional ovarian tissue. In Stein–Leventhal syndrome, the ovaries form multiple cysts, which interfere with normal ovulation. Other endocrine problems may interfere with implantation or maintenance of the early pregnancy.

STRUCTURAL DISORDERS. Although they are rarer, structural or anatomic problems can contribute to difficulties in conception and maintenance of a pregnancy. An easily corrected condition is that of the rigid hymen, which does not permit penetration by the male. Rarely, there is total congenital absence of the uterus; more often it is malformed. Other conditions include large fibroid tumors of the uterus, and the "incompetent" cervix—a leading cause of second trimester spontaneous abortion.

PROBLEMS IN THE MALE

Unlike the female, whose entire supply of immature ova is established in the ovary prior to her birth, the male is capable of continuous sperm production throughout adult life. A normal ejaculate contains about 40 to 500 million active sperm in a volume of 2 to 5 cc of semen; however, a count of 20 million or more, with good morphology and motility, may be quite adequate for conception.[2]

Problems may arise in the production of adequate numbers of sperm, in the transport of sperm through the male reproductive system, and in the deposition of sperm within the vagina.

Problems in Sperm Production. Any infection associated with high fever can be responsible for diminished sperm production temporarily. Mumps in adulthood may cause permanent damage to the testes. Varicocoele (a varicose vein in the testicle), prolonged elevation of the temperature of the scrotum, exposure to radiation, certain drugs and industrial chemicals, excessive smoking and alcohol intake may possibly influence sperm production adversely. In congenital disorders, such as Klinefelter syndrome, there is no functional sperm-producing tissue. Failure to correct undescended testes in early childhood may also lead to an irreversible inability to produce sperm.

Problems in Sperm Motility (or Capacity to Fertilize an Ovum). The motility of the sperm may be adversely affected by hormonal factors, prostate disease, or, theoretically, by an autoimmune response in which a man produces antibodies against his own sperm.

Problems in Sperm Transport. Sperm transport within the male reproductive system can be blocked by scars formed as a consequence of venereal disease, accidental injury to the vas deferens, or vasectomy.

Inadequate deposition of sperm in the female can be related to impotence, ejaculatory difficulties, and disabilities that impair male sexual functioning (such as spinal cord injury). In retrograde ejaculation, sperm flow backward, into the bladder.

Combined Problems

Each partner may have an individual problem, to a lesser or greater degree, or some factor may prevent the couple as a unit from conceiving.

Probably the most remediable cause of infertility in a couple as a unit is faulty sexual technique or improper timing of sexual relations. For example, certain positions in intercourse favor the delivery of sperm to the cervical opening; one that is known to do so is where the woman lies on her back, with her hips flexed or elevated on a pillow. She then remains in that position for ten or fifteen minutes following intercourse. The fertile period may be missed each month because of misinformation (e.g., the rise in basal body temperature usually occurs one or two days after ovulation, so that the couple who wait for this rise before having intercourse will miss ovulation regularly), or because of religious prohibitions (in Orthodox Judaism, a couple is required to abstain from intercourse for a week following the cessation of menstrual flow). Very frequent intercourse (more than once a day) may diminish the number of sperm per ejaculate, and very infrequent intercourse may diminish the motility of sperm.[2]

Sexual dysfunction based on psychological conflicts may, in rare instances, result in vaginismus in the female (spasm of the vaginal muscles which prevents penetration by the penis), or impotence or ejaculatory problems in the male. Conception can and does occur in the absence of orgasm in the woman, but if the problem exists, it deserves attention in its own right.

Another important factor in combined infertility is that of the immunologic response. Some women produce antisperm antibodies, which cause sperm (from any man) to clump and die. The antibody levels seem to increase with the woman's exposure to sperm.

THE INFERTILITY STUDY

Traditionally, the gynecologist is approached by his/her female patient when help with an infertility problem is sought, but it is important that both partners be seen early in the investigation in order to obtain adequate histories, to listen to what their separate and joint concerns may be, and to explain to both what the workup may entail. Often the husband is referred to a urologist for his physical examination and semen analysis. Good communication among the members of the medical team is essential.

The initial investigation requires a thorough medical, sexual, and social history, physical examination of both partners, and routine laboratory tests to ascertain the general state of their health. Because of the complex and multifactorial nature of the problem, a finding in one partner does not exclude the possibility of problems in the other.

The woman's history includes a detailed menstrual history (onset, regularity, etc.), history of previous pregnancies, use of birth control techniques, and history of venereal disease. The man's history includes the history of his sexual development, pregnancies resulting from other relationships, and any illness, trauma, surgical procedure, or hazardous chemical or radiation exposure that might affect his ability to produce sperm.

The sequence and number of diagnostic tests vary with the situation and the doctor's preference. The underlying rationale is to establish whether ova and sperm are being produced and whether there is some barrier to their union.

The tests most commonly conducted at the outset of the investigation are the basal body temperature chart, to establish whether, when, and how regularly the woman ovulates, and the semen analysis, to establish the quantity and quality of the man's sperm.

For basal body temperature charting, the woman takes her temperature daily, immediately upon arising, in order to determine the body temperature at total rest. If she is ovulating normally, a lower basal temperature is characteristic of the preovulatory phase of the cycle. Shortly after ovulation, the production of increased amounts of progesterone causes the temperature to rise about 0.4° F. or more, and this higher level is maintained until the next menstruation begins (a sustained rise for longer than two weeks is suggestive of pregnancy). If the woman does not ovulate, the chart shows a variable, uniphasic pattern. Often a woman must chart three or four cycles before a pattern emerges. The charts are significant in planning further tests, which often need to be done at certain stages of the cycle, and in planning intercourse so as to maximize the chances for conception (i.e., on alternate days for three or four days before and after ovulation). The demands placed on both partners by the very act of temperature charting itself are stressful and anxiety-provoking; often the charting is discontinued if the woman is found to have regular ovulatory cycles. Having sexual relations on schedule is difficult for most people. As one man expressed it:

> The most difficult part of my infertility experience has been, ironically, in the bedroom. I feel I must *produce* at a specified, clinical, predetermined moment, when the act of sharing love with a wife is something that should be natural, unplanned . . . spontaneous. I must constantly remind myself that this is necessary if we ever hope to accomplish our goal of pregnancy.[1:126]

As for the semen analysis, it is obviously a threatening experience for a man to have to produce a specimen on command, with the knowledge that his production will be "counted" or "graded." Usually two or three analyses, several weeks apart, are performed before a diagnosis of an inadequate sperm count is made.

Other tests often performed in the doctor's office include an examination of the cervical mucus and an endometrial biopsy, both indicators of ovulation in the woman, and of the response of her tissues to her own hormones. The postcoital test, an examination of the cervical mucus within a few hours after intercourse, demonstrates how well the sperm survive within the vaginal and cervical secretions.

If ovulation and sperm production are normal, the next step in the investigation is usually a study of tubal patency in the woman. The Rubin test, tubal insufflation with carbon dioxide gas passed into the uterus, has been largely replaced by the hysterosalpingogram (tubogram), in which a radiopaque dye is passed into the uterus and its flow out through the tubes is followed by means of X-ray pictures and fluoroscopy. If the test indicates tubal blockage or shows other evidence of scarring, the doctor usually proceeds to a study in which the pelvic organs can be visualized directly. The most commonly used approach is the insertion of a fiberoptic instrument through the abdominal wall, close to the navel (laparoscopy). Laparoscopy affords a clear view of the pelvic organs, and is almost always done by the doctor who will perform the corrective surgery, if that is indicated.

Depending on the nature of the problem, other specialized tests may be required. Sophisticated hormone assays, immunologic tests, and chromosome studies may be required for one or both partners. For the male, testicular biopsy or vasography may be indicated.

Treatment may be medical, requiring long trials of various drugs to promote ovulation; results of efforts to enhance sperm production have not been very successful, but research in this area is still quite new. Or the treatment may be surgical, as in the repair of blocked tubes. Apart from the repair of a varicocoele, relatively few surgical procedures exist to correct male infertility.

PSYCHOLOGICAL ASPECTS OF THE INFERTILITY INVESTIGATION

The couple undergoing an infertility investigation enters a world of complicated tests and procedures in which a special language, full of medical terms, is spoken. The process may last for several years, with moments of hope and moments of despair. The timing of the tests and of sexual intercourse itself is so critical that other aspects of living must often be subordinated to the infertility study. Patients must expose not only their bodies for examination and manipulation, but also the intimate details of their sexual lives, and the private wishes and fears surrounding their motivation for a pregnancy.

The infertility study is a long-term project requiring an unusually high degree of patient participation and cooperation. Physicians and other professionals working with the infertile patient must be attuned to psychological conflicts, transference issues, and countertransference feelings.

The old practice of beginning the investigation with the woman and postponing the evaluation of the man is usually both medically and psychologically unsound. As one woman expressed her feelings:

> After a month of testing me, my doctor thought my husband should also be tested. He urged me to handle this with utmost care. His message was clear; go easy on his self-esteem and sense of masculinity. It was clear he felt my husband's feelings were more important than my own. I had to

shoulder the burden of responsibility—and protect my husband from
threatened feelings. My feelings were not considered. I felt alone and even
guilty that my husband had to have tests done.[1:31]

Because of the highly emotionally charged nature of the history-
taking, it is essential that husband and wife be interviewed separately
as well as together. The doctor may learn that one spouse has a secret,
such as a history of venereal disease, a child by a previous relationship, a previous abortion, which he or she has been unable to
discuss with the other. Some form of individual or couple psychotherapy may be indicated to help the couple deal with that aspect of
their problem.

A couple may wait several years before seeking medical attention
because of their own difficulties in acknowledging the problem or
revealing it to outsiders. Other couples may be very anxious to start an
infertility study after only a few months of trying to achieve a pregnancy. Sometimes there is a realistic basis for their concern, for example, the woman with endometriosis, or the man with a history of
mumps in adulthood. Sometimes the anxiety reflects the concern of
one or both partners about his or her sexual adequacy, or about the
status of the marriage. Women may feel that they have a deadline to
meet—that postponing childbearing past the age of thirty or thirty-
five means great risks to the mother or markedly increases the likelihood of producing a defective child.* The couple's anxieties may be
somewhat alleviated by careful explanations from the physician.

Because of the nearly 85 percent chance that a spontaneous pregnancy will occur within a year of trying to conceive, some doctors will
not take the patient seriously until a year has elapsed. This is not particularly helpful to the patient, nor does it inspire a good relationship
later on, when tests are undertaken. A couple seeking help with an infertility problem, even a self-defined one, already feels perplexed, inadequate, and angry. They have an extra need for support and explanation throughout the infertility study. It is the physician's
responsibility to communicate clearly that he/she is no magician, despite the patient's wish for magic. If a patient knows others who have
been helped to achieve a pregnancy, she may become angry with the
doctor for withholding the treasure from her; the doctor may be perceived as a powerful parental figure who may grant or deny the power
to make babies. The physician must be prepared to deal with the pa-

---

*While there is good evidence that a woman's chances of having a child with Down
syndrome increase past the age of thirty-five, it is possible to detect the condition early
enough in pregnancy, by means of amniocentesis, to allow the couple to decide
whether or not to terminate the pregnancy.

tient's anger when the magical expectations are not fulfilled. Some patients express their anger overtly, and others run from one doctor to another in hopes that the next one will be the miracle-worker.

Frequently a physician's efforts to reassure a patient may be perceived as a rebuff, or as a trivialization of her feelings. The infertility patient is very sensitive to anything that sounds as if she is being infantilized.

One of the most helpful defenses against the assaultive, intrusive nature of the infertility study is the use of information. Many patients become experts in their areas of special concern, and this helps them to feel like active, respected participants in a joint endeavor to solve a problem. The doctor who feels threatened, or who takes a patronizing "don't worry—leave it to me" attitude when his/her patients confront him/her with information from other sources, may not be aware of how helpless the patient feels.

Many infertility specialists agree that they should restrict their practices to the investigation of infertility problems. Many of the tests require careful timing, and a general obstetrician-gynecologist cannot always be available to the infertility patient. The patient's sense of being a failure may be augmented by seeing many pregnant patients in the waiting room, or having the doctor rush off to a delivery during her appointment time. The infertility specialist often refers those patients who become pregnant to another doctor for prenatal and obstetrical care, except under unusual circumstances.

The Psychological Aspects of Infertility Problems

People confronted with an infertility problem suffer narcissistic injuries at many levels of ego integration, as well as concerns about relationships with others in a personal and social context. Old conflicts are reactivated, and the resolution of the problem depends as much on the psychological strengths and vulnerabilities a person brings to the situation as on the actual outcome, that is, whether and by what means pregnancy or parenthood is achieved.

Menning[1] describes the initial reaction of surprise experienced by many people when they discover that they have an infertility problem. Underlying the surprise, I believe, is the feeling that a dreaded fear has come true. Despite the conventional presumption that everyone is fertile, and the social acceptability of discussing fears about unwanted pregnancies, the concern about infertility is universal. Single women, and married women who are not overtly planning to become pregnant, often voice their secret apprehensions about infertility even

148 MIRIAM D. MAZOR

when there are no objective reasons for special concern. In my own clinical experience, some of these women become pregnant "accidentally" in order to test out their own fertility. As one patient put it:

> My body wants to become pregnant, even though my head tells me I shouldn't . . . I've had two abortions because I had to know if I could get pregnant if I wanted to.

Another important aspect of the initial reaction to an infertility problem is the sense of losing control over one's life plans. Most people plan, or try to plan, whether and when they will marry and have children, how long they will prepare for their careers, and how much time they need to explore various lifestyles and potential partners. Hence, it comes as a rude shock to most people that although the use of birth control may prevent unwanted pregnancies with a fairly high degree of success, there are no guarantees that they can have children if they want them. The process of making the decision about whether or when to have children may be difficult, but the elimination of any option is not accepted without resentment. An initial indignation may mobilize some people to want to do something right away. Those who attempt to handle the problem by denying it may take a long time to come for medical attention. They may rationalize their position by saying that they are not ready for children yet, or that they have chosen not to have any, but somewhere inside there is a painful awareness that the choice was not really theirs to make.

The infertile woman, regardless of the cause of her infertility, is concerned about her bodily integrity and intactness. She experiences a profound depression over the loss of her reproductive function, and feels herself to be damaged or defective, as the following quotations demonstrate:

> It is more than I can bear to think of myself as barren. It's like having leprosy. I feel "unclean" and defective . . .[1:122]
> I feel empty. It's like within me, where a uterus ought to be, there is a "black hole" of space. I feel mutilated and yet I am told I am lucky to be free of my pain. I do not feel lucky. I feel terribly, terribly depressed.[1:133]

In his discussion of patients with physical disabilities, Wright[4] discusses the phenomenon of "spread," in which feelings about a specific physical disability spread to encompass the individual's overall sense of self-worth and body image. For the infertile patient, the defect is usually invisible to others and is most commonly *not* associated with a life-threatening or even health-threatening situation. The patient may have difficulty in asking for or accepting the kinds of support afforded to people with "real" handicaps, but nonetheless struggles with the feeling that her body is "bad." The sense of defectiveness does not remain confined to reproductive function alone, but spreads to encompass sexual function and desirability, physical appearance, and performance in other spheres as well.

The infertile woman worries seriously about her sexuality and her sexual desirability. She may feel that she does not deserve to enjoy sex, or that she could not perform adequately as a sexual partner, since the possibility of producing a baby no longer exists:

> I always felt that sex had other functions than procreation. I used birth control for many years before my infertility was discovered. But at the back of my mind, when my husband and I made love, was that happy knowledge that someday, when the time and circumstances were right, this was the way we would create a baby. For a long time after the diagnosis we didn't feel like making love. In part, it was because of our general depression. In part, it was because of my new feelings of defectiveness (there was something so drastically wrong with my sexual equipment—how could anyone want to make love to me?). But lurking behind it was also the feeling, "Why bother?" "What for?"[1:130]

It is not at all uncommon to experience some loss of sexual desire or capacity for orgasm during the course of the infertility investigation or after the diagnosis has been reached. It may compound the feeling of undesirability. The necessity for sexual relations at specified times during the woman's cycle, the concern about whether this time will be successful in terms of conception, add external pressures that inhibit the spontaneous enjoyment of sex. It becomes a task, even a mission, for the couple who are still trying to conceive, and a reminder of their failure for those who know they have no chance. Episodes of impotence are common, regardless of which partner is infertile, and it is helpful for the couple to understand that this problem is usually temporary, related to stress and depression.

There is also a tremendous buildup of hope and tension toward the end of the woman's cycle, as the couple await the onset of the next menstrual period. The woman is acutely aware of the changes in her body, and may become preoccupied with searching for signs of pregnancy. Physiological changes during this portion (luteal phase) of her cycle may intensify her anxiety and emotional lability. Drugs such as Clomid, used to stimulate ovulation, may prolong the luteal phase and increase the patient's hope that she is pregnant. When the menstrual flow begins, many women are plunged into a deep, acute depression, verging on despair. The recurrent barren cycles and attendant emotional turmoil may become exhausting. The intensity of the monthly disappointment may diminish with time, and often reflects the patient's general level of anxiety. One patient described the onset of each menstrual period as a kind of personal reproach—"My body is laughing at me and my efforts." She noted, however, that during her summer vacation her period came and went uneventfully—"I guess I decided to take a vacation from working to get pregnant, too."

Many women fear that their husbands will abandon them for a fertile woman or, even worse, will remain with them and harbor resentment against them. Some will make an open offer of divorce, and may continue to test and provoke their husbands to a point where they are tempted to take up the offer. In their discussion of single women with infertility problems, Williams and Power[5] describe some of these women as retreating from relationships with men altogether. It is not unusual for a patient, on meeting other women with infertility problems, to express surprise that the others look so attractive and normal, while she herself feels so unattractive and abnormal. Sometimes a woman feels compelled to restore her sense of sexual worth by calling special attention to her sexy external appearance, or by behaving in inappropriately seductive ways with men.

Some women feel that since they cannot produce a baby, they are unable to produce anything of worth. Or they become so preoccupied with their infertility or with the evaluation that they allow their careers and other pursuits to suffer, and point to this as further proof of their inadequacy. One patient, a graduate student in her early thirties, was unable to proceed with her doctoral dissertation after discovering that she had an infertility problem. She complained that her mind was "sterile," too. Psychotherapy helped her to sort out the issues so that she could write creatively again.

The patient may focus on her infertility as the source of *all* her feelings of inadequacy and discontent, in order to avoid confronting other issues. In the case mentioned above, the graduate student was able to acknowledge that she had many doubts about her ability to hold her own in the male-dominated academic world; jobs had become harder to find and the pressure to do research and publish had become more intense. Prior to the discovery of her infertility problem, she had always felt that having a baby would be a respectable way to get out of the "academic rat race." When this option was no longer the easy "cop-out" she had hoped for, she became seriously depressed and sought psychiatric help.

Associated with the feeling of being inadequate and defective is a heavy load of guilt that the infertile patient bears. Sometimes it is focused on a past event, such as a previous pregnancy or abortion or an episode of venereal disease, which may or may not be related to her current infertility problem. De Brovner and Shubin-Stein[6] describe the lengths to which some patients will go to find some past event to explain their infertility. More commonly the guilt is experienced in a general way—guilt about masturbation, sexual fantasies, incestuous wishes, or sexual desires of any kind. The guilt may be felt as a global sense of "badness." The patient's infertility is then viewed as a punishment for her sins or her unworthiness, and she may begin to think magically about bargaining with God—about undergoing a certain amount of suffering in exchange for a pregnancy. The tests and procedures involved in the infertility workup may suit that purpose well. The physician should be aware of these dynamics in the patient who is too eager to do anything to become pregnant, to participate in any kind of experimental procedure. Special care should be taken to let such patients know what the risks and chances of success in any treatment procedure may be, and to help her deal with her guilt more adaptively, instead of offering procedures as instruments for expiation.

At some point the patient will no longer be able to bear the attacks on herself, and her anger will be directed outward—at the situation, at physicians, at members of the family, at the fertile world in general. It may be focused on the doctor and other members of the medical team for real or perceived insults or insensitivities, for the inconvenience, pain, and indignities associated with the diagnostic procedures. It may be focused on the husband if he appears to be less motivated toward achieving a pregnancy.

The patient's family may become a special target for anger, especially if family members are pressuring her to produce a grandchild, or if they have their own theories about why she is infertile. Old rivalries with the woman's mother may be rekindled with a new intensity; after all, she has been successful in achieving a pregnancy and bearing a child. One patient described her feelings as follows:

> When the doctor suggested that maybe I was too neurotic to get pregnant, I blew up. I told him that if he thought I was uptight, he should meet my mother! My grandmother was even worse, and she had eight children. I come from a long line of uptight fertile women!

Some patients feel betrayed and cheated by their mothers, who "promised" them that they would be able to have babies when they grew up. Others have elaborate fantasies, sometimes based on a grain of reality, that their infertility is somehow the product of their mother's revenge:*

> My appendix was removed when I was twelve. I had just begun to menstruate, and after the surgery I didn't have another period for a year. I

---

* Feelings like these, I believe, are at the root of the folklore about witches (i.e., bad mothers) who cause women to become barren, and saints or goddesses (i.e., good mothers) who enable women to become pregnant.

guess it's common at that age, but somehow I thought that my mother
didn't like the idea of my growing up, that she had arranged with the doctor to have my female insides removed along with my appendix.

Old conflicts about sibling rivalry may be reawakened, especially if
the siblings have been able to provide the parents with the much-
desired grandchildren. Jealousy of friends who become pregnant or
bitter feelings toward friends who have children may seriously restrict
the patient's social relationships; she may rationalize her withdrawal
from friendships by saying that she has "nothing in common" with
friends who have children. She may attempt to channel her anger in
the service of causes against those who appear to take their fertility for
granted, or who seem to conspire against her chances to adopt a
child—for example, she may ally herself with the antiabortion movement because of her bitterness, rather than on ethical or religious
grounds.

MOTIVATIONS FOR PREGNANCY AND PARENTHOOD

Motivations for pregnancy and parenthood are multiple and complex. For the couple with an infertility problem, these motivations are
probably subject to more self-examination and scrutiny by others than
is true in the general population; the issues, however, are much the
same. To some extent, everyone is ambivalent about parenthood. Most
people expect to have children, and parenthood may be viewed as an
essential part of the process of becoming an adult. It is, however, an
awesome responsibility, requiring a major reorganization of lifestyles
and goals. For a woman, the childbearing experience itself can be
viewed as an idealized fulfillment of her role, and also as an uncomfortable, even frightening experience that limits her activities and
drains her inner resources. In addition to the personal, inner conflicts
about having children, she must also contend with a variety of pressures from family, friends, and society. Economic factors appear to
play a significant role in determining the number of children considered desirable.

Traditionally, a highly positive value has been placed on having
children. Even the Zero Population Growth movement "allows" a couple 2.11 children. In recent times, however, the increased emphasis on
self-fulfillment and creativity in other areas has created its own pressure against having children.

Despite her reputation for extolling motherhood, or a close equiv-
alent (such as a "mothering" profession), as the culmination of a
woman's development, Helene Deutsch says:

> It is difficult to judge to what extent woman's will to motherhood, her
> desire for a child, is influenced by external circumstances, to what extent it

has passively and plastically adjusted to the wishes and ideas of men, and
to what extent it corresponds to a primary tendency composed of motives
both conscious and unconscious.[7:25]

The intrapsychic and social forces affecting a woman's attitude toward
pregnancy and motherhood are probably so integrated that it is almost impossible to separate them. In contemporary America, even the
cultural message is mixed. At the same time that women are encouraged to free themselves of the "burdens" of child-bearing and
child-rearing in favor of more diverse, "interesting" work, the experiences of pregnancy, labor, and delivery are more idealized and roman-
ticized than ever. Natural childbirth, delivery at home, and breast-
feeding are emphasized as experiences no one should miss. Fathers
are eager to share in these experiences to the greatest extent possible,
and to participate in child-rearing as partners with their wives.

The infertile woman may feel incredibly left out, and she is especially prone to idealize the pregnant state. She may view it as a visible
symbol of her sexual adequacy or desirability, just as in many cultures
it is viewed as a sign of the man's virility. She may focus on the narcissistic aspects of pregnancy—the sense of "completeness" she thinks
it will bestow on her, the radiant face and blooming belly, the joy of
feeling the baby move inside. For the moment she disregards the dis-
comforts, the nausea, heartburn, backaches, and hemorrhoids that so
often accompany a real pregnancy. She may inflate beyond all realistic
proportions the privileged status of the pregnant woman as a person
to be cared for and catered to. And the experience of childbirth may be
fantasized in grandiose terms:

> When I was in the midst of my infertility workup, I began dreaming
> about giving birth. These were no small dreams—they were gigantic Cecil
> B. DeMille productions, with a cast of thousands. I was always at the cen-
> ter, very beautiful and in control. My husband was standing at my side
> and I labored (sweating ever so slightly) very briefly, then had a wonderful
> birth. The baby was perfect, and everyone cheered and praised me for how
> well I had done. My husband was crying and telling me how much he
> loved me.[1:158]

For some patients, the wish for a child is closely linked to their
wish to participate in a state of symbiotic closeness with a very young
baby, to receive nurturance by nurturing, to enjoy the comfortable
regression to infancy that is an essential part of mothering:

> My worst despair came over thoughts about breastfeeding—an experi-
> ence I had always wanted. I bought a print of Picasso's mother and child
> and became very bitter at the thought I might not be able to duplicate that
> scene myself.[1:102]

The child may be perceived as a means of avoiding loneliness and
emptiness, filling up a void in the patient's life, as someone she can

count on to be hers. Or the child may represent a chance to be reborn, to create an idealized version of oneself, someone to live out parental hopes and dreams, or to compensate for parental disappointments.

The child may be viewed as the product of one's efforts, a living symbol of the parents' usefulness and worth. This attitude may be more prevalent among women who have serious doubts about their ability to perform and produce in other areas. Having a child may appear to be the only way for such women to achieve full adult status. As Angela Barron McBride says:

> For a woman to be considered fully "grown-up" in much of American society, she has to have children. If she wants people to listen to her as a responsible person, she has to be able to show her credentials—Tom, Ann, Billy, Wendy, and so forth.[8:17]

In his paper on womb-envy in boys, Nelson[9] suggests that for very young children in our society, the *mother* is initially perceived as the more powerful and productive parent. Toddlers traditionally spend more time in her company, and see what she can actually do. She is the wielder of the mighty vacuum cleaner, and she has an impressive capacity to make babies. Only later do children come to understand and appreciate what their fathers do, the source of their power and productivity. Children of both sexes feel small and inadequate in comparison to their giantess-mother; they fantasize about growing babies inside themselves, too. Little girls take comfort in the knowledge that they will grow up and have babies; little boys learn that other paths to "greatness" are available to them. Hence, the infertile woman who has been brought up to believe that motherhood is the only legitimate goal for a woman suffers an even greater blow to her self-esteem than does the woman who has been prepared to value and use her other capabilities. Even in contemporary America, with its changing attitudes toward women's roles, where barren wives are no longer cast aside, many women still feel that motherhood is the only sure guarantee of love and approval from their spouses, parents, friends, and society:

> I married into the fourth generation of a family that came over on the Mayflower. After three attempts at pelvic and tubal surgery for endometriosis, I now know that I can never bear children. The pressure had been so great, my pain so intense that I offered my husband a divorce if he truly wanted one. Our marriage is not happy. I don't know what we will do. I think I know how Princess Soroya felt when she could not produce an heir for the Shah of Iran.[1:101]

An important aspect of the wish to become a parent is the wish to foster the growth of the next generation, to transmit the cultural and personal messages we feel to be significant in our own lives. Erikson[10] defines the failure to reach the level of generativity as a state of stagnation, characterized by self-absorption. He emphasizes that the mere fact of having, or wanting to have, children does not mean that a person has necessarily achieved this level of development, and that there are many ways in which the drive to foster development of the young can be expressed. However, for the woman with an infertility problem, it may be difficult to find alternatives to mothering her own biological children. Some feel that their infertility is a sentence passed upon them as being unfit or too immature for parenthood. They feel that the world views them as objects of pity and scorn. If the fact of their infertility is not generally known, they may feel that others view them as self-centered or irresponsible. They may doubt their right to own a house or to make some other major adult investment. Men, too, are judged to be more respectable and solid, better qualified for responsible jobs or elected office if they are "family men." If a couple is in the process of applying for a child through an adoption agency, the agency's evaluation and screening procedure may intensify the feeling of being tried and found wanting.

Related to the wish to foster the development of the next generation is the wish to leave something of oneself in the world beyond one's own lifetime. In this sense, the child is a kind of link with immortality. Persons facing infertility must inevitably comes to grips with their own mortality.

MOURNING AND GRIEF

Even if the diagnosis of infertility is not absolute and there remains a lingering chance to have a child, at some point the couple will go through a period of mourning for the children they never had, for the dreams and aspirations that must be relinquished. Sometimes a dramatic event, such as a hysterectomy, or a series of events, such as a succession of miscarriages or unsuccessful operations, will mark the loss. But in many instances, recognition of the loss is gradual. The couple may need a "marker" in order to give themselves permission to grieve, to experience in a unique, personal way the meaning of their loss. This mourning period seems to be essential to recovery, to getting on with the business of living and making decisions about whether to pursue alternate routes to parenthood. Some patients feel that they have no right to grieve precisely because the loss they experience is so potential and vague:

> My fertile years were over before they began. The loss was somehow unreal, confusing, because it was a loss not of something concrete, but of something potential . . . . it felt like a bad dream. Nothing had changed in

my everyday life: no one had died, no one was sick, everyone looked the same. *Yet everything had changed.*[1:111]

One woman described her need for a "catalyst" to help her get started on the work of mourning:

> It was almost a year since I'd had my last tube surgery. The doctor had told me that either I'd conceive in six months or I'd better forget about having a baby. But I was stubborn and kept on trying, charting my temperature, having sex at the right times, in the right position. . . . I passed a bookstore on my way home from work, and they were featuring a book called *Pregnancy: The Best State of the Union.*[11] I *had* to stop and stare at it, and I remember that something inside me told me that it was all right to cry. I cried right there, in the bookstore, and it felt wonderful! I didn't care what anybody thought—I'd been waiting a long time for that cry.

The couple for whom no definitive diagnosis is reached remain in a prolonged state of cyclic hope and despair, and may have much more difficulty in acknowledging their loss. There may be significant differences of opinion between the man and woman, or between the couple and their doctor, about when to call a halt to the investigation. The statistical chances for conception are meaningful only in the context of the interpretation the patients put on them.[12] Some couples choose to use birth control as a means of ending their chronic tension and anxiety, and to give themselves an opportunity to work through their grief. The lingering doubts about who is "responsible" for the couple's infertility may put even greater strains on a marriage than in situations where a conclusive diagnosis is reached.*

In cases where one partner has a confirmed infertility problem, it is important that the fertile spouse also be given an opportunity to mourn the loss of the children they could not have together. All too often, the fertile spouse feels that he or she must preserve a front of unswerving love and support for the "afflicted" partner. This may only intensify the infertile spouse's feelings of guilt and unworthiness. The wife of an infertile man often feels obligated to go to great lengths to boost his sense of masculinity and prove how sexually attractive she finds him. Usually the husband sees through these efforts and recognizes that they are an attempt to cover up her disappointment and anger. An honest discussion of her feelings often does more to improve their relationship and maintain his self-esteem.

The couple with secondary infertility may also feel that they have no right to grieve, since they already have a child. Family and friends may not even be aware that the problem exists, and may be quite

---

* In some situations, couples for whom no conclusive diagnosis was reached divorced, remarried, and each had children by their subsequent partner. (Dr. Hilton A. Salhanick, personal communication).

vocal in their disapproval of the couple for having an only child. The couple may feel guilty, too, and have difficulty explaining to the child why they cannot provide him/her with a brother or sister. It is hard to deal with a child's anger and disappointment; only children often feel that they were themselves unwanted, or that they turned out so badly that their parents chose not to repeat the experience. Sometimes the couple become overly protective and fearful of losing the irreplaceable child they have; they may overinvest him/her with all their hopes and dreams, to the detriment of the child's unique development.

The infertile couple are usually very isolated in their grief. There are few social supports, and no formal rituals to assist the "bereaved"—no funerals, wakes, or graves to visit. People unaffected by the problem do not want to hear much about it. Well-meaning friends and relatives are quick to suggest easy solutions (everybody knows someone who adopted a baby and got pregnant right away)* in an effort to circumvent the sadness of the infertile couple.

SOLUTIONS AND NEW PROBLEMS

Each couple must come to terms with their infertility problem in their own way, and at their own pace. There are no easy solutions.

The traditional solution has been adoption. However, this decision must be made on its own, taking into consideration the problems involved in adopting older children, racially mixed children, children with physical, mental, or emotional disabilities, and children from abroad. Adoption presents a whole new series of tests and challenges, whether done through an agency or privately, in the United States or the Far East or Latin America. Macnamera's *The Adoption Advisor*[13] presents a comprehensive account of current resources for adoption; for a discussion of adoption of children with special needs, see Anderson's *Children of Special Value*.[14]

Adoption does not restore the patient's fertility, and she cannot successfully avoid the process of grieving for the pregnancy and childbirth she did not have, for the genetic children she never bore. If she is capable of mourning those losses, she will be much better able to enjoy her adopted children and more confident about her capacity to mother them.

A couple may wait for as long as five years to adopt a child, and then find the "delivery" somewhat precipitous. They receive a phone

---

* In fact, the incidence of pregnancy is no higher among couples who adopt than among those who do not; statistics may become skewed because those who become pregnant during the waiting period for adoption may withdraw their applications or become ineligible to adopt a child.

call, and suddenly they are parents. The reality may not live up to the long-cherished fantasies, and they may expect themselves (or the child) to fall in love at first sight! They may not allow themselves the normal "getting-to-know-you" period that parents go through with their biological newborns in the process of forming close affectional bonds.

Similarly, the couple who finally conceive, whether as a result of treatment or by a spontaneous stroke of luck, may feel that they have no right to complain or express ambivalent feelings about pregnancy, delivery, or parenting, when those experiences fail to measure up to their long-cherished fantasies. The pregnancy is felt to be very special by the couple and the doctor, and the fear of taking risks during labor may contribute to the higher than average rate of cesarean sections among formerly infertile women. The couple may tend to overprotect their miraculous child, or have great expectations for him/her. They may be reluctant to use birth control after the child is born, for fear that they will not be able to have another, only to find themselves overwhelmed by a second baby before they are really ready.

If the husband's sperm count is low, or if there is a combined problem, artificial insemination with the husband's sperm in a concentrated form may be used. The couple may harbor feelings of guilt and shame about the child conceived under such "unnatural" circumstances.

For couples with an infertile male and a fertile female, artificial insemination by donor (AID) is a possibility. This raises a host of medical, legal, ethical, and personal issues, which require a separate discussion in their own right. Attempts are made to match the donor to the husband in terms of certain genetic traits, and the husband's semen is often mixed in with the donor's, in order to preserve some feeling that the child *could be* his genetic child. Usually several treatment cycles are required for conception to occur, and the procedure is not always successful.[1] A great deal of secrecy and shame is still associated with AID in the minds of some people. They may view it as a form of technologically-assisted adultery or have science fiction-type fantasies about "test-tube babies." However, those couples who have had AID children and who choose to speak openly about it tend to feel positive about the experience.[1]

Some couples may elect the alternative of child-free living. They may feel that the exhausting efforts to achieve a pregnancy or to adopt a child exact too great a toll on themselves or on their relationship. They may reassess their initial motivations for wanting children and find that other goals have become more important in their lives. Social support for not having children, or not feeling obligated to have them, is certainly growing.[15] However, the couple who has been through an infertility study is not in quite the same position as the couple who elect not to have chidlren. The infertile couple must deal with their frustration, disappointment, and grief; they must accept the fact that their decision is at least partially determined by forces beyond their control.

Whatever alternative a couple may choose or find themselves faced with, it is important for them to acknowledge and experience their feelings honestly. Peer support groups for infertile people offer some an opportunity to share their feelings with others who are facing similar issues. Counseling or psychotherapy may be helpful for those who wish to explore their feelings privately or in greater depth, or for those who are more deeply troubled. The therapist working with such patients should have a basic understanding of the objective difficulties and internal struggles that infertile people face, as well as an understanding of the issues that take on special significance in terms of a particular patient's history, social background, characterological makeup, and expectations. If therapy is to focus on the infertility issue, an important goal may be to help the patient discover and appreciate inner sources of self-esteem independent of her capacity for reproduction. Another major goal is to help such patients with their grief and to put the problem into perspective. The losses may be remourned, but with less acute pain:

> My infertility resides in my heart as an old friend. I do not hear from it for weeks at a time, and then, a moment, a thought, a baby announcement or some such thing, and I will feel the tug—maybe even be sad or shed a few tears. And I think, "There's my old friend." It will always be part of me. . . .[1:117]

REFERENCES

1. Menning B: *Infertility: a guide for the childless couple.* Englewood Cliffs, New Jersey, Prentice-Hall, 1977.
2. Behrman S, Kistner R: *Progress in infertility.* Second edition. Boston, Little, Brown, 1975.
3. Boston Hospital for Women: Fertility and Endocrine Unit booklet. Affiliated Hospitals Center, Inc., 1976.
4. Wright B: *Physical disability—A psychological approach,* New York, Harper & Row, 1960.
5. Williams L, Power P: The emotional impact of infertility in single women: some implications for counselling. *Journal of the American Medical Women's Association* 32:327–333, 1977.
6. De Brovner C, Shubin-Stein R: Sexual problems in the infertile couple. *Medical Aspects of Human Sexuality* 9:140–150, 1975.
7. Deutsch H: *The psychology of women: volume II—motherhood.* New York, Grune & Stratton, 1945. New York, Bantam, 1973.

8. McBride A: *The growth and development of mothers.* New York, Harper & Row, 1973.
9. Nelson J: Anlage of productiveness in boys—womb envy. *Journal of the American Academy of Child Psychiatry* 6:213–225, 1967.
10. Erikson E: *Childhood and Society.* New York, WW Norton, 1950.
11. Fielding W: *Pregnancy: the best state of the union.* Porter's Landing, Freeport, Maine, The Bond Wheelwright Company, 1972.
12. Wicks S: The effects of non-conclusive infertility diagnosis on married couples: an exploratory study. Boston University School of Social Work, master's thesis, May 1977.
13. Macnamera J: *The adoption advisor.* New York, Hawthorn Books, 1975.
14. Anderson D: *Children of special value.* New York, St. Martin's Press, 1971.
15. Peck E, Senderowitz J: *Pronatalism: the myth of mom and apple pie.* New York, Thomas Y Crowell, 1974.

Chapter 12

A Historical Understanding
of Contraception

Peter Reich

Potions, pessaries, magic rituals, and infusions to prevent conception or cause abortion have been used since the days of the Pharaohs. The folklore of many cultures includes practices, generally relegated to women, that today seem dangerous, bizarre, and perhaps even erotic. Insertion of some sort of barrier—dung, lard, beeswax, silver balls—was frequently described. A number of nineteenth-century historians were particularly intrigued by a practice reported in some primitive cultures of women ejecting sperm with violent thrusts of the pelvis. In Western culture, transmission of contraceptive information was carried on largely by midwives, who dominated birthing until the eighteenth century. The preferred method at that time was a sponge or cotton tampon soaked in spermicide and attached to a string for retrieval.

Birth control did not become an issue until mortality rates permitted it. When Edward Gibbon was born in 1737, the chances of a child surviving to regenerate the family line were so slim that Gibbon's father gave the name Edward to several sons to ensure continuance of the name. For the remainder of the eighteenth century, however, the death rate dropped while the birth rate remained relatively constant. As more children survived, they were put to work. During the Industrial Revolution in Britain, child labor abuses increased, and it was not until laws regulating child labor went into effect that family limitation became acceptable.[1] To this day, the possibility of deriving income from a large family remains a significant factor in family size for migrant workers in the United States.

Peter Reich, B.A. • Department of Socio-Medical Sciences, Boston University School of Medicine, Boston, Massachusetts 02118.

The philosophical base for birth control came from Thomas R. Malthus, who warned in 1798 that population would someday outstrip the capacity to feed. Although he advocated little more than "moral restraint," Malthus laid the groundwork for vigorous birth control campaigns in Britain during the nineteenth century.

CONTRACEPTION IN EARLY AMERICA

In the United States, medicine's control of contraceptive devices and the dominance of law in moral issues combined to make birth control illegal, illicit, and improper for over a century.

The establishment of university chairs of midwifery for physicians in the eighteenth century cut deeply into the influence of midwives and gave physicians prerogative. Although these men proved innovative in developing contraceptive technology, laws rooted in strict religious dogma prevented widespread use of contraception. Statutory law was generally reactionary, gaining impact in direct proportion to increased availability of literature and, finally, technology. Common law whittled away at the statutes in a manner that focused on the middlemen, physicians and pharmacists, leaving the consumer and manufacturer in a blurry, ill-defined position. The complexity of medical and legal issues made birth control what one historian has called "an excellent example of a social problem which has severely challenged the ability of legal institutions to respond creatively to social change." [2]

Earliest legal activity in the United States relating to contraception occurred on the issue of obscene literature. Although tampons and folkloric methods were commonly used, there was no marketable, taxable, or regulatable contraceptive commodity. Public outrage over publication of a book dealing specifically with contraception led to action by the Massachusetts legislature in 1836. *The Fruits of Philosophy,* by Dr. Charles Knowlton (1800–1850), distressed proper Bostonians with its detailed descriptions of douches. The statute adopted to curb such literature was included in "Offences against Chastity, Morality and Decency" in the criminal code and stated:

> If any person shall import, print, publish, sell or distribute any book or any pamphlet, ballad, printed paper or any other thing manifestly tending to the corruption of the morals of youth . . . he shall be punished by imprisonment in the state prison, not more than five years, or imprisonment in the county jail, not more than two years, and a fine not exceeding one thousand dollars. [3]

The Fruits of Philosophy enjoyed wide circulation in Britain four decades later, when its distribution was the issue in the famous Bradlaugh-Besant trial (1877–1879), which prompted the first large-scale publicity about contraception. A dramatic decline in the British birth rate is attributed to publicity from the trial. In the United States, however, the book's sale was limited and impact minimal. Chastity, morality, and decency, firmly buttressed by common and statutory law, continued their crusade into America's industrial revolution toward a confrontation with technology.

Technology and the Comstock Law

In 1844, Charles Goodyear revolutionized the rubber industry by inventing vulcanization. This enabled birth control-minded physicians to experiment with and develop the rubber diaphragm, condom, and stem pessary. This new technology, coupled with concepts of family planning that grew out of Malthusianism and child labor abuses, clashed with the American notion of moral propriety and precipitated "a deliberate public policy making contraception per se a crime."[2:4]

In March 1873, the U.S. Congress enacted a bill that dominated public access to birth control for the next sixty years. The Comstock Law, named after its fervent originator, Anthony Comstock, used every verb and adjective imaginable to suppress—especially in the U.S. mail—"trade in and circulation of obscene literature and articles of immoral use."[4] In the years that followed, twenty-two states adopted similar statutes, some more stringent, others less. Curiously and inexplicably, a clause excepting physicians was deleted from the final version of the federal law. New York State managed to include such an exception for physicians (1879), providing a wedge for the court decisions that eventually redefined the federal law in the 1930s.

Unaffected by the tough language of the law, research and development continued, and manufacturers were proud enough of the rubber condom to present it at the Centennial Exposition in Philadelphia in 1876. Prior to this dramatic entry into the ranks of industrial successes, condoms maintained a relatively low profile. History is curiously vague about this masculine method of contraception. Fallopius is credited with invention of a linen sheath in 1564; the condom appears in literature in the seventeenth century, but its use appears to have been confined largely to the privileged classes for prevention of disease. That physicians used sheep caeca as a rudimentary surgical "glove" in 1750 leads one to believe it might also have been employed as a condom; such "skins" are regarded today as the most sensitive of condoms. It is significant that mass production of a simple and relatively effective rubber condom coincided with such a strict law as the Comstock Law.

The law's most enthusiastic implementor was Anthony Comstock himself, who, as Special Agent for the New York Society for The Prevention of Vice, was personally responsible for the arrest and conviction of 2,911 individuals.[5] It is especially fitting that Mr. Comstock caught cold at the 1915 trial of William Sanger, husband of Comstock's most formidable adversary, and died shortly thereafter.

EFFECT OF LIBERALIZED PUBLIC ATTITUDES

Another event of 1873 was to have an enormous impact on the lives of women: the Remington Firearms Company brought out its Model I typewriter and the modern secretary was invented. With jobs opening up and feminine reform in the air, women went to work. Between 1870 and 1900, the number of women in jobs outside the home rose from 1,800,000 to 5,300,000.[5:76] The movement gathered steam and while suffragettes took to the streets to give women the vote, Margaret Sanger and others opened clinics to give them birth control information and devices. More often than not, Mrs. Sanger ended up in jail.

Convicted in 1917 for distributing birth control information and devices in New York, Mrs. Sanger appealed, arguing that the law was an unreasonable police regulation preventing a *physician* from giving contraceptives to patients and was thus unconstitutional. The court held that Mrs. Sanger was not a physician and since "no one can plead the unconstitutionality of a law except the person affected thereby," dismissed the constitutional question and upheld her conviction.[6]

Inasmuch as cases such as this test and realign outer limits of the law, this case is important because the court showed marked deference to that curious clause in the New York statute that excepted physicians. This laid the foundation for later opinions that expanded on the physician's role. It also set a precedent for what would be a long, arduous debate over strict physician control versus paraprofessional activity in clinics.

Undaunted, Mrs. Sanger continued her campaign at an international level, and in 1925 the International Congress on birth control and family planning, which had been held in Europe since 1900, convened in New York. Historically, Mrs. Sanger is associated with the move to legalize abortion, although she did not favor it. Surgical techniques had advanced dramatically in the mid-nineteenth century with the safety of asepsis, painlessness of anesthesia, and precision of improved surgical steels, but abortion remained sub rosa in this country for decades until the reform of the 1960s.

Despite strict interpretation of the law, business in contraceptive devices flourished, and by the 1929 Depression, it was a multimillion dollar industry. Women, obviously taking advantage of devices available in the privacy of a doctor's office, continued to opt for careers rather than motherhood. By 1930, 10,752,000 women were earning their own living in whole or in part.[1:274] Women had complete dominance in telephone operation, nursing, and office work, and caught the attention of *Fortune* magazine because of their increasingly significant buying power. The popular and widespread use of contraceptives by working women led to what historian Norman Himes describes as the "Democratization of birth control" that occurred in the 1930s.

In the years that followed, the birth rate dropped from 21.3 per 1,000 in 1930 to a low of 18.4 in 1936. This decline was due largely to the legalization of birth control in a court decision involving condoms. The discovery of synthetic rubber in the early twenties had been a breakthrough in the manufacture of condoms and diaphragms; sales boomed during the twenties. In a case involving the famous Trojans trademark, the U.S. Court of Appeals for the Second Circuit held in 1930 that sale of contraceptives was not in all cases illegal. The court essentially redefined the Comstock law to include the clause about physicians that had been omitted fifty-seven years earlier. Citing the same New York statute that convicted Margaret Sanger in 1918, the court applied New York's statutory exception for physicians against the federal law, asserting that "the intention to prevent a *proper medical use* of drugs and articles merely because they are capable of illegal use is not likely to be ascribed to Congress."[7] This decision put even more responsibility in the hands of doctors, and although it led to wider dissemination of contraceptives, it left the question of clinics and paraprofessionals unresolved and untested.

At the time, Youngs Rubber Corp. was selling about 20 million condoms a year to druggists; within five years total output of the fifteen principal manufacturers was put at a million and a half a day. [1:201] Sales of condoms and diaphragms represented $250,000,000 worth of business by 1936, with diaphragms far outselling condoms.[8]

Birth control advocates were indeed ecstatic over the decision, and as more and more clinics opened their doors across the nation, physicians began taking a more active role. Alan Guttmacher and Robert Latou Dickinson were among the physicians who helped Margaret Sanger establish a *Journal of Contraception* in 1935. One of the objectives of the *Journal* was to encourage the medical community to recognize contraception as an alternative to abortion and to encourage research for "a simple, harmless and efficient chemical contraceptive."[9]

At its annual meeting in 1935, the American Medical Association appointed a committee to examine the issue. Its first report, presented in May 1935, showed little enthusiasm; it reported that "no evidence was found which would indicate that wider dissemination of contraceptive *information* [emphasis supplied] would tend to establish a better social and economic equilibrium in society."[10] Nor was evidence found "to justify the broad claim that dissemination of contraceptive information will improve the economic status of lower income groups."[10] Reserving comment on contraceptive devices, the committee did give cautious approval to the rhythm method. It also recommended that a committee be formed to develop standards for judging contraceptives and noted its disapproval of lay organizations, deploring "the support of such agencies by members of the medical profession."[10] Commenting on the "first actual consideration of the subject of birth control by the AMA after many years of evasion," the *Journal of Contraception* criticized the "mental confusion and the conservative hesitancy of the medical profession on the subject."[11]

A number of factors account for the reluctance of organized medicine to jump on the family planning bandwagon. A key issue was health and safety. Puerperal fever, which had been epidemic in the seventeenth and eighteenth centuries, was still a woman killer, ranking second after tuberculosis. Despite innovations in sterile technique, maternal mortality remained relatively constant during the years 1915–1930, while infant mortality increased.[12] There is no doubt that physicians were extremely wary of risks of infection by women or paraprofessionals inserting objects into their vaginas.

While the debate continued, the birth rate continued to plummet, and in 1936, the Comstock Law had another overhaul. In U.S. v. One Package of Rubber Pessaries, Dr. Hannah Stone was accused of violating the Tariff Act of 1930 and the Comstock Law when she received a package of new experimental rubber devices in the mail from Japan. In a decision that reopened the U.S. Mail to articles of contraception, the U.S. Court of Appeals for the Second Circuit expanded on the concept of "proper medical use" enunciated earlier, and clarified the legal standing of physicians. In its correction of the U.S. Congress, the court held that the Comstock Law and the Tariff Act

> embraced only such articles as Congress would have denounced as immoral if it had understood all the conditions under which they were to be used. Its design, in our opinion, was not to prevent the importation, sale or carriage by mail of things which might intelligently be employed by conscientious and competent physicians for the purpose of saving life or promoting the well being of their patients.[13]

By extending the physician's prerogative to include not only lifesaving measures, but a sense of "well being," the court did everything but hand medicine a carte blanche.

Margaret Sanger was elated. "The field is cleared for the discovery of inexpensive, reliable methods for the control of human fertility," she wrote, adding that "contraceptive research in both the laboratory and the clinic is now free to pursue its course emancipated from the stigma of prejudice."[14]

The AMA wasn't so sure. "The decision," grumbled *JAMA*, "has nothing to do with the practice of contraception within any state except as that practice may introduce foreign and interstate commerce or use of the mails."[15] Despite the AMA's conservative interpretation of the law, or what the *Journal of Contraception* called the AMA's "ostrich policy," pressure continued to build within the medical profession. The AMA was urged "to consider seriously the inroads that are being made on the prestige of organized medicine by the rapid advance of popular thought . . . it has come to the pass at which the road for medical advance is blazed by laymen assisted by the law."[16]

The public was indeed ready for large-scale, organized family planning. *Fortune* had extended its newly devised Quarterly Survey to the birth control business and reported in July 1936 that 63 percent of the American people, including two-thirds of the Catholics, believed in "the teaching and practice of birth control."[17] With board rooms abuzz with projections of sales in a more benevolent legal climate, *Fortune* called for federal legislation to supersede statutes in many states that still allowed no exception for physicians, and criticized the Judiciary Committee of the U.S. Congress for shelving numerous bills to do just that. By its failure to bring these bills out of committee, said *Fortune*, the committee was "thwarting the will of an overwhelming majority of the people."[17:158] Applauding the business survey's revelation of public interest, the *Ladies Home Journal* noted that "From farm and village and city and from every geographical section of the nation rose the affirmative chorus for birth control."[18]

In 1938, the U.S. Court of Appeals for the Second Circuit slapped a final coat of liberal reform on the cracked and peeling Comstock Law by affirming the right of physicians to receive birth control literature in the U.S. Mail.[19] A year later, the AMA grudgingly admitted, "there is a definite need to inform the medical profession of the facts."[20] The facts in 1939 were 478 birth control centers in the nation, 158 supported in whole or in part by public funds, 82 in hospitals, 97 part of city and county health departments.[21] In 1936, the national birth rate was 18.4 per 1,000, a low that would not again be equaled until 1966 (during the war years it rose to a high of 26.5 in 1947).

THE LEGAL STRUGGLE

The results of a decade of democratization were impressive, but the battle was not won. The new interpretation of the law, with its reliance on the role of physicians, was only valid in states with the provision excepting them. In the wake of the liberal decisions of the thirties, some states adopted even more stringent statutes. Massachusetts, Connecticut, and six other states had statutes, newly revised or left over from the days of Anthony Comstock, that attempted complete suppression of contraceptives. The dream of bringing large-scale family planning to the public was thwarted not only by these statutes, but also by the war and the political climate that followed. Although research on progesterone, which had been isolated in 1938, continued toward a rendezvous in Puerto Rico in 1956, medical research on contraception dwindled during the war years. Interestingly, the Cumulated Index Medicus shows that remarkably few studies were conducted during the McCarthy period.

Some states, notably Oregon and North Carolina, had popular and smoothly running clinics by the late 1930s; but in most of the nation, family planning was still illicit, if not illegal, and birth controllers fought to extend the law's ambivalent shadow of approval.

The battleground was primarily the Massachusetts and Connecticut courts, and the battle dragged on for years, with occasional attempts at a Supreme Court ruling that would overturn the strict statutes.

The Massachusetts statute, Chapter 272, Section 21, made giving or selling contraceptives a felony. In 1937, the North Shore Mothers' Health Office in Salem was raided and a physician, a nurse, and two social workers were charged with violating the statute. Convicted of the charge, they alleged exceptions and appealed. There was no argument over the facts of the case, and the court even agreed that it was "sound and generally accepted medical practice to prescribe contraceptives to protect life and health."[22] That wasn't the issue. The issue was that under the statute, providing contraceptives to a married woman, even by a physician, was illegal. The appellants argued that excluding physicians denied them constitutional rights.

But the court stuck adamantly by the law in remarkably firm language. The terms of the statute were "plain, unequivocal and peremptory. They contain no exceptions. They are sweeping, absolute and devoid of ambiguity. They are directed with undeviating explicitness against the prevention of contraception by any means specified."[22] The court referred to the Sanger case of 1918 and to the more recent decisions revising the Comstock Law, pointing out that those cases were all based on that curious clause in the New York Statute that *did* except physicians. The absence of that clause in the Bay State meant that in no uncertain terms, birth control was against the law for everyone. On appeal to the U.S. Supreme Court, the case was dismissed per curiam "for want of a federal question."[23]

As numerous clinics in Massachusetts shut down because of the decision, groundwork was being laid for a continuing attack based on the constitutional rights of physicians. The *Journal of Contraception* anticipated the successful parry by roughly a quarter of a century when it stated in 1939,

> If contraceptives are generally conceded by physicians to have a legitimate medical use and their denial to a patient would involve injury to health, it is believed that these cases indicate that a denial to the physician of the right to prescribe contraceptives is deprivation of life or liberty within the fourteenth amendment.[24]

It was a matter of the right idea at the wrong time.

The constitutional question arose in Connecticut, too, where the state made *use* of contraceptives illegal. In a raid on a New Haven clinic in 1939, a nurse and two physicians were charged with violating a section of the general statutes outlawing use of "medicinal articles or instruments" to prevent conception. They were found not guilty in Superior Court of New Haven County. On appeal by the state, the appellees argued that the statute interfered with individual liberty and deprived them of due process. Furthermore, they claimed that by not making an exception for physicians, the statute obstructed his right to care for the health of his patients.[25]

In a detailed argument, the court maintained that the intent of the legislation had not changed, and that judicial modification was not in order, especially in view of the Supreme Court's decision in Commonwealth v. Gardner. Social and moral wrongs, the court held, were in the legislative realm of police powers, and it was up to the legislature to make the kinds of changes involved. Much of the appellees' argument was on a rhetorical issue: the wording "medicinal article or instrument" was construed to mean that even a calendar to calculate the rhythm method might be unconstitutional, as a medicinal instrument. But the court ruled that the adjective "medicinal" modified article, not instrument. The court upheld the statute, and remanded the case to Superior Court with directions to overrrule the demurrers. Across the state, clinics closed their doors.

The Connecticut statute came before the Supreme Court in 1943, when, in Tileston v. Ullman, a physician argued that the statute was an infringement of his and his patients' rights under the fourteenth amendment. The High Court refused to strike down the statute, holding that the physician's patients "are not parties to the proceedings and there is no basis on which we can say he has standing to secure an adjudication in his patients' constitutional right to life, which they do not assert in their own behalf."[26]

Even in 1961, the Supreme Court refused to strike down the Connecticut statute, an act that would have rendered contraceptives available to women in states with similar statutes. In Poe v. Ullman, it became clear that while contraceptives might be administered in the privacy of a doctor's office, the decision to make contraceptives available on a larger scale was up to the legislature. Lack of sufficient adversary action at the state level weakened the case:

> The fact that Connecticut has not chosen to press the enforcement of this statute deprives these controversies of the immediacy which is an indispensable condition to constitutional adjudication. This court cannot be umpire to debates concerning harmless, empty shadows.[27]

Dissent from this opinion was strident and lengthy. While Justice Douglas hinted at the light he would soon cast on those shadows, Justice Harlan complained about the state "asserting its right to enforce its moral judgment by intruding upon the most intimate details of the marital relationship with full power of criminal law." [27:508]

This case is significant because it involved a couple who had undergone three pregnancies, all terminating in births of infants who died shortly thereafter of congenital defects; it added the issue of rights of married couples to that of physicians' rights. The case against the statute was still not strong enough but it now had a broader base.

Four years later, Justice Douglas was finally able to illuminate those "harmless, empty shadows" with an intense and benevolent light that attracted constitutional lawyers like moths. Writing the majority opinion in Griswold v. Connecticut (1965), Justice Douglas finally struck down the Connecticut statute and made it legal for physicians to prescribe contraceptives for married women. In his opinion, he focused on "specific guarantees" in the Bill of Rights. Those rights of the first, third, fourth, fifth, and ninth amendments, as applied to the states by the fourteenth, he wrote, "have penumbras, formed by emanations from those guarantees that help give them life and substance." [28]

CURRENT LEGAL STATUS

The extension of constitutional rights by the Supreme Court in the decision would prove to be a key factor in the rights movements of the next decade. Seven years after the decision, the Supreme Court held that a Massachusetts statute permitting married persons to obtain contraceptives but prohibiting distribution to single persons violated the equal protection clause, and the Supreme Court legalized birth control for unmarried persons.[29] As of 1976, with the national birth rate at an all-time low of 14.8 per thousand, and with attendance at family planning clinics at an all-time high and increasing, the dream of mass availability of contraception envisioned by the courageous pioneers of the 1930s has come true—almost.

Teenagers now have a birth rate of nearly sixty per thousand, roughly four times the national figure. *Family Planning Perspectives* estimates 3.9 million women aged fifteen to nineteen are at risk of unwanted pregnancy, with an estimated half a million women under fifteen facing the same risks.[30] With abortion looming as the de facto method of birth control for many of these youngsters, critics of family planning might argue that morality, chastity, and decency have crumbled in our permissive society; meanwhile, family planners are attempting renewed efforts to make birth control an accessible, practical alternative.

Presently, twenty-six states and the District of Columbia have statutes or judicial decisions affirming minors' rights to contraceptives without parental consent. In states such as Massachusetts, without such legal protection, the law is vague enough to discourage ambitious programs to deal with the teenage problem. Technically, a physician could be charged with battery for examining a teenage woman to prescribe contraceptives. However, in view of two Supreme Court decisions of July 1976, dealing with parental consent to abortions for minors, it appears unlikely that a physician would be prosecuted for prescribing contraceptives in order to obviate the need for abortion. But it is unfortunate that medicine had to get that dubious protection from a law relating to abortion.

Since the earliest days of popularization of birth control, its advocates have called for widespread education programs on the subject. But throughout the years a tight rein has been held on this subject; public schools and airwaves (for advertising) are still forbidden territory. The issue, at its core, is one of protecting morality. Concurring in Poe v. Ullman, Justice Brennan pointed out that there were no real obstacles to married couples obtaining and using contraceptives, and that the real issue was "opening of birth control clinics on a large scale," and provision of easy access.

The question is, what can be done to make contraception for teenagers acceptable, accessible, and guilt-free? Birth control advocates have for generations asserted the importance of contraception in industrialized society as an alternative and deterrent to abortion; in retrospect, one cannot help but wonder if abortion would be the issue it is today had a more enlightened view prevailed a generation ago.

REFERENCES

1. Himes E: *Medical history of contraception.* New York, Schocken Books, 1970, p 219.
2. Dienes: *Law politics and birth control.* Urbana, University of Illinois Press, 1972, p 4.
3. Mass. Rev. Stats. Chap. 130, Sec. 10 (1836)
4. 18 USC 1461–1462 (1873)
5. Fryer P: *The birth controllers.* London, Secker & Warburg, 1965, p 193.
6. 118 NE 1107 (1918)
7. 45 F2d 103 (1930)
8. *Fortune* 42(2):84, Feb. 1938.
9. *Journal of Contraception* 1(1):4, Nov. 1935.
10. *Journal of the American Medical Association* 102(22):1191, May 30, 1936.
11. *Journal of Contraception* 1(8):108, June–July 1936.
12. Wertz, DC, Wertz, RW: *Lying in: a history of childbirth in America.* New York, Free Press, 1977.
13. 86 F2d 737 at 739 (1936)
14. *Journal of Contraception* 2(1):4, Jan. 1937.
15. *Journal of the American Medical Association* 108(14):1179, April 3, 1937.
16. *Journal of the American Medical Association* 108(26):2213, June 26, 1937.
17. *Fortune* 11(1):158, June 1936.
18. *Ladies Home Journal* 55(3):14, March 1938.
19. 97 F2d 510 (1938)
20. *Journal of the American Medical Association* 12(14):1311, April 1939.
21. *Journal of Contraception* 2(4):43, February 1939.
22. 300 Mass. 373 at 374
23. 305 US 559 (1940)
24. *Journal of Contraception* 4(1):155, January 1939.
25. 126 Conn. 412 (1940)
26. 318 US 44 at 46 (1943)
27. 367 US 497 at 508 (1961)
28. 381 US 479 at 484 (1965)
29. 92 S. Ct. 1029 (1971)
30. *Family Planning Perspectives* 8(4):167, July–August 1976.

Chapter 13

The Emotional Impact
of Abortion

CAROL C. NADELSON

Recent controversy about who should have access to abortion has renewed claims that abortion should be looked upon as a psychologically damaging procedure.[1] Before 1960 professionals held this view, believing that guilt and shame resulting from abortion would lead to serious depression and disturbance in relationships with men.[2] In addition, physicians and other health professionals opposed abortion because it was not seen as a safe medical procedure, and also because it violated the Hippocratic Oath, which contained the phrase, "I will not give to a woman an instrument to produce abortion." This prohibition was in fact supported by the high mortality rate for abortion. As medical techniques improved and resulted in a revisal of mortality rates, so that childbirth carried a greater risk than abortion, medical risk was no longer a viable argument.[3] Likewise, psychological evidence has not borne out the claims that serious repercussions follow abortion.

PSYCHOLOGICAL DAMAGE RELATED TO ABORTION: MYTHS AND REALITY

Prior to 1973, in most states, abortions were "therapeutic." When they were done the indications were to preserve the life and/or health of the mother. Most states differed on grounds and indications, and hospitals as well as physicians accepted different criteria. For example,

CAROL C. NADELSON, M.D. • Psychiatrist, Beth Israel Hospital; Associate Professor of Psychiatry, Harvard Medical School; Director, Medical Student Education, Department of Psychiatry, Beth Israel Hospital, Boston, Massachusetts 02215.

174   CAROL C. NADELSON

in one hospital a woman would have been required to have made a suicide attempt in order for the pregnancy to be considered a danger to her life; whereas in another hospital a statement of suicidal intent was sufficient. There were few abortions performed for medical reasons, because the technical ability to preserve life through pregnancy had improved to the extent that disorders which would threaten life during pregnancy were rare. Thus, the vast number of therapeutic abortions were performed for psychiatric reasons, although guidelines and criteria were vague, and poorly defined.[4]

The myth of psychological damage related to abortion persisted despite Ekblad's 1955 study of 479 women who had legal abortions in Sweden for psychiatric reasons. This was the first report providing evidence that abortion was not necessarily detrimental to emotional health. He found that 74 percent of the women he followed had no regrets or self-reproach, 14 percent experienced some regret and only 11 percent regretted having had an abortion. Of the 1 percent who had demonstrated emotional consequences, all had had previous histories of emotional disorders. Ekblad concluded that there was little evidence that abortion had serious effects on the mental health of women. Furthermore, he stated, "The problem of abortion for psychiatric reasons is far more often the question of judging the effect of the addition of another child to a household or mother or both, under stress, than predicting the likelihood of madness or suicide."[5]

This report did not evoke much interest until a 1963 study in the United States confirmed Ekblad's findings. Kummer, in a survey of 32 psychiatrists who frequently saw women postabortion, found that 75 percent of them stated that they had never seen severe, emotional sequelae, and 25 percent stated that it rarely occurred.[6]

Subsequently other studies began to challenge the views which had been so pervasive and to develop methodologies for more careful investigation. Peck and Marcus found that women who had already been diagnosed as psychologically ill, benefitted from the procedure. They found that symptoms of depression and anxiety, precipitated by the pregnancy, were relieved, and new symptoms were mild and self-limited.[7] Another study reported that women who were psychologically healthy, as well as those who were ill, responded to abortion with transient symptoms, but were generally improved following the procedure. In fact this study found an increased risk of neurotic or depressive illness if an unwanted pregnancy was not terminated.[8]

In 1969 the Group for the Advancement of Psychiatry published a monograph which reviewed the moral, ethical, psychological, and medical issues involved in abortion. They recommended that the decision for termination of a pregnancy rested primarily with the pregnant woman. They noted the lack of serious postabortion complications and recommended that the physician explore the motivation for the decision with the woman and be able to recommend or provide counseling.[9]

At this time other psychiatric groups took similar positions.[10,11] They all emphasized the need to clarify motivation. One report noted that psychiatrists were unable to predict which women would suffer from emotional disturbances if therapeutic abortion was denied, and recommended that the woman and her family, not the psychiatrist, make the decision.[12] Another stated that, "there are no unequivocal psychiatric indications for therapeutic abortion."[13]

Studies from Britain following the changes in their law refocused the issue on the stress of bearing an unwanted child. They reported that psychiatric symptoms were more likely to occur in the overburdened multipara and the single woman without support, and found that women who had a pregnancy terminated had little psychiatric disturbance.[14]

THE UNWANTED CHILD

Meanwhile, although far too little attention was paid to the discovery, it was becoming clear that psychiatric risks must also be considered in light of preventative gains for the mother as well as the child. In 1954 Caplan had reported that special problems were apt to develop between mother and child when an unsuccessful attempt at abortion had been made during the pregnancy.[15]

Hook studied 213 children born to women who had been refused therapeutic abortion and found that unwanted children were both physically and mentally impaired.[16]

In their classic study Forssman and Thuwe followed, for twenty-one years, 120 children who were born after an application for a therapeutic abortion was refused. These children were matched with controls of the same sex born in the same hospital or district on the same day. The results indicated that the unwanted children fared worse in almost every way. They had a higher incidence of psychiatric disorder, delinquency, criminal behavior, and alcoholism. They were more often receiving public assistance, they were often exempted from military service, and they had less schooling than the control group. The study concluded that the very fact that a woman applies for a legal abortion means that the prospective child has greater difficulty in having to surmount social and mental handicaps, than his peers.[17] The authors recommended that these factors be seriously considered when recommendations for therapeutic abortion were made. Subsequent studies of child abuse and neglect repeat these warnings about the fate of unwanted children.[18,19]

THE EFFECT OF LEGALIZATION OF ABORTION

As the climate of opinion about abortion began to change and some states revised their laws, investigations began to focus on counseling and crisis intervention in the decision making process. Senay emphasized counseling particularly when a woman seemed to be pressured toward an abortion decision by her family or friends;[20] Marder reported his observation that negative attitudes on the part of hospital personnel and inadequate counseling contributed directly to the incidence of postabortion guilt, remorse, and depression.[21]

Others reported that for most women abortion was indeed therapeutic when they had made a decision that this was the best course of action for them.[22-25] One study found that "tired mothers," who often requested sterilization were particularly benefited by abortion. These women reported that they found new meaning in life when they were no longer in the position of having obligatory pregnancies.[26]

Another study speculated that under legal conditions requiring severe prior psychiatric illness one would find a group least likely to respond favorably to abortion as a therapeutic procedure. Of the 207 women followed in this study (average age 18) the reasons for seeking abortion included depressive feelings (most frequently), guilt, anxiety, fears (hurting parents, having and raising a child), social stigma, rejection, malformed fetus, and losing a job. Seventy-four of this group were contraceptive failures. Naiveté was prominent in many (e.g., you can't become pregnant the first time). The reports of the women in this study indicated that 98 percent of them felt their general health was the same or better and 94 percent felt that their emotional health was the same or better. Most of the symptoms reported (depression, anxiety, and guilt) decreased with time. The authors found very few patients who required psychiatric treatment. In fact a history of previous psychiatric symptoms or illness did not predict those who had a negative emotional response to abortion.[27]

A report from the Peter Bent Brigham Hospital in Boston, Massachusetts emphasized that healthier, more knowledgeable women were able to get therapeutic abortions rather than those who were disturbed, because the latter had difficulty negotiating the process.[28]

In a recent study which measured anxiety, depression, anger, guilt, and shame preabortion and postabortion, the investigators found that the pattern of response was similar to that of other instances of crisis reaction and crisis resolution. In the 24-hour postabortion observation period, relief and feelings of well being predominated. Over the six month period the absence of grief, sadness or depression suggested that abortion was not experienced as a major loss to most women. Those women who were most vulnerable to conflict following abortion were those with:

1. A previous history of mental illness or serious emotional conflict.
2. Immature interpersonal relationships or an unstable, conflicted relationship with men.
3. A negative relationship with their mothers.
4. Strong ambivalence or uncertainty and helplessness with regard to abortion.
5. Religious or cultural background where there were negative attitudes toward abortion.

In addition, single women, especially those who had not borne children were more susceptible to conflict following abortion. The authors caution, however, that these factors are not to be interpreted as contraindications to abortion. They point out that women in the vulnerable groups believed, at their six-month follow-up evaluation, that their decision for abortion was the right one. They conclude that the opportunity to play an active role in resolving the crisis of an unwanted pregnancy, and to choose or reject abortion, promotes successful adjustment and maturation. Thus, rather than making a decision for or against abortion, on tenuous grounds, a variety of crisis intervention and therapeutic techniques may be most beneficial to the woman seeking an abortion.[33]

In another report, Freeman considered the implications of abortion to women from another perspective.[29] She found that the women she studied did not perceive themselves to be active and instrumental in their own lives and thus chose abortion out of "necessity." Postabortion, however, these women felt that the experience resulted in a "different awareness about themselves," especially since for many it was their first experience with a major individual decision where the consequences were important and affected others as well as themselves. The author also confirmed reports of others that contraceptive use increases postabortion.[30,31,32,33]

Although in 1973 the United States Supreme Court eliminated the "reason" for abortion and the necessity for psychiatrists to "approve" a "therapeutic" abortion, the belief that abortion was psychologically damaging persisted. While the evidence runs counter to this view it is also clear that abortion cannot be seen as a minor procedure without significance to the individual. It is the result of an unwanted pregnancy, a crisis situation for a woman. The decision for abortion is an important one, requiring careful consideration, which may be facilitated with counseling. For many women this may extend into the postabortion period. When counseling is provided in an atmosphere where a woman's decision is respected and her right to make that decision is not interferred with by socioeconomic or any other externally imposed restrictions, fewer adverse reactions are to be expected.

REFERENCES

1. Pasnau RO: Psychiatric complications of therapeutic abortion. *Obstetrics and Gynecology* 40(2):252–256, 1972.
2. Deutsch H: *The psychology of women*. Vol II. New York: Grune & Stratton, 1945.
3. Tietze C: Somatic consequences of abortion. Paper presented at the NICHD/NIMH Workshop on Abortion, Bethesda, Maryland, December 15–16, 1969 (National Institute of Child Health and Human Development, and National Institutes of Mental Health).
4. Nadelson C: Psychological issues in therapeutic abortion. *Journal of the American Medical Women's Association* 27:1, 1972.
5. Ekblad N: Induced abortion on psychiatric grounds. *Acta Psychiatrica Scandinavica Supplementum 99*, 1955.
6. Kummer J: Post abortion psychiatric illness—a myth? *American Journal of Psychiatry* 119:980–983, 1963.
7. Peck A, Marcus H: Psychiatric sequelae of therapeutic interruption of pregnancy. *Journal of Nervous and Mental Disease* 143:417–425, 1966.
8. Simon N, Senturia A, Rothman D: Psychiatric illness following therapeutic abortion. *American Journal of Psychiatry* 124:59–65, 1967.
9. Group for the Advancement of Psychiatry, No. 75. October 1969.
10. American Psychiatric Association Postion Statement on Abortion. *American Journal of Psychiatry* 126:1554, 1970.
11. American Psychoanalytical Association. Position Statement on Abortion. San Francisco, California, 1970.
12. Whittington H: Evaluation of therapeutic abortion as an element of preventive psychiatry. *American Journal of Psychiatry* 126:1224–1229, 1970.
13. Sloane RB: The unwanted pregnancy. *New England Journal of Medicine* 22:1206–1213, 1969.
14. Pare CMB, Raven H: Follow up of patients referred for termination of pregnancy. *Lancet*, March 28, 1970, pp. 635–638.
15. Caplan G: The disturbance of the mother-child relationship by unsuccessful attempts at abortion. *Mental Hygiene* 38:67–80, 1954.
16. Hook K: Refused abortion. A follow-up study of two hundred and forty-nine women whose applications were refused by the national board of health in Sweden. *Acta Psychiatrica Scandinavica Supplementum 168*, 1963.
17. Forssman H, Thuwe I: One hundred and twenty children born after application for therapeutic abortion refused: their mental health, social adjustment and educational level up to the age of 21. *Acta Psychiatrica Scandinavica* 42:71–88, 1966.
18. Resnick PJ: Child murder by parents. a psychiatric review of filicide. *American Journal of Psychiatry* 126:(3)325–334, 1969.
19. Kempe CH: Approaches to preventing child abuse: a health visitor's concept. *American Journal of Diseases of Children* 130:941, 1976.

20. Senay E: Therapeutic abortion. *Archives of General Psychiatry* 23:408–415, 1970.
21. Marder L: Psychiatric experience with a liberalized therapeutic abortion law. *American Journal of Psychiatry* 126:1230–1236, 1970.
22. Ford C, Castelnvono-Tedesca P, Long K: Is abortion a therapeutic procedure in psychiatry? *Journal of the American Medical Association* 218:1173–1178, 1971.
23. Kravitz A, Notman M, Anderson J, Payne E: Outcome following therapeutic abortion. *Archives of General Psychiatry* 33:725–733, 1976.
24. Osofsky J, Osofsky H: The psychological reaction of patients to legalized abortion. *American Journal of Orthopsychiatry* 42(1):48–60, 1972.
25. Osofsky H, Osofsky J: *The abortion experience: psychological and medical impact.* Hagerstown, MD, Harper & Row, 1973.
26. Ford C, Atkinson R, Bugonier J: Therapeutic abortion: who needs a psychiatrist? *Obstetrics and Gynecology* 38:206–213, 1971.
27. Partridge JR, Spiegel TM, Rouse BA, Ewing JA: Therapeutic abortion: a study of psychiatric applicants at North Carolina memorial hospital. *North Carolina Medical Journal* 32:132–136, 1971.
28. Morris T, Jr: Abortion: psychiatric implication. *Progress in Gynecology* 5:249–256, 1970.
29. Freeman E: Influence of personality attributes on abortion experiences. *American Journal of Orthopsychiatry* 47(3):503–513, 1977.
30. Dauher H, Zalar M, Goldstein P: Abortion counselling and behavioral change. *Family Planning Perspective* 4(2):23–27, 1972.
31. Margolis A, Rindfuss R, Coghland P, Rochat, R: Contraception after abortion. *Family Planning Perspective* 6:55–60, 1974.
32. Smith E: A follow-up study of women who request abortion. *American Journal of Orthopsychiatry* 43(4):574–585, 1973.
33. Tietze C: Contraceptive practice in the context of a nonrestrictive abortion law. *Family Planning Perspective* 7(3):197–202, 1975.

Chapter 14

Medical Gynecology: Problems and Patients

GAY GUZINSKI

Medical gynecology is that field of medicine that concerns itself with both the external and internal organs of the female reproductive tract. The visible genital structures called the vulva (Figure 1) are the introitus, the urethral meatus, the clitoris, the labia minora, and the labia majora. The openings of the paired vulvovaginal or Bartholin's glands are also found in this area. The internal organs of reproduction (Figure 2) are the vagina, the uterus, the Fallopian tubes, and the ovaries (the lower portion of the uterus is the cervix). These organs are covered with a thin layer of tissue called the peritoneum, and are supported by several fibrous ligaments.

The normal function of these reproductive organs is under the control of the central nervous system. In general terms, a portion of the brain sends hormonal messengers (gonadotropins) to the ovary, causing the ovary to produce an ovum (egg). The ovary also produces hormones (steroids) which prepare the uterine lining to receive a fertilized egg, and which inhibit further stimulation from the brain centers. If conception does not occur, the ovarian hormone production declines drastically, and the brain is free to begin stimulating the ovary with hormones again. The total normal cyclic interaction of these hormones produces the physiologic changes we call the menstrual cycle. This interaction is outlined in the accompanying diagram (Figure 3) and discussed in more detail in the following paragraph.

The menstrual cycle begins on the first day of vaginal bleeding. At this time an area of the brain called the hypothalamus initiates the

GAY GUZINSKI, M.D. ● Assistant Professor of Obstetrics-Gynecology; Director, Division of Women's Health Care, University of Washington, Seattle, Washington 98195.

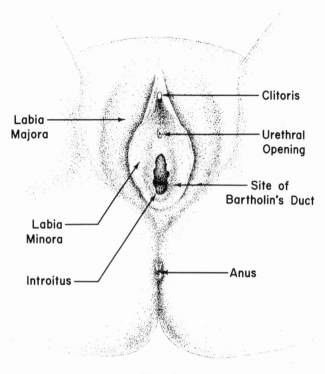

Clitoris

Labia Majora

Urethral Opening

Site of Bartholin's Duct

Labia Minora

Introitus

Anus

Figure 1

cycle by secreting releasing factors. These chemicals travel in a special system of blood vessels to an adjacent gland in the brain called the pituitary. The anterior portion of this gland then produces the gonadotropins follicle stimulating hormone (FSH) and leuteinizing hormone (LH) which pass into the general circulatory system. This hypothalamic activity can be influenced by higher brain centers as well as by "short loop" feedback from the gonadotropins themselves. The gonadotropins stimulate a germ cell in the ovary to grow and mature into a follicle, and cause certain cells of this follicle (theca lutein cells) to produce the steroid estrogen. High levels of estrogen inhibit the hypothalamus (long loop feedback) from production of certain releasing factors, and this results in a decrease of pituitary production of FSH.

Very high levels of estrogen are produced at midcycle, and this has a positive effect on the hypothalamic-pituitary axis resulting in a surge of LH. Ovulation then occurs from the mature follicle and after ovulation the remaining cells from that follicle coalesce to form a yellow body in the ovary called the corpus luteum. These cells then produce high levels of another steroid hormone, progesterone. Estrogen and progesterone produce the secondary sex characteristics, and inhibit the hypothalamus from producing releasing factors, as the reproductive organs are held in readiness to receive a conceptus. The level of progesterone reaches its peak in approximately 9 days. If fertilization of the egg and implantation do not occur, the progesterone and estrogen levels drop as the corpus luteum ceases to function and begins to deteriorate. When deterioration is sufficient, and hormone levels are low enough, menstruation begins. The low levels of estrogen then allow the hypothalamus to produce releasing factors and the cycle begins again.[1]

The successful interaction of the central nervous system with the reproductive organs results in these physiologic events which periodically ready the whole organism for sexual reproduction. The ovarian hormones cause the uterine lining to increase in thickness and glandular activity in preparation for implantation of the zygote. If this does not occur, the endometrium begins to degenerate and slough off pieces of lining together with blood. This process is called menstruation. All the components of this system are present in the pubertal female, and their successful interaction leads to the visible sign of

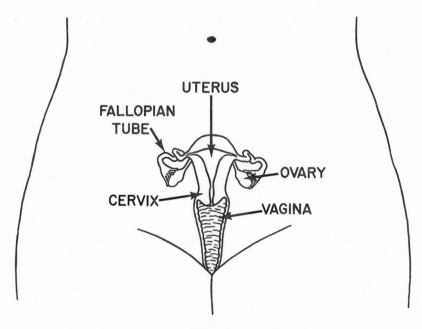

Figure 2

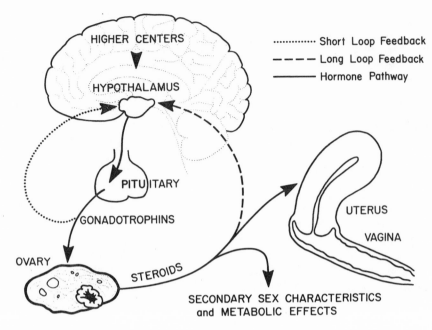

Figure 3

menstrual bleeding which marks the entrance of the female into her reproductive years. During the first years of reproductive activity, the menstrual cycle may be quite irregular as ovulation does not occur regularly. Then, as the interaction of nervous system and reproductive organs becomes more firmly established, ovulation and menstruation occur at more predictable intervals. The typical menstrual cycle lasts 28 days; however, there are variations in cycle length among women, and cycles in any one woman may vary by as much as 8 or 9 days and still be considered within the normal range.

COMMON PROBLEMS OF THE MENSTRUAL CYCLE

The menstrual cycle itself is divided into three phases which are represented in the accompanying diagram (Figure 4). Menses, or the menstrual phase, is first. It may be as short as 2 days or as long as 8 days without being considered pathologic, although the average length is 4–6 days. The second phase is from the end of the menstrual phase to ovulation and this is termed the proliferative phase. During this time estrogen causes the uterine lining to increase in thickness due to growth of glands, connective tissue, and blood vessels. This phase may vary significantly in length between women and from cycle to cycle in a single woman, but is usually 7–11 days. Ovulation marks the beginning of the third and final phase called the secretory phase. During this time, the glands in the uterine lining are affected by estrogen and progesterone. The cells become filled with glycogen, and the connective tissue becomes more swollen. This phase is controlled by the corpus luteum in the ovary, and since the life of that structure is approximately 14 days, the secretory phase of the menstrual cycle is usually less variable, with an average variation among women of 12–16 days.

Thus, there is room for considerable variation within what may be described as the normal menstrual cycle. Beyond these normal limits, the two problems most commonly confronted are those of abnormal bleeding and pain.

ABNORMAL BLEEDING. Variations in the normal bleeding pattern can range from total absence of uterine bleeding to a complaint of almost continuous vaginal bleeding. In treating this problem it is most important to ascertain what the patient is concerned about. She may be worried that she is pregnant or she may need information on con-

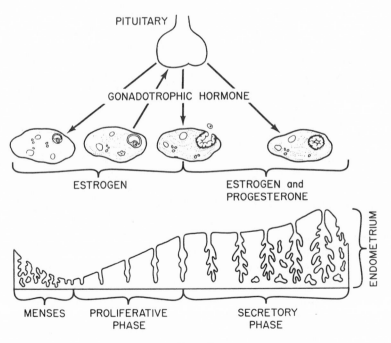

Figure 4

traception. She may want "normal" monthly cycles or just the reassurance that no life-threatening problem is present.

Prepubertal Years. Vaginal bleeding in prepubertal females is not common, and any vaginal bleeding should be considered abnormal. A pelvic examination is required to determine the cause of bleeding. This may be infection, foreign bodies in the vagina, or tumor. Bleeding from an irritating foreign body generally stops upon removal of the object. Tumors are not common in this age group, but when they do occur they have a poor prognosis.

Lack of menstrual function in the young female is often a cause for concern although the complete workup for primary amenorrhea is not mandatory until age 18.[2:652] The physician can often detect developmental anomalies in the young patient which may preclude menstruation. Appropriate genetic studies can then be instituted or the patient reassured that the physical condition of her pelvic organs is normal.

Reproductive Age. Amenorrhea is called secondary when menstrual function ceases for more than 3 months. Oligomenorrhea is defined as reduced frequency of menses with an interval between bleeding greater than 38 days. These two complaints together have been estimated to comprise approximately 5 percent of the problems seen in a general gynecologic practice.

Since menstruation is the end result of the successful interaction of the hypothalamus, pituitary, ovary, and uterus, amenorrhea and oligomenorrhea can result from deranged functioning of any component of this system.

If the patient has no symptoms other than absent or very infrequent menses, the first step in evaluation is testing the capability of the uterus to respond to a progesterone challenge. If bleeding occurs, the ovary is producing enough estrogen to prime the uterus, and if no bleeding occurs estrogen production is too low. Further investigations of hypothalamic pituitary and ovarian function must be carried out to determine the exact nature of the defect. In addition, disorders of the whole organism like chronic illness, emotional stress, malnutrition, and disturbances of thyroid, pancreas, and adrenal glands should be considered.

Treatment must be based both on the etiology of the amenorrhea and the woman's desires. Patients who do not ovulate regularly and wish to become pregnant can be given a chemical to cause egg production. Patients not desiring contraception should have an induced period of bleeding once every two or three months using a progesterone to counteract the effects of their high continuous estrogen production.

Hypomenorrhea is a reduction in the amount or number of days of menstrual flow, and many of the derangements previously discussed can produce this symptom. In addition, hypomenorrhea may develop while the patient is taking oral contraceptives. This symptom does not have any documented serious consequences, but patients may become concerned about pregnancy if monthly bleeding does not occur.

Complaints of "too much bleeding" are nearly as common as too little. Polymenorrhea is regular cyclic menstruation with an interval of less than 21 days. Metrorrhagia is irregular uterine bleeding, and menorrhagia is abnormally heavy vaginal bleeding at regular intervals. Diagnosis of these problems involves a careful history with special attention to specific days and amounts of bleeding. Bleeding can be quantified by "number of pads or tampons used," use of double pads and/or tampons and pads, degree of saturation or "bleeding through."

Anatomical disorders which can lead to heavy irregular bleeding include benign or malignant tumors of the reproductive organs, and pregnancy-related problems such as retention of products of conception, ectopic pregnancy, and placental tumors (trophoblastic tumors). Infections of the internal genitalia can cause irregular but usually light vaginal bleeding.

If no anatomical cause can be detected, the bleeding problem is called dysfunctional. It is rarely life threatening, but can be very disabling to the patient. This problem is poorly understood and usually difficult to treat. Therapy must be designed in collaboration with the patient's wishes regarding regular vaginal bleeding and her desires for child-bearing. For example, a patient who feels her femininity is related to her possession of a uterus may be distraught at its removal even though she is socially embarrassed and sexually immobilized by her metrorrhagia. Another patient who has a firm desire to forego all future possibilities of pregnancy may be inappropriately selected for a trial of hormonal therapy.

Menopausal Age. Ovulation may occur less regularly in the woman approaching menopause. Bleeding in some perimenopausal women may therefore be very irregular, and need not always trigger an intensive diagnostic work-up. Some authorities have suggested that a woman in the menopausal age range with a normal pelvic exam should have six months of irregular bleeding before further studies are done to determine the cause of the bleeding. This should be modified depending on other factors such as those which place the patient at high risk for development of cancer of the uterine lining.

Bleeding in the postmenopausal woman—that is, bleeding which occurs in a woman over age 45 who has had no vaginal bleeding for a period of 12 consecutive months—is always a cause for further diagnostic investigation. This should always include evaluating the lining of the uterine cavity where cancer may develop. This can be done in a clinic setting if no enlargement of the endocervical canal is necessary, but it may require a procedure in the operating room to dilate the canal and scrape out the uterine lining (a D and C). Treatment should be based on the results of this investigation.

PAIN. Pain is another common gynecologic complaint. It is a highly subjective, culturally and environmentally influenced sensation which is difficult to define and quantify. It can be acute or chronic, mild or severe, tolerable or intolerable. Whatever the patient claims it to be, it is irrefutable because no one but the individual herself can actually experience it.

Mild Pain. In the mild pain category Mittelschmerz and dysmenorrhea are most common. Mittelschmerz is pain which occurs at mid-cycle, and is thought to be an accompaniment of ovulation. The actual mechanism of pain is unknown, but measures which suppress ovulation generally abolish the pain. Dysmenorrhea or painful menstruation is more difficult to diagnose and treat. Ovulation again is thought to be related to dysmenorrhea, and suppression of ovulation may produce relief. Tension and anticipatory anxiety (i.e., menses have been painful in the past and will be painful again) have been postulated as a cause of dysmenorrhea. This is the basis for recommending measures that produce relaxation, such as hot baths, locally applied heating pads, and minimal oral alcohol intake. Swelling is thought to play a role, either by local compression with excitation of nerve endings or by central nervous system swelling leading to increased irritability and lowered threshold for pain. Diuretics and salt restriction have been prescribed for this reason. More recently, the hormone prostaglandin which causes smooth muscle contraction has been implicated in dysmenorrhea. This is released by the uterine lining, and causes contraction of uterine muscles and blood vessels with resultant pain. It may even be released into the circulatory system and produce characteristic nausea, diarrhea, and flushing. Some investigators have obtained good results in treating dysmenorrhea with the prostaglandin antagonists, aspirin and indomethecin, but results are still preliminary.[2:725] Acetylsalicylic acid (aspirin) is listed as an analgesic; it does, however, have significant "anti-prostaglandin" effects, as discussed in several more recent publications. A very small percentage of women who complain of dysmenorrhea will have endometriosis (implantation of tissue which normally lines the inside of the uterus in an extra-uterine position). A variety of hormonal regimens have been recommended, and may result in the relief of pain when it is caused by endometriosis.

Acute Severe Pain. The common causes of acute, severe pelvic pain are pelvic infection, ruptured or twisted ovarian cysts, incomplete or infected abortion, and ruptured ectopic pregnancies. If the patient has fever, chills, and a history of pelvic infection, repeat infection is the most likely. Signs and symptoms of pregnancy, sexual activity without contraception, and irregular vaginal bleeding make an accident of pregnancy more likely. The diagnosis and treatment in each case will depend on a careful history and physical examination as well as supporting laboratory data.

Chronic Pain. Chronic pelvic pain is more difficult to evaluate and treat. It has been estimated that as many as 25 percent of gynecologic patients bring this complaint to the physician for evaluation. These patients commonly receive massive doses of hormones to suppress poorly diagnosed endometriosis. They are frequently treated with large amounts of antibiotics for "pelvic inflammatory disease" which is not documented by history, physical, or laboratory findings. Finally, they may have their internal pelvic organs removed even though they are visibly and palpably normal, or have abnormalities too mild to account for the degree of pain. Since the late 1800s physicians have recognized that many patients with this complaint also have significant psychological disturbances. However, the published studies of patients with chronic pelvic pain fail to establish a definite etiology either organic or psychic for the problem. The numbers of patients are statistically small, the periods of follow-up brief, and the control groups poorly matched. The major studies, however, all agree that psychologic problems are present to a significant degree in this group of patients.[3,4,5] Further studies of these patients will be necessary to arrive at a more accurate method of diagnosis and treatment for this group of women.

Common Problems of the Female Genital Organs

As far as the female genital organs themselves are concerned, two of the most common problems are those associated with infections and with screening for cancer.

Infections. Infections vary in severity and may occur acutely or be present for many years.

Vulva. The external genitalia are particularly sensitive in some women and their anatomic location produces conditions of warmth, darkness, and moisture which favor infection. Treatment of vulvar infection involves determination by history, physical, and laboratory data if a specific infectious agent is present. *Monilia* (yeast or fungus) can grow on the vulva and is readily identified under the microscope.

The herpes virus produces painful ulcers which harbor viral particles, and absolute diagnosis rests on culturing this virus in the laboratory. A virus is also thought to be responsible for warts of the vulva, vagina, and cervix. Infestation of the vulvar hair and skin by parasites such as scabes or lice is also seen.

All of these infections except herpes will respond to appropriately selected chemotherapeutic agents. Additionally, general measures to keep the vulva clean and dry, including wearing loose fitting garments, will aid in decreasing symptoms and accelerating the healing processes.

Vagina. Vaginal infections can cause internal itching or burning as well as irritation of the vulva. The diagnosis of vaginal infections should be based on examination of vaginal discharge and culture where appropriate. Monilial discharge is curdy white and the fungus can clearly be seen on a wet-mount preparation, especially if KOH is added to the fluid. The protozoan *Trichomonas vaginalis* causes the production of a foamy yellow-green discharge and the trichomonad can also be detected on a wet-mount. A variety of other organisms ranging from bacteria like *Haemophilus vaginalis* to *chlamydia* and mycoplasmas have been implicated in "nonspecific vaginal infection."

Treatment of vaginal infections is again by the use of specific chemicals designed to eradicate a known infectious agent, and meticulous perineal cleanliness sometimes including the use of a tampon to absorb discharge and prevent it from soiling the vulva.

It is not always possible to find a specific infectious agent, however, and many patients need reassurance that some vaginal discharge is normal, and does not always signify an infection. Douching is not a necessary activity in normal women because the vaginal lining is continually renewed. If the patient prefers to douche she should use only a mild vinegar solution or a commercial preparation to avoid injury to herself.

Cervix. The cervix may be infected by any of the agents listed above. Chronic cervicitis may lead to abnormal or atypical Pap smears and a chronic vaginal discharge. Frequently, no specific infectious agent can be cultured from the cervix; however, the gonococcus can be cultured from asymptomatic women and should be treated if found.

Uterus. Endometritis, the infection of the lining of the uterine cavity, occurs most commonly as an isolated event after a full-term pregnancy or an abortion. The uterine cavity provides conditions which are ideal for growth, particularly of anaerobic or non-oxygen-requiring organisms. These are difficult to culture and they may not immediately be detected in a diagnostic workup. Infections of the uterus can produce cramping, mild to moderately severe lower abdominal pain, and a temperature elevation. This infection may respond to antibiotic therapy alone, however, removing the infected lining tissue by D and C may be necessary.

Tubes and Ovaries. Acute pelvic inflammatory disease is a relatively common medical problem in a young sexually active population. The first episode is usually gonococcal. Infection in these cases involves the cervix, uterus, tubes, ovaries, and sometimes the lining of the pelvic cavity, and may result in symptoms which range from mild lower abdominal cramping to severe lower abdominal pain with nausea and vomiting. This infection may remain localized to the pelvis or it may spread throughout the entire abdominal cavity. It may also lead to formation of an abscess which can be life threatening. Treatment of this condition is designed to localize the infection to the pelvis and eliminate the causative organism with antibiotics.

A first episode of acute pelvic inflammatory disease usually resolves quickly with the appropriate therapy. This episode and each subsequent one may leave scarring and damage which predisposes the woman to still another infection. Since the woman who acquires an initial pelvic inflammatory disease is often exposed again to the same infectious agents, many develop chronic pelvic inflammatory disease. Chronic changes involve further scarring and distortion of the internal pelvic organs and may result in complete closure of the open end of the tube with development of a pus- or fluid-filled tube. Pain and infertility are common presenting complaints. Therapy for this problem may involve low doses of suppressive antibiotics over a protracted period of time to decrease pain and discomfort. Ultimate therapy in the form of removal of all previously infected tissue (the uterus, tubes, and ovaries) must be based on the patient's ability to tolerate discomfort from her condition, and her wishes for preservation of her internal genital organs.

CANCER SCREENING. Tumors of the female genitalia account for about 25 percent of all malignant disease in women and tumors of the breast account for approximately another 25 percent of malignancies.[6] The routine yearly checkup should include a breast examination, Pap smear, and physical examination of the internal and external genitalia and can detect early signs of malignancy in the breasts and pelvic organs.

Pap Smears. Detection of pelvic malignancies involves visualization and palpation of the external and internal genitalia. The Pap smear is used primarily to detect cancer of the cervix. (In rare cases tumors of the uterus, tubes, or ovaries may be suggested on Pap smear.)

Even with correct sampling techniques, slide preparation, and cell interpretation, the Pap smear is not infallible for cancer detection. For example, with a cancer of the lining of the uterus, 75 percent of the time the Pap smear from the vaginal pool will show identifiable cancer cells, and 15 percent of the time it will show an abnormal pattern which is suggestive of cancer. This adds up to an overall accuracy of detection of only 90 percent. With a proven cervical cancer, vaginal pool cells will be positive for cancer in only 90 percent of the cases and in 97 percent when the cells come from the endo-cervical canal.[7] In the best series then, the false negative Pap smears (smears which were negative when the patient actually has a cancer) may be as low as 3 percent, although in other series the false negative rate may be as high as 20 percent. The false positive rate (smears which are "conclusive of the presence of cancer" and no cancer can be detected on exhaustive attempts) may be as high as 16 to 20 percent. These data indicate that the Pap smear is only a screening device and should always be used with the physical examination as a guide to further evaluation. Many classifications of Pap smears are currently in use in the United States, emphasizing numbers (I–IV), grades (I–IV), or words (normal to positive). For simplification we will discuss management of Pap smears which are normal, atypical (mildly abnormal but not suspicious for malignancy), suspicious for malignancy (dysplastic), and positive for malignancy.

If the patient's Pap smear is returned as negative, a yearly pelvic examination and repeat Pap smear is routine. If the Pap smear is atypical, it should be repeated within a reasonable interval (two months), and if a specific infectious agent is present on the smear, the patient should be treated before her smear is repeated. If no specific agent is identified, some authorities recommend treatment for nonspecific vaginitis before the Pap smear is repeated. If the repeat Pap smear is atypical, colposcopy should generally be performed. If the Pap smear is suspicious (dysplastic) or positive, colposcopy should be performed without repeating the smear first. Further diagnostic steps and therapy should be based on the findings.

Diethylstilbestrol (DES). Pap smears and colposcopy can be used to advantage in the examination of another group of patients of considerable recent interest to the gynecologist, those exposed in utero to diethylstilbestrol. The synthetic estrogen, diethylstilbestrol (DES), was used by physicians from the mid-1940s through about 1970 in an attempt to prevent pregnancy loss from spontaneous abortion. It has been estimated that 1 to 2 million women received this drug during pregnancy. Certain changes have recently been observed in some of the offspring of these women. One study reported a variety of abnormalities occurring in the genitalia of about 10 percent of the male offspring who were DES exposed in utero, and further studies from that team of investigators report abnormal sperm counts in some 30 percent of that group. Information on male offspring is still scanty, however, compared to the volume of material published on the effects of DES on female children.[8] The genital abnormalities in female offspring exposed to DES appear now to be related to the time during pregnancy when the drug was given. Several changes have been detected in these patients although the significance of all the abnormalities has yet to be determined. First, a very rare form of cancer of the cervix and vagina, clear cell adenocarcinoma, has been reported in some 290 females, two-thirds of whom had a definite history of exposure to DES or similar compounds while in utero. Second, anatomical changes in the vagina and cervix have been noted in some DES-exposed female children: the vagina may grow in a collar around the cervix or a hood or a cockscomb over the cervix; additionally, glandular (columnar) tissue usually found in the endocervical canal, may be seen on the vaginal portion of the cervix (called ectropion or "erosion") or upper portion of the vagina (called adenosis) in place of the usual smooth (squamous) tissue. This adenomatous tissue undergoes typical changes into squamous epithelium and this process can be observed over a period of time. The area where this is occurring is called the transformation zone. As yet, there are no documented cases in which a clear cell cancer has developed from a previously identified area of glandular tissue in the vagina (adenosis).

Recommended Examination Procedures. The examination procedures in DES-exposed women are done to identify clear cell carcinomas, to observe and record abnormalities in the cervix and vagina of individual patients, and to observe and record changes in these abnormalities over time. The natural history of this problem is unknown as there are yet no reports of statistically significant numbers of patients followed over a long period of time. There is still considerable controversy even among the experts regarding the appropriate diagnostic and therapeutic approach to this problem.

Clear cell cancers have been reported in some very young children, although, since the large majority of cases are reported in females over the age of 14, authorities recommend initial examination of DES-exposed females after menarche or by age 14 if menses have not yet begun. Examination of the virginal female can be facilitated by instructing her to use tampons for two or three months prior to the exam. If the changes are small and Pap smears are negative, repeat examinations can be done at yearly intervals. However, if extensive changes are observed or Pap smears or biopsies are abnormal, follow-up should be individualized based on these reports.

There are six methods available for examining these patients: visual inspection; Pap smears; iodine staining; palpation; colposcopy; and biopsy. Visual inspection is inexpensive, requires no special skills, and reveals structural abnormalities of the vagina, but it does not always reveal the extent of the abnormal cells and the transformation zone. A Pap smear may reveal abnormalities of squamous cells from the area of the scrape, but it does not give information about cells on the vaginal side walls which are not sampled (it is not useful in evaluating columnar cells since clear cell carcinomas usually produce columnar cells which look normal by themselves). Iodine staining does reveal nonstaining areas which correspond to the presence of adenosis and transformation zone, although no information is obtained about surface tissue or blood vessels in the transformation zone. Palpation usually indicates the presence of an abnormality in the vaginal mucosa even if one cannot be seen (almost all of the carcinomas have been palpable), but it does require a careful and thorough examination of the entire vagina. Colposcopy gives accurate information about the distribution of glandular tissue and the transformation zones as well as more specific information about the surface epithelium, but it requires an expensive instrument and a skilled operator. In addition, it is time-consuming and visible changes have not yet been correlated with deeper tissue changes. Biopsies give tissue evidence of adenosis, metaplasia, and dysplasia, but they increase the pain and cost of examination. The recommended examination should include visual inspection with accurate reporting of the findings, Pap smears from the cervix and from the four vaginal side walls, iodine staining with accurate recording of nonstaining areas, palpation of the entire vaginal canal and cervix. (Colposcopy can be done instead of iodine staining if the evaluation is done in a teaching center where the instrument and operator are available.) Tissue should be taken on the first visit only if a highly suspicious area is noted by palpation or colposcopy and a biopsy done on return visits if Pap smears or colposcopy indicate a suspicious area. At the present time, no specific treatment is recommended. There is a central registry for clear cell cancer, and many university centers maintain a registry of patients with DES exposure in order to obtain more information about the natural history of this disease, and to keep records of patients for notification purposes should further developments make this necessary.

GYNECOLOGY IN CHANGE

The actual diagnosis and treatment of gynecologic problems is most often carried out by a physician who specializes in this area.

Both the care of the pregnant woman and the handling of problems in the female reproductive system are currently assigned to the surgical subspecialty known as obstetrics and gynecology.

HISTORICAL PERSPECTIVES. Originally the care of the pregnant woman was not in the hands of the surgeon but rather the midwife, whose function was to assist at delivery. This position was generally occupied by women, and it was not until the 17th century that men became appreciably involved in the practice of obstetrics. During the 1600s English physicians in the Chamberlain family invented obstetrical forceps for live delivery of an infant who did not deliver spontaneously. Variations of their instruments are still used today.

Historically, both obstetrics and gynecology were included in surgery, which together with the basic science of anatomy, constituted an academic field in which one could earn the title of "professor." In the United States, during the first part of the 19th century obstetrics was divorced from the professional chair of surgery, but gynecology was much slower to be identified as a subspecialty. "Gynecologic" operations were performed throughout the 1800s in several countries, but they increased considerably in popularity with the introduction of asepsis and anesthesia. In the 1850s Dr. Sims became the first president of the American Gynecologic Society, and gynecology was firmly established as a distinct surgical subspecialty in 1889 by Howard Kelly. He founded the division of gynecology at the Johns Hopkins University, publishing *Operative Gynecology* and establishing a long-term program for the training of residents. Obstetrics and Gynecology as we know it has been in existence for approximately 85 years, but the specialty certification from the American Board of Obstetrics and Gynecology became available in 1930, just 30 years ago.[9]

Physicians entering this specialty, then, were predominantly surgical subspecialists whose interest in nonoperative problems grew slowly. The basic training remains oriented to teaching care of the acute surgical and medical problems related to the reproductive organs and portions of the urinary tract. Formal residency programs still require four years of medical school education, which is then followed by four years of specialty training with long hours, minimal pay, and moderate to poor supervision. There have been few opportunities to modify this training program since participants in anything less than the full program are still regarded as weaker individuals who cannot take the rigors of night call and operating room. The training period has now been extended by the establishment of subspecialty boards. An individual with a particular interest in genital cancer, female hormones, or high-risk pregnancy may take two additional years of fellowship in these areas.

There is still no formal requirement for training in human sexuality, psychosocial issues, or communication skills. Few programs offer the resident an opportunity to examine bioethical issues, discuss and decide the responsibilities of the physician both to patients and to self, or gain an understanding of psychosomatic problems. Yet the practitioner of obstetrics and gynecology is supposed to be an expert in all these areas, and is frequently called upon to make significant decisions on these issues in the care of patients.

TRADITIONAL ROLE OF GYNECOLOGY PATIENTS. The traditional role of the woman seeking obstetric and gynecologic care was determined both by society and the physician who provided that care. Many unverified suppositions about the female reproductive organs have been held throughout recorded history, such as the belief that certain behavior states in women were due to a wandering uterus or "hysteria." Some primitive myths about childbirth and menstrual periods persist in barely altered form in our present day such as pica, the custom of ice, clay, or starch eating during pregnancy and the familiar designation of menses as a sickness or curse.

Ignorance of bodily function was socially acceptable for women and culturally enforced during the 1800s. When Elizabeth Blackwell went to medical school in the 1840s there was great concern by school officials about the propriety of a lady's learning the requisite information about bodily organs and functions. Queen Victoria in England epitomized the ideal genteel lady who maintained a proper ignorance and disinterest in matters of sexuality and reproduction. This attitude was prevalent in the continental United States during the early 1900s when obstetrics and gynecology was emerging as a subspecialty, and existed into the mid 1900s when "well-bred" ladies and gentlemen publicly protested the sale of explicitly sexual books like *Lady Chatterley's Lover* and later *Tropic of Cancer*.

Socially acceptable roles for middle-class women during the late 1800s and early 1900s centered around the home and family unit. Women married early and depended on a husband to provide an income. There were few labor-saving devices and housekeeping demanded hard work and constant attention. This was a period of tremendous economic growth and geographic expansion during which children were regarded as a valuable resource. A woman submitted to the sexual demands of her husband and welcomed whatever children came of this union partly from a sense of duty and partly because the perinatal mortality rate was high and large families were welcome.

When a woman was acutely ill or pregnant, she sought care from a physician and literally placed herself in his hands. The physician's training encouraged him to assume the responsibility for patient care at all times, and always before his own personal needs, to be worthy of belonging to the "elite class of dedicated humans" called doctors.[10] This degree of self-sacrifice seldom allowed the patient any role other than that of passive recipient of the doctor's dearly bought medical skills. Since the physician was always available and certainly more knowledgeable about the reproductive organs, he saw no need for the patient to make decisions about her health care. He regarded himself as rightfully protecting her from unpleasant particulars about her body. Older ob-gyn textbooks offer ample documentation that the physician's orientation was not toward the patient's needs, but toward those of her husband to have a good wife, responsive sexual partner, and affectionate mother of his children.[11]

The physician covered his ignorance about certain female reproductive problems by several tactics. He dismissed a wide variety of complaints as psychosomatic and therefore not worthy of scientific investigation.[12] He made woman's sexuality totally dependent on her relationship with a man, in spite of lack of facts about the nature of the female sexual response.[13] Finally, like Dr. Edgar F. Berman, one of Senator Hubert H. Humphrey's advisors, in 1970 he believed that women could be unstable and unreliable due to periodic raging storms of female hormones.

MEDICAL AND SOCIAL CHANGES. Several things both in society and in medicine happened which changed the role women were willing to play as consumers of health care. First, a true sexual revolution occurred during which women were liberated from the position that enjoyment of sexuality was the exclusive domain of the male. The Kinsey Report in the 1950s gave facts about women's sexual behavior, and the work of Masters and Johnson in the 1960s and 1970s made the physical aspects of human sexual response a legitimate topic for scientific inquiry.

Second, woman's roles in the social order gradually changed. The coming of washing machines, vacuums, commercially canned foods, and ready-made garments vastly decreased the amount of time a woman needed to spend on domestic tasks. The participation of women in higher education and in the labor force exposed them to horizons beyond those of the home, and gave them the satisfaction of being paid for working. The decline in mortality rates of children of all ages decreased the pressure on a woman to have an enormous family, and the decline in maternal mortality and rise in life expectancy meant that more women survived childbirth and lived past the age when their children were dependent. These things contributed to woman's rejection of the stereotyped image of wife and mother and the pursuit of more meaningful ways to express generative and nurturing capabilities.

From the medical point of view, there were other significant changes. The development of the Pap smear in the 1940s by Papanicolaou and Trout made low-cost, relatively painless screening available for cervical cancer, one of the most common and deadly tumors that afflict women. The discovery and use of effective antimicrobial agents beginning also in the 1940s made effective medical treatment of gynecologic infections available. Additionally, understanding of egg production in the female and the synthesis in the 1950s of relatively safe, orally active steroids to control function, made contraception nearly 100 percent effective for the first time. These medical advances along with others have vastly improved our understanding of the human body and its functions.

The women's liberation movement in the late 1960s and early 1970s made many of the social changes more noticeable. It allowed women to identify their problems and express their needs as members of a large group rather than as individuals. Women became a visible, vocal consumer group, at first requesting, then demanding new services and attitudes from the health care system. Among these were the desire to have more knowledge and control over their bodies, particularly their reproductive functions. Women also wished to have health care maintenance as well as treatment during acute illness. The liberated woman wanted to be treated as an equal, intelligent adult by her physician, not subjected to patronizing, moralizing, or protective attitudes.[14]

PROBLEMS AND DIRECTIONS. These social and medical changes have resulted in problems when physicians have attempted to maintain traditional doctor–patient roles. One area of conflict is in physician attitudes toward women. The contemporary patient wishes to be treated with dignity and respect particularly by the gynecologist who examines her body in the most vulnerable of positions and deals with some of the most sensitive issues in her life—sexuality and reproduction.[15] The message that medical education gives at both a graduate and postgraduate level is still at variance with this point of view.[16]

Another problem relates to the control of reproduction functions. More patients today are requesting complete information about their reproductive functioning and unlimited access to contraception, abortion, and sterilization. They do not wish decisions in these areas to depend on their husbands, their doctors, or the government. Although such information is more readily available today, and most states no longer require the husband's consent for sterilization, control is not completely in the hands of the patient. Discussion of these areas is often cursory and the patient usually accepts what the doctor recommends rather than work out which benefits are most important and what risks she is willing to take. This is partially because the physician may be unwilling or unable to spend the time in a complete discussion and also because the patient may be unwilling to accept the responsibility of making the decision. Finances may also enter the picture, since government regulation of funds for dependent patients may affect the quality of care a woman can obtain and limit her options. For example, the current funding for abortions may change the availability of this procedure for low-income women. This could have profound medical and social implications if illegal abortions again flourish.

A third area in which patient expectations are not being met is in health care maintenance. A recent article indicates that of the specialists in ob-gyn graduating from 1955 to 1964, more than 50 percent treat common nonobstetric gynecologic disorders in their own patients and spend about 20 percent of their time providing that care.[17] Yet the residency training programs provide little instruction on diagnosing and treating common medical problems. The gynecologist in private practice makes the bulk of his income in delivering babies and performing operations and may thus resent the patient who occupies his time with problems unrelated to pregnancy or operative care.

Another time-consuming problem area is that of counseling. The patient with sexual maladjustment, chronic pain problems, or menopausal difficulties may require a great deal of physician time in the diagnosis and treatment. Not only is the physician's fund of knowledge in these areas lacking, but the time used in handling them is inordinate compared with the revenue generated. The physician may cover his ignorance and dislike of these patients by prescribing multiple medications, performing poorly indicated operations, or simply referring them elsewhere when he can no longer cope with them.

Finally, the tremendous advances made in our understanding of the causes of disease, the functioning of the human body, and the technology of scientific instruments have lead to the popular misconception that medicine is capable of defining and righting all bodily ills. The patient may have the conviction that medicine can and should be able to render a knowledgeable diagnosis and permanent cure for her every complaint, or she may expect a "magical" cure from medicine and surgery. These unrealistic expectations may cause her to go from physician to physician in her belief that previous ones were either ignorant or deliberately withholding appropriate therapy. The doctor may fall prey to this assumption as well, and fully believe that he is equipped with healing powers. In this guise he may resent the patient who questions his treatment or fails to respond to it.

SOLUTIONS. A variety of solutions to these problems have been proposed and tried. Patients themselves have formed self-help groups, in which a number of women get together to share their experiences, feelings, and knowledge of their bodies. This may involve vaginal examination using speculums and mirrors so the participants can see their own and others' genitalia. These groups fill a definite need that many contemporary women feel to explore their own feelings and bodies with other women who can understand and sympathize with the problems. Formal medical personnel are often rejected because they are seen as basically unsympathetic to the patient's desire to know about her body and to understand her feelings.

A related response has been the establishment of feminist women's health centers or clinics. These clinics are organized, administered, and staffed exclusively by and for women. They represent the liberated woman's challenge to the established health care system—that it either develop care responsive to her needs or she will care for herself and cease to need the system. Basic information about family planning, nutrition, sexuality, and cancer detection is usually provided. Prenatal education and childbirth classes may be held, and menstrual extractions and abortions by vacuum curettage may be done. As yet, these clinics are confined to the large urban centers, but their popularity may result in a wider distribution.

Another answer to the problem has been to train nonphysician paramedical people as "women's health care specialists." These women work under the close supervision of a physician who is available to check their findings and answer patient questions. These paramedical professionals largely take over the function of the maintenance of health by routine examination. They also participate in patient education, both by teaching classes and instructing individual patients.

The desired change in physician attitudes toward women has been and will be a more difficult one to achieve. The conviction that appropriate "masculine" and "feminine" behavior is determined biologically by hormones and not by culture is strong and persistent in our society,[18] in spite of evidence by several writers that cultural forces are the major factors.[19,20] The recruitment of more women physicians is only a partial answer since many women become "one of the boys" in order to survive the rigors of a surgical training program. Following that, they have very traditional attitudes toward their female patients similar to those of their male colleagues.

Our knowledge of the functions of the human reproductive system both in health and disease states is continually increasing. Medical and surgical care for women is currently better than at any other time in history. Our understanding of health care maintenance is improving and should result in more comprehensive and easily available preventive care. The social and medical changes that have taken place in the last 100 years are currently having a widespread impact on the practice of medicine. Attitudinal changes will be slow, but the force of women as consumers of health care will place continuing pressure on the system. What is now just an awakening to change will hopefully expand into deeper understanding, and ultimately more humanistic, patient-oriented medical services.

REFERENCES

1. Speroff L, Glass RH, Kase NG: Clinical gynecologic endocrinology and infertility, Baltimore, Williams & Wilkins, 1976.
2. Novak ER, Jones GS, Jones, HU: Novak's textbook of gynecology, Ninth edition. Baltimore, Williams & Wilkins, 1975.
3. Duncan CH, Taylor HC Jr: A psychosomatic study of pelvic congestion. American Journal of Obstetrics and Gynecology 64:1, 1952.
4. Gidro-Frank L, Gordon T, Taylor HC Jr: Pelvic pain and female identity: a survey of emotional factors in 40 patients. American Journal of Obstetrics and Gynecology 79:1184, 1960.
5. Castelnuovo-Tedesco P, Krout BM: Psychosomatic aspects of chronic pelvic pain. Psychological Medicine 1:109, 1970.
6. Romney SL, Gray MJ, Little AB, Merrill JA, Quilligan EJ, Stender R: Gynecology and obstetrics: the health care of women. New York, McGraw-Hill, 1975.
7. Novak ER, Woodruff JD: Novak's gynecologic and obstetric pathology. Philadelphia, WB Saunders, 1967.
8. Manber MM: Diethylstilbestrol. Medical World News. Aug. 23, 1976.
9. TeLinde R, Mattingly R: Operative gynecology, Philadelphia, JB Lippincott, 1970.
10. Telinde R, Mattingly R: Why more women are choosing careers in ob-gyn. Contemporary Ob/Gyn 3:21, 1976.
11. Heimbach DM: Letter regarding reduced surgical clerkships. Written to female medical student, University of Washington, circulated to all Department Chairmen in medical school, 1976.
12. Lennane KJ, Lennane RJ: Alleged psychogenic disorders in women—a possible manifestation of sexual prejudice. New England Journal of Medicine 288:288, 1973.
13. Wy ML: What's behind women's wrath toward gynecologists. Modern Medicine, October 14, 1974, p. 17.
14. Boston Women's Health Book Collective, ed: Our bodies ourselves, New York, Simon & Schuster, 1971.
15. Kaiser BL, Kaiser IH: The challenge of the women's movement to American gynecology. American Journal of Obstetrics and Gynecology 120:652–665, 1974.
16. Howell MC: What medical schools teach about women. New England Journal of Medicine 291:304–307, 1974.
17. Willson JR, Burkons DM: Obstetricians-gynecologists are primary physicians to women. American Journal Obstetrics and Gynecology 126:627, 1976.

18. Serban, G: *Psychopathology of human adaptation*, New York, Plenum Press, 1976.
19. Mead M: *Sex and temperament in three primitive societies*. New York, William Morrow, 1950.
20. Rosaldo MZ, Lamphere L (eds): *Woman, culture and society*. Stanford, Calif., Stanford University Press, 1974.

Chapter 15

Surgical Gynecology

Ann B. Barnes and Caroline B. Tinkham

The prospect of undergoing surgery is a particularly stressful moment in an individual's life. This is especially true when an operation involves the sexual and reproductive organs or when the question of malignancy arises. The basic responses of male and female are not fundamentally different. Moreover, the manner in which fear is expressed varies according to male–female role conditioning and the expectations of society. To be rendered unconscious and cut with knives is in itself a devastating idea and this anxiety is further exacerbated by the complete surrender of control which surgery implies.

In one regard, women do have an advantage over men since society has traditionally allowed them to express their emotions much more openly. Females have been given a kind of tacit permission to verbalize their feelings of fear, insecurity, grief, dependency, and anxiety. The implication is that less is expected of women in a crisis. At difficult moments they have been encouraged to lean on men and to draw their strength and support from them. At the same time, these attitudes have made it possible for women to be more in touch with their feelings and to be more comfortable with them than most men.

The patient must mobilize her defenses in order to meet the onslaught of surgery and to deal with the impact of a threatening diagnosis. With various techniques ranging from denial, to anger, to depression and finally to a degree of acceptance marked by fleeting moments of panic, each individual reacts in her own characteristic way.

The hospital environment with its unfamiliarity, strange ma-

Ann Barnes, M.D. and Caroline B. Tinkham, M.S.W. ● Vincent Memorial Hospital (Gynecology Service, The Massachusetts General Hospital); Harvard Medical School, Boston, Massachusetts 02114.

chines, and aura of depersonalization underscores the patient's feelings of helplessness. The medical setting accentuates one's perception of herself as a pawn on a chessboard. The microscopic examinations, the probing questions, and the uncomfortable diagnostic procedures all combine to increase anxiety. The patient, who is regressed because of illness and passivity, feels subjugated and at times overwhelmed by the authoritative physicians and nurses who suddenly take charge of her. In addition, many doctors readily admit that they are in a position to ask a question in such a way as to elicit the response they desire. Accordingly, the patient's sense of being manipulated sometimes becomes a reality.

Within the hospital itself patients may find themselves categorized as "good" or "bad" as determined by the caretakers. The "good" patient is controlled, relatively uncomplaining, cooperative, reasonably intelligent, personally clean, and with anxiety under control. "Bad" patients are unduly dependent, regressed, demanding, or hostile with free-floating anxiety. On the whole, patients tend to react to current stress in much the same way they have reacted to past crises and personal losses. Well-established patterns of behavior repeat themselves at such critical moments. The following is an example of an unusual situation in which this is so.

A sixty-eight year old retired missionary of the Pentecostal Church underwent pelvic exenteration for a Stage IV carcinoma of the cervix. She was left with a colostomy and an ileal bladder. She was wheeled to the operating room praying loudly and chanting, "Praise the Lord." During her lengthy hospitalization, the staff on the Gynecology Ward came to know her well. She continually pondered the "reasons" why she had developed cervical cancer and she related to the diagnosis, which had sexual connotations for her, with a strong sense of sin. She made a particular point of telling the ward social worker, who visited her regularly, that she had been celibate throughout a forty-year marriage to another Pentecostal minister. She said she married because she was "a delicate girl" and needed a man to help her do her religious work. "He has never touched me," she said with pride, "and I have lived like a nun with him." She could not understand how a woman, who had been so pure and had never had sexual relations or given birth to a child, could be stricken with extensive cancer of the reproductive organs. The patient put a tremendous emphasis on cleanliness and this made her colostomy and ileal bladder an even greater burden on her than it would be for most people. She hated the needles the doctors and nurses gave her, but she said they made her think of the nails which were driven through the hands and feet of Christ and she was able to endure her suffering better when she thought of it in this way.

Surgeons tend to be activists rather than empathetic listeners and many of them need to distance themselves from the patient's feelings and fears as a kind of protective insulation against the things they see every day. Some do not "hear" the patient and instead relate to a uterus or a breast or an appendix and not a human being in distress. At times one observes a kind of "cut and run" syndrome in some surgeon–patient relationships. There are also doctors with a tendency to react to their patient's problems in terms of their own personal and moral value systems.

Hotlines, handbooks, and the various women's liberation groups together with Planned Parenthood organizations are disseminating information about where and to whom a woman may go to obtain the kind of services she is seeking. Some hospitals and health facilities are providing patient advocates who serve as liason people between doctors, patients, and families to make sure that channels of communication are kept open and to resolve misunderstandings should they occur.

This has proved to be very helpful to patients who have little or no idea what their rights or entitlements are. Many such people are reluctant "to rock the boat" or to do or say anything controversial during their hospital experience.

As a result of this insecurity and combined with a kind of magical thinking, some patients feel it is necessary to play the game of "bargaining" with the physician. Such patients, who view their doctor as an omnipotent figure with the power of life and death in his or her hands, feel a need to placate this caretaker as a way of warding off imagined reprisals or rejection and also as a means of achieving their desired ends, that is, to be cured and not to be abandoned. Feelings of timidity in the presence of this powerful person often make patients reluctant to ask their doctors questions or to take too much of the physician's time. This failure in two-way communication can pose unnecessary problems and increase the patient's anxiety.

Hysterectomy for a fibroid uterus is a case in point. Fibroids (leiomyoma uteri) are noncancerous growths (tumor) of fibrous tissue and uterine muscle. In some instances, a pattern of inheritance has been demonstrated. Fibroids are a common uterine tumor. Many women have them and do not know it and live happily, having the family they desired. At menopause, the fibroid may become smaller. Birth control pills or menopausal estrogens may stimulate the growth of fibroids. If the fibroid grows near the lining of the uterus, distorting

206 ANN B. BARNES AND CAROLINE B. TINKHAM

blood vessels, it may increase menstrual flow or cause floods between menstrual periods. The fibroids may grow so large as to feel heavy or to put pressure on other organs, the rectum, bladder, ureter, back, or nerves, causing symptoms. Thus, a woman with a fibroid uterus may want or need a hysterectomy or the fibroid may be an incidental finding of no consequence. Alternately, it may be hard to differentiate a large fibroid uterus from a mass of similar size which is an ovarian cancer. Ovarian cancer, however, is rare and fibroids common. One lethal, the other only troublesome. Using just the diagnosis of fibroid uterus, the necessity of hysterectomy cannot be established and unfortunately the qualifying phrases which will appropriately indicate the need for hysterectomy are an area of controversy.[1] In Saskatchewan, the number of hysterectomies dropped as a result of discussion about possible unnecessary hysterectomies. Without any significant alterations of those diagnoses indicating the need for hysterectomies, the changes could be accounted for by changes in the definitions of the necessity for hysterectomy in women with fibroids.[2]

Another communications problem is presented by the abnormal Pap smear. No one dies from cervical dysplasia or carcinoma-in-situ, yet to call them premalignant and to do expensive time-consuming procedures appears justified to extricate the uterus that harbors such lesions.[3] Few women are quoted the risk of dying from hysterectomy when such a procedure is advocated for a disease which is not life threatening at the time.[4] In fact, most dysplasias disappear on their own. Only very few ever become a life-threatening invasive cancer, and the risk of the general anesthesia required for hysterectomy may be higher.

The patient, not the physician, may actively seek hysterectomy or other types of surgery in the mistaken belief that it will relieve her of her anxieties and may somehow ameliorate her life situation, or be the only sure escape from childbearing.

In the context of malignant disease of the uterus, tubes, ovaries, or in vaginal cancer, the patient is faced with the overwhelming threat which the diagnosis triggers. To be in touch with one's deeper feelings at a time like this is to confront one's own mortality. The most frightening kinds of fantasies about cancer and its causes may assail a patient.[5]

> Mrs. P. was a 52-year-old, separated mother of a 20-year old daughter. She was admitted to the hospital with advanced uterine cancer. She had ignored her progressing illness until heavy bleeding, nausea, and diarrhea had forced her to seek help. Talks with the ward social worker revealed the following:
> The patient had worked as a waitress and then as a restaurant cook prior to her marriage. She had always had a number of men friends. At the

age of 31 she had married a man twenty years her senior. Mrs. P. described him as "a good man, old fashioned and practical, not the glamour type." Her husband believed that women belonged in the home doing the domestic tasks and caring for the children. As a result, the patient gave up her job and became a full-time housewife and mother to their child born one year later. Things went along reasonably well for some time. Mrs. P. said she had security in her life but no excitement.

As her daughter progressed in school and spent more time with her own friends, the patient became increasingly aware of her own feelings of boredom and isolation. Her husband had continued his previous pattern of spending most of his time and energy at work. Mrs. P. felt neglected emotionally and she became restless.

She took a part-time job as a waitress and began going out with other men. Eventually, her husband found out about her activities. He never discussed it with her, but it was the end of their marriage. He made her leave the house and he retained custody of their daughter. After this, the patient lived alone.

Mrs. P. told the social worker that her actions which resulted in the breakup of her marriage and her home had been the single greatest mistake of her life. She always hoped that her husband would finally forgive her and allow her to return. She wondered whether her illness would make him change his mind.

Through a long and painful ordeal, Mrs. P almost never complained and assumed a stoical attitude bearing all her suffering with dignity and acceptance. Without ever using the word cancer she spoke of "the tumor which is eating my life away." It was as if she felt she deserved all this as a punishment for her sexual "acting out." She appeared to have adopted her husband's evaluation of her as a faithless wife and sinful woman and her great personal guilt expressed itself in a martyr-like resignation in the face of impending death. On an unconscious level, she saw her cancer was the expression of a judgment against her. Through the efforts of the doctor, the social worker and her daughter, a kind of reconciliation was finally effected between Mr. and Mrs. P. and she returned to her husband's home to live with him until her terminal hospital admission.

Perhaps this woman's fateful delay in seeking treatment for her disease when the symptoms first appeared was a reflection of her loneliness and her depression and her lack of interest in preserving her life.

STERILIZATION

There comes a time for many women when they know their potential for childbearing is no longer essential. For some, this is at age 25 with three children, for others it may be at 27 with none, or at 35 with one. For many women, such a time never comes. However, when a woman does know childbearing is no longer a necessity for her, she will often seek sterilization as the easiest form of contraception. Menopause may only be months away, but there is no reliable method for its prediction. Male vasectomy is a quick, effective, office procedure, costing half the price or less of a laparoscopic tubal division for a woman. Some husbands readily have a vasectomy much to the wife's relief or worry. Other men find vasectomy a threat and the woman bears total responsibility for family planning. For some women, even those with chronic illness, the wish to perpetuate themselves is important, and for them sterilization, wise as it may seem, will be unacceptable. Sterilizing the healthier partner in such a setting seems unduly limiting but many such partners will demonstrate their affection by undergoing permanent sterilization.

For those who have attained their desired family, sterilization of one partner is an increasingly common choice. There are many methods for sterilizing women today. At delivery, a small abdominal incision may be made and the Fallopian tubes divided. When carefully done so the two ends of the tubes are widely separated, the failure rate is less than 1 percent. However, if the tube is just knuckled or kinked-tied and the knuckle portion cut off (Pomeroy method), a 2 percent failure rate may occur. The sterilization may add one or two days to the postpartum stay. Occasionally, bleeding, infection, or anesthetic complications may occur but these are very rare.

At any time, tubal division may be accomplished by laparoscopy, minilaparotomy, or vaginal colpotomy: all one-day procedures. Sterilization will also be a by-product of hysterectomy for prolapsing uterus, bladder, or rectum as well as benign or malignant disease.

Since the mid 1970s, various silastic and plastic bands have been devised which would occlude the tube. Their advantage is that cautery is not needed. Cautery always has the small but significant risk of inadvertently damaging bowel or other abdominal structures, resulting in emergency major surgery. The disadvantage of these plastic rings and clips is that they hurt while going on and for several days thereafter. Furthermore, the natural history of the plastic is not known. Anyone who buys a plastic waste basket knows that they become brittle and fracture eventually. What would be worse than to find twenty years from now the same fate for these gadgets. At about 55 years of age after thinking one was sterile for the past 20–30 years, it would be more calamity than surprise to find tubal patency had returned!

Tubal division by cautery under local or, more usually, general anesthesia is at present the most common method of sterilization in the United States. Women of all ages request sterilization. In one report from a Northeastern urban center,[6] most were married with a mean of 5 pregnancies, 3.8 living children. Forty-six percent of the patients had a therapeutic abortion at the same time, reflecting the local referral pattern as well as the effect of abortion in helping women to focus on their needs. Nearly half of the women had learned about "band-aid" surgery (laparoscopic tubal division) from nonmedical sources. The others had heard about the procedure from doctors, nurses, or Planned Parenthood. The time elapsing between the moment when the patient had reached the decision to be sterilized until she undertook the procedure varied from weeks to years.

The patients' feelings afterward about their decision was not influenced by that time span. Most of the women followed in this report wished they had had the procedure sooner. About a fifth had been denied sterilization earlier because of their physician's religious convictions or because of arbitrary age or parity limits set by the physician. A few had only been offered operative procedures requiring many days away from home or work. The major reason most women gave for sterilization was "enough children." Some women underwent sterilization for socioeconomic reasons and were a bit angry that their economic situation rather than their perception of enough children was the dominant factor in their decision.

Even those 12 percent who had ambivalent feelings about sterilization said they still would have had the procedure if they had the choice again and would have even had it done earlier. For those few who felt regret, the major reason was of altered self-image, negative reaction of their partner, and concern about the health of an existing child.

Those with ambivalent feelings had more complaints of menstrual disorders, diminished sexual satisfaction, or found their partners unhappy. Nearly all the women felt their femininity had not been altered.

The decision for sterilization belongs to the individual. Medical personnel can offer information on general hazards or specific risks if concurrent disease exists. However, like abortion, medical personnel should be wary of asserting their own religious and moral beliefs and failing to consider their patient's views.

Untying tubes by cutting the sutured or cauterized sections and reanastomosing the tubes under optical magnification (microsurgery) has become popular amongst both gynecologists and urologists. To date, the overall success rate in terms of subsequent births for either men or women appears to be about 33 percent under optimal circumstances. As only good news is reported in such surgical endeavors, tubal surgery for sterilization on men or women should be presented as an irrevocable decision.

ABORTION

American women in the 1970s are confronted by a social milieu condoning small families and yet permitting broad sexual experience. Value systems further confound women's problems by contradictory assessment of what is considered good and bad. An effective surgical operation (abortion) in this era of cost-benefit determination is considered morally "bad" yet oral contraceptives are acceptable. The risk of death from oral contraceptives for certain groups of women far exceeds that of abortion.[7,8] Morbidity from thromboembolic disease, hypertension, and hepatomas is clearly increased. The balance of risk results from far more complicated interplay of social forces than a physician–patient interchange.[9]

The birth rate in the United States has fallen amongst all age cohorts of women except teenagers, where it is rising. These young women are the least prepared biologically or socially for pregnancy and childbearing and many, in fact, do not want a child. It is estimated that 10 percent of all women under twenty become pregnant each year. About two-thirds of the estimated 600,000 pregnancies are unintended.[10] Most studies show that women coming for abortion are not using effective contraception.[11] The number of motor vehicle accidents to young men, and the attendant deaths and medical expenses, are 100 percent unintended. These deaths and expenses continue to be borne by society with little discussion while federal and state authorities readily evade the cost of these young men's adolescent activities which result in pregnancy. That young women are confused about their role in society and how to be "responsible" is not surprising. Just like their male counterparts, they believe "it will never happen to me." The one getting killed by driving too fast, the other getting pregnant.

Many teenage patients who have come for abortion are in the second trimester of pregnancy and require the saline, prostaglandin, or late suction procedure. These young girls deny the early symptoms of pregnancy and are extremely reluctant to face their problem and confide in a parent or older friend who might be able to give them specific guidance and to steer them toward resources which the community has provided. Some of these girls say they felt that if they were careful not to think about the possibility of pregnancy or discuss it (face it), then somehow it might go away.

Fifteen-year-old Karen S. is illustrative of this kind of turmoil. Her father died several years ago and her mother was recently placed in a nursing home. Mrs. S. is suffering from a progressive neurological disease. Karen makes her home with her older brother, his wife, two nieces, and a three-month-old nephew to whom she feels very close. She is pregnant by her 18-year-old boyfriend who lives in another city. She cares for him but feels they have been drifting apart emotionally and she does not want to tell him of her pregnancy since he is still in school and in no position to marry. They have not used contraceptives and would not have known how to obtain them even if they had thought about it. Intercourse was unplanned and spontaneous after they had been dating for a number of months.

Karen admits to ambivalent feelings about her pregancy. She was depressed over her mother's illness, the breaking up of their home, and the separation which occurred when it became necessary for her mother to go to the nursing home. She loves children, and her nieces and nephew in particular. She has been active in helping care for them. They meet many of her maternal needs and perhaps have stimulated these needs as well. They may also be a kind of replacement for the major emotional losses she has experienced recently.

Karen described her delay in coming to the clinic to discuss the abortion issue. She told us that when she missed her first period she wondered momentarily whether she might be pregnant, but would not allow herself to dwell on it. She then missed her second period and again became suspicious but quickly denied the reality of what was happening. It was only after missing her third period that she faced the truth and contacted a women's health service. She was then referred to an abortion clinic where she was examined and found to be in the second trimester of pregnancy and a candidate for a saline abortion in a hospital. Karen realized she had mixed emotions and had made things more difficult for herself, but she said reality was so painful she could not face it any earlier and needed to take additional time in order to move.

Summing up her feelings about the abortion, Karen said, "If I really wanted to have this baby, nobody in the world could talk me out of it." She sees the abortion as being the most appropriate alternative for her. In her present social situation and with no husband and no money and at the age of 15 she feels she has very little to give a baby. The quality of the life she would be offering is a matter of great concern to her. She felt she could never go through with the pregnancy and then "give the baby away to strangers."

There is an unending effort by persons of some persuasions to prove the psychological damage abortion incurs. This issue is discussed in detail in this volume. The negative evidence of psychological damage is supported by Brewer who points out that the incidence of puerperal psychosis (around the time of delivery) is more frequent than postabortal psychosis.[12]

In the United States, it is estimated that between 250,000 and 300,000 married women each year have unwanted births. Thus, it is not surprising that abortion advocates continue to call for more facilities and easier access. Since the 1973 Supreme Court ruling, many facilities have emerged to provide safe abortions.

About half the abortions are performed in specialized clinics while 42% took place in hospitals. Of the nation's non-Catholic private hospitals, only

one in three reported even one abortion in 1975. Of the nation's public
hospitals, only 18% reported performing any abortions.[4]

The disparity in access is greatest in low-income women whose main
source of care is the public hospital. In 1976, it is estimated about one
in three pregnancies ended in induced abortions. In many industrialized countries, the ratio is one to one.

The danger of childbirth, the increased awareness of the hazards
of birth control pills and of the IUD make it unlikely the need for safe
abortions will diminish in the near future.

DIETHYLSTILBESTROL (DES) EXPOSURE IN UTERO

Diethylstilbestrol (DES) fell into disuse in most areas of the
United States when, clinically, it appeared not to be effective.[13,14] Two
articles clearly detailing its ineffectiveness were published in the late
1950s; yet its use continued in certain areas for nearly twenty years.
The efficacy of a drug or treatment was not required to be demonstrated by the manufacturer or distributor until Senator Kefauver
pushed such legislation through Congress in the mid-1960s.

In the last few years the risks of drugs like DES have been detailed.
Following the use of diethylstilbestrol, progesterone treatment was
advocated, then abandoned. This was followed by the use of alcohol
infusion for stopping premature labor. Each therapy was based on
limited animal experiments with extensive extrapolation to the human
situation. Each was found to be invalid and, in fact, harmful.

In 1968 and 1969, a cluster of seven cases of clear cell adenocarcinoma of the vagina and cervix in young women was reported.[15] The
tumor had previously been recognized in only one young patient at
that hospital. At the suggestion of one of the patient's mothers, an association with DES administration during pregnancy was considered,
and a careful epidemiologic study confirmed the association.[16]

Further studies revealed an even more common association with
physical deformity in the cervix and abnormal location of normal tissue in the vagina and cervix.[17] As evidence has been collected by a
registry and through government-funded cooperative projects across
the country, the cancer risk appears very small. Pregnancy, driving an
automobile, and smoking cigarettes are probably ten times as dangerous. Of the one to two million girls possibly exposed, around 300 have
had a clear cell adenocarcinoma. A few clear cell carcinomas of the cervix have sporadically occurred in the past, so not all the cases reported
have had documented association with DES exposure. Most of the
cancers have occurred in girls aged 14–24, one in a girl as young as
nine, and one woman was as old as 27.[18]

The noncancerous changes tend to appear after menstruation begins and slowly seem to undergo spontaneous healing and transformation into more normal-appearing upper vagina and cervix.[19] Investigators who were curious about the extent of DES effect on female reproductive organs asked enrollees in a research project to undergo x-ray studies of their uterus. Some structural changes were found in the uterus in association with extensive cervical changes.[20] Women have borne children with many abnormalities of the uterus, and so the significance of these findings is probably very limited, and, in fact, most women who suffered DES exposure have had the families that they wish to have and continue to do so.[21]

Medical uncertainty as to the natural history of DES exposure leads to speculation amongst physicians which is interpreted by the public and the press as an imminent threat. The anxiety generated by physicians wishing to learn the natural history by frequent observation has lead to a sustained state of worry, often unfounded, amongst the patients and their families. The following are two examples where anxiety led to medical contact but with poor psychological support and needless stress.

History I

M.S. is a 15½-year-old high school student. Her father is a pediatrician, and her mother cares for six other children, of whom she is the oldest. She was taken out of school for the day and brought seventy miles to a special clinic without any explanation from either parent. The parents enjoined the physician not to disclose the nature of their concern. However, it was pointed out that M.S. might misunderstand their intent and believe that they thought that she was fooling around, and that they were just trying to check up on her. It was also pointed out that she would need to undergo the examinations either as part of the research study or for her own benefit as she got older. Reluctantly, the family agreed to have the physician explain the situation to M.S.

Her first response was in fact that her family thought that she was sexually active. She eventually understood that they were upset and concerned. The findings were typical of many girls whose mothers had taken stilbestrol. Over the course of the next three years, M.S. came first at six-month intervals for one year and then yearly. Photographs revealed spontaneous healing. M.S. recognized that the physician was interested in her welfare as well as allaying her mother's apprehensions. She asked for birth control pills, comfortable that her request would not be transmitted beyond the examining doors. Her mother or father accompanied her to each visit, and the simple comment that, "Everything looks all right or is improving," made them feel relieved and greatly reassured.

History II

G.W. is a 22-year-old girl who was first seen in a Western city after her mother called her to tell her that she had taken DES and suggest that she had better have a checkup. G.W. was seen in the college infirmary. Since

reddish tissue in the upper part of the vagina was observed, she was referred to a local gynecologist. She was promptly admitted to the hospital
for removal of some of the tissue. No mention was made as to whether she
could enjoy sexual activities or what her fertility was. She was simply told
that she would be all right.

When she called for follow-up appointments, she was told that none
were available for the next twelve weeks. In desperation, she called her
mother, who made an appointment for her with a hometown gynecologist,
who took extensive photographs and put vinegar and an iodine solution
(which burned) in her vagina. After looking with great interest, he told her
that she probably ought to be seen in three months, and that he might
need to do some cauterization.

As G.W. thought she had had enough treatment to her vagina, she
was not seen by anyone for the next three years. Finally, afflicted by a
vaginal infection, she went to the hospital outpatient clinic, where her
vagina was recognized to be abnormal. She finally unburdened herself of
her concerns about her femininity and her fears about having children. She
admitted that contracting vaginal infections was part of her continued need
to reassure herself of her femininity and sexuality, and that, in fact, she
found little pleasure in the company of the many young men with whom
she associated. Her records and her mother's records were all collected over
the course of the next few months, and when she returned for an exam, she
was reassured that she most likely could have children just like any other
woman.

After talking with the same interviewers and nurses and seeing the
same physician over time, she slowly came to the realization that life might
not be over at any moment. She called several times to talk with the interviewers as personal crises arose.

Slowly, G.W.'s fear turned to anger. When she received a brochure
from a group of other DES-exposed girls, she eagerly sacrificed her meager
earnings to join in a class-action suit against the manufacturers of DES repeatedly asking, "Why is it they don't sue the doctors?"

G.W. now attends clinic regularly. This response of anger reflects the
reaction to her vulnerability which many women in these circumstances
feel.

REFERENCES

1. Rodgers J: Rush to surgery. *New York Times Magazine*, December 1975.
2. Dyck FJ et al: Effect of surveillance on the number of hysterectomies in the province
   of Saskatchewan. *New England Journal of Medicine 296*:1326–1328, 1977.
3. Barnes BA, Barnes AB: Evaluation of surgical therapy by cost-benefit analysis.
   Surgery 82:21–32, July 1977.
4. Bunker JP, McPherson, K, Henneman P: Elective hysterectomy, in *Costs, risks, and
   benefits of surgery*. Edited by Bunker JP, Barnes BA, Mosteller F. New York, Oxford
   Press, 1977.
5. Abrams RD: *Not alone with cancer*. Springfield, Illinois, Charles C Thomas, 1974.
6. Kopit S, Barnes AB: Patient's response to tubal division. *Journal of the American Medical Association 236*(4):2761–2763, December 13, 1976.
7. Bernal V, Kay CR: *Lancet 2*:8 October 1977.
8. Vessey MP, McPherson K, Johnson B: *Lancet 2*:8 October 1977.

9. Editorial, *Lancet 2*:727, 8 October 1977.
10. Planned births, the future of the family and the quality of American life. Position paper, June 1977, Alan Guttmacher Institute.
11. Barnes AB, Cohen, E, Stoeckle JD, McGuire MT: Therapeutic abortion medical and social sequels. *Annals of Internal Medicine 75*:881–886, 1971.
12. Brewer C: Incidence of post-abortion psychosis: a prospective study. *British Medical Journal 1:* 476, 1977.
13. Ferguson JH: Effect of stilbestrol on pregnancy compared to the effect of a placebo, *American Journal of Obstetrics and Gynecology 65:* 592–601, 1953.
14. Dieckmann WJ, Davis ME, Rynkiewicz LM, et al: Does the administration of diethylstilbestrol during pregnancy have therapeutic value? *American Journal of Obstetrics and Gynecology 66*:102, 1953.
15. Palumbo L Jr, Shingleton HM, Fishburne JI et al: Primary carcinoma of the vagina. *Southern Medical Journal 62*:1048–1053, 1969.
16. Herbst AL, Ulfelder H, Poskanzer D: Adenocarcinoma of the vagina: association of maternal stilbestrol therapy with tumor appearance in young women. *New England Journal of Medicine 284*(16):878–881, April 22, 1971.
17. Herbst AL, Kurman RJ, Scully RE, Poskanzer DC: Clear-cell adenocarcinoma of the genital tract in young females. *New England Journal of Medicine 287*:1259, 1972.
18. Herbst AL, Cole P, Colton T, Robbou S.J, Scully R: Age incidence and risk of DES-related adenocarcinoma of the vagina and cervix. *American Journal of Obstetrics and Gynecology 128*:43–50, 1977.
19. Burke L, Antonioli D, Knapp RC et al. Vaginal adenosis: correlation of colposcopic and pathologic findings. *Obstetrical Gynecology 44*:257–264, 1974.
20. Kaufman R, Binder G, Gray P Jr., Adam E: Upper genital tract changes associated with exposure in utero to diethylstilbestrol. *American Journal of Obstetrics and Gynecology 128*:51–59, 1977.
21. National Cooperative DES-Vaginal Adenosis Project. The DESAD project: a study of genital tract anomalies and cancer in female offspring exposed in utero to synthetic estrogens—design and preliminary observations. *Obstetrics and Gynecology 51*:453–458, 1978.

Chapter 16

Hysterectomy and Other Gynecological Surgeries: A Psychological View

Nancy C. A. Roeske

The theory which equates the presence and stability of the uterus with a woman's identity has its origins in antiquity. The Egyptians and the Greeks attributed emotional disturbance in women to the peregrinations of a disturbed womb. The Greek word for the uterus was *hystra*. An indication of the temporary importance of this word which symbolizes femininity is the use of the term hysteria. Hysteria describes a type of personality structure (usually attributed to women) characterized by emotional excitability, suggestability, dramatism, and narcissism.

Opposite Attitudes toward Hysterectomy

Ambivalent medical and social attitudes toward a woman's uterus and toward a hysterectomy are recorded in the literature of the past century. Opinions have varied between two extremes: one position equates the presence of the uterus with womanhood, motherhood, and sexuality, and another equates the uterus with intractable hysteria. Those individuals who espouse the first position state that, regardless of the justification for surgery (even though it may result in saving a woman's life), the fact remains that in the human market place, the hysterectomized woman is damaged goods, even if no evidence of the operation is apparent on the surface. Individuals who

Nancy C. A. Roeske, M.D. ● Professor, Director of Undergraduate Curriculum, Coordinator of Medical Education, Department of Psychiatry, Indiana University School of Medicine, Riley Hospital, Indianapolis, Indiana 46202.

maintain the other position and equate the uterus with intractable hysteria, which includes a wide variety of physical, emotional, and behavioral symptoms, recommend a hysterectomy as a potential cure for the hysteria.

Today, the emotionally charged controversy continues in spite of the reduction in surgical mortality, improved surgical technology, and new knowledge about endocrinology, physiology, and the female sexual response. The necessity of the uterus is perhaps a more controversial subject than ever before in American history. This situation seems to have occurred because of women's general heightened self-awareness and their questions about the rationale and the decisions of male surgeons who perform hysterectomies. Women patients and male physicians do not always have opposing opinions, however. A number of both women patients and male physicians share the attitude that, if a woman wishes to have either no children or no more children, a hysterectomy relieves her of a useless bleeding organ which may become cancerous. The contraceptive effectiveness of the procedure, as well as the act of removing a potential source of cancer, are regarded as an improvement in the quality of a woman's life. At the other extreme, some women and men think that American surgeons are doing too many hysterectomies, since more hysterectomies are done in the United States (700,000 per year) than in any other country in the world. This surgical procedure ranks second to tonsillectomy in frequency. The financial remuneration for the surgeon and the ease with which the physician may abuse insurance programs are cited as major variables influencing the large number of hysterectomies.

Extreme position statements tend, by definition, to disregard (or pay superficial attention to) the familial, educational, vocational, social, and cultural factors which influence the choice of the operation, as well as the complex nuances of meaning of the uterus and its function to the individual woman. The investigation of these factors, and of the effects of the operation on a woman's psychological adjustment, has not received the scientific scrutiny it merits. The majority of studies that have been done suffer from inadequate definitions of terms, confusing terminology, poor methodology, and a lack of meaningful statistical analyses. In spite of these liabilities, the studies do indicate that a woman's self-concept can be disrupted by this operation. However, women differ significantly, one from another, in their attitudes toward their uterus and their response to a hysterectomy, even when they are well informed about the surgery and its sequelae.

In general, the following factors are often cited as being potentially related to a woman's poor prognosis for mental health after hysterectomy: the woman's gender identity (the intimate sense of herself as a woman); previous adverse reactions to stress; previous depressive episodes as a reaction to anxiety and stressful situations; depression or other mental illness in her family of origin; a history of multiple physical complaints (especially chronic low back pain); numerous hospitalizations and surgeries; age at time of hysterectomy (less than 35 years); a wish for a child or more children; anticipation that the surgery will produce a loss of interest in and satisfaction from coitus; husband's or another significant person's negative attitude toward a woman's hysterectomy; marital dissatisfaction and instability; disapproving cultural and religious attitudes; and lack of vocational or avocational involvement. Research studies indicate that, if a woman experiences many of these internal and external factors, she is highly vulnerable to serious psychopathology between three months and three years postsurgery.

THE DEVELOPMENT OF GENITAL FUNCTION AND GENDER-ROLE IDENTITY

INFANCY AND CHILDHOOD. A cultural blueprint for a feminine gender role is set in motion with the appearance of the external genitalia at birth. The biological sexual identity is the crucial stimulus for the parents' behavior in anticipation of the baby's eventual gender role. The type and variety of experiences offered a girl in infancy and childhood depend upon the concept of her gender role by parents and the reinforcement of these attitudes and behaviors by the extended social environment. From the interaction of the girl's awareness of physical attributes and her gender-role experiences, she develops a gender identity which continues to evolve throughout her life.

The difference in appearance of the external sexual characteristics leads to significant differences in the evolution of a boy's and a girl's gender identity. The visibility of the penis and testes and the invisibility of the uterus and ovaries are important factors in the incorporation of the physical attributes into a core gender identity. The crucial nature of this core identity has been demonstrated in most attempts to change the gender role and identity of a child from female to male or vice versa after age three. John Money et al. have verified that the result is usually a seriously emotionally disturbed person.[1]

The boy can see and touch his genitals. He can watch and feel the sensations from their function. Thus he has many obvious experiences with his genitals which aid in his incorporating them into his gender identity. The integration of their appearance and function are repeatedly demonstrated and verified by him. In contrast, the young girl must be told about this important organ. She may have a picture drawn about her "insides" which include the place where "babies can grow." The secret hiddenness of the uterus, which she can neither see nor feel, stimulates fantasies about the appearance of her genitals. Fantasies about the uterus' function (a place where babies grow) are stimulated to an even greater extent by significant people in her environment. Furthermore, from the first mention of her role as a girl, her potential function as a mother is described. Thus girls are encouraged to focus on the function rather than on the appearance of their genitals.

MENSTRUATION. In contrast to boys' early and multiple experiences with their genitalia, a girl must wait many years for verification of the existence of her uterus. Menstruation is the first visible sign of the functioning uterus and corroborates its existence. Ambivalence about wanting to fulfill the baby-bearing function and the prerequisite sexual intercourse are expressed in descriptions of menstruation as "the plague" or "the mess." Yet menstruation is also equated with "monthly cleansing" and subsequent feelings of vigor, energy, and healthy normalcy. To the extent that the uterus is viewed by a girl as an excretory organ, the attitude toward the bladder and rectum may be part of the attitude toward uterine functioning. Menstruation may be used by an adolescent girl or a grown woman to regulate her sexual functioning, work schedule, and social life. To the extent that the uterus is viewed as a monthly clock or regulator of bodily functions, its irregularity or loss may disrupt other life patterns.

UTERUS AND GENDER IDENTITY. Women vary markedly in their dependency upon the presence and function of the uterus for an adequate self-concept. The degree to which a woman's self-concept depends upon the uterus is determined by two major factors: the regularity of her biological functioning, and her beliefs about children and about the relationship between sexual intercourse and the inherent possibility of pregnancy. Menstrual irregularities or pain can heighten the woman's focus on her menses and the uterus. It may be viewed as a burden or a less esteemed part of self. If a woman's parents or spouse perceive children as a sign of health, vigor, or wealth, then sexual intercourse may be considered pleasurable mainly or only if childbirth is a possibility. If, on the other hand, a woman's mother presented the model of fatigue and unhappiness because of the burden of children and of sexual intercourse, the woman may also incorporate this concept into her self-image.

HYSTERECTOMY AND GENDER IDENTITY. A woman's gender identity is usually not consciously reviewed by her unless there is a specific reason for questioning her sources of self-concept. The possibility or actuality of a hysterectomy can stimulate a woman, for the first time, to consciously formulate her attitudes toward her uterus and ovaries. She finds she has definite feelings and beliefs about their anatomy, their physiology, and the value of these particular organs in her life adjustment.

All women have feelings about the cessation of menstruation (if hysterectomy occurs premenopausally), childbearing, and the effects of a hysterectomy upon sexual functioning and general physical strength and health.[2-8] It seems logical that a premenopausal woman would mourn the sudden surgical cessation of menses regardless of the discomfort or disruption of her life which may have occurred because of the uterus. Furthermore, she may retain fantasies of the uterus and ovaries no matter how dysfunctional and diseased they might be. Yet, some women express relief at the removal of a uterus and adnexa which have shown evidence of anatomical pathology. Now there is actual proof of previous problems including infertility or pathological menses. These findings relieve the guilt for feelings of abnormality. Yet, even for a woman who has demonstrated organic pathology, the issue of a loss of gender identity is still present. The pathology may have served to heighten the awareness that the uterus and ovaries did exist, and even the distressing symptoms may be missed and mourned through dreams, fantasies, and sensations similar to those ascribed to a phantom limb.

A woman's dreams and fantasies can express the manifest and latent psychological meaning of the uterus and its functioning. The following dreams and fantasies are examples of various women's reactions to a hysterectomy: a myomatous (tumors of muscular tissue) uterus may be dreamt about as smooth and beautiful; disseminated endometriosis may be symbolized by the search for a lost and favored orange and red dress; a woman may dream of a car accident in which her face is scarred and made unattractive; she may hear an infant's cries and wake up at night with a desire to care for the baby; or she may dream of a sensation of abdominal distention and pregnancy. Women who comment about experiencing pregnancy or having more children in their dreams, as those who describe sensitivity to the distress of children whom they see, are most likely to be less than 40 years old and to have either desired more children or highly valued the maternal role.[9-12]

The woman who has the diagnosis of cancer of the cervix, uterus, or ovaries may experience the least difficulty in mourning the loss of the organs since they are now a bad or undesirable part of herself. Nevertheless, the confrontation with issues of life and death arouses thoughts and feelings regarding separation from family, occupation, and other meaningful aspects of a woman's life. Dreams and behavior will often indicate how the woman is coping with the threat to her life.[5,12]

In conclusion, most premenopausal women express some form of ambivalence about giving up a valued part of self. Women have difficulty in assigning negative connotations to the internal sex organs, and thus rationalizing their loss.

VARIABLES AFFECTING A WOMAN'S REACTION

VOCATIONAL AND AVOCATIONAL INVOLVEMENT. Prospective studies are needed to increase our understanding of women's feelings after a hysterectomy. However, depression symptoms in reaction to hysterectomy have been related to education, socioeconomic class, satisfaction with number of children, marital stability, and husband's attitude. In spite of the fact that the majority of women under age 50 are employed, data is needed about the relationship between employment and reactions to hysterectomy. It may be that negative reactions are alleviated by part-time or full-time employment, volunteer community involvement, and the personal satisfaction that comes from these activities. In a small (21 women) study by the author, it was found that 19 of the women felt better after the hysterectomy than before it. Eighteen of the women were married; all of the single women were employed. All of the women were in the middle and upper middle social-economic class. With four exceptions, the women had a hysterectomy between the ages of 40 and 50 and were operated on because of benign myomata and menorrhagia (excessive bleeding) and metrorrhagia (profuse bleeding between periods). (Two women were less than 40; two women were over 50). Eighteen of the women were employed full-time or part-time; the other three women were involved on a voluntary basis in community projects. The spontaneous expression of feeling "better than ever" and "glad to get it over with," as well as the relief from fear of pregnancy, enabled the woman to invest herself in, and find gratification from, her vocational and avocational interests. For these women, the uterus was no longer as highly valued as during their childbearing years. They had other sources for self-esteem which had, in the past, been sometimes limited by child care and by the internal sexual organs' pathology. Physiological reactions of fatigue, constipation, gastritis, hot flashes, and insomnia were common during the first six to twelve months postsurgery. However, their intensity varied and was not incapacitating. For most women, the exact length and characteristics of the mourning process are unclear. But meaningful involvement in vocational and avocational areas was mentioned as increased or improved, thereby probably modifying the mourning period.

SOCIOECONOMIC CLASS. Socioeconomic class has been reported as influencing a woman's thoughts about having a hysterectomy. For the purpose of contraception, educated and/or middle class women with children are more apt to request or agree to a hysterectomy than lower class or minority group (black and Mexican) women. Rodgers and D'Esopo point out that an active financially secure woman, who has completed her family, seeks a hysterectomy.[13,14] On the other hand, there is some evidence, according to Rodgers, that minority group women, who are evaluated in large municipal hospitals, are encouraged to have a hysterectomy without adequate evidence of pathology.[13] The former group of women are less likely than the latter to link the presence of the uterus with sexual function and general physical health. There is a direct correlation between socioeconomic class and the sense of relief from the negative, confining, and disruptive effects of pelvic pathology on a woman's life. Minority group women express more concern about the effect of surgery upon their general physical health and upon their marital relationship, the major bond of which was viewed as coital. The following statements cited by Williams by black women are examples of feelings about general health: "I don't want my womb out because it makes a person old, like a refrigerator with no heat to the body like a dead person. . . . I want nothing out because this might injure my body, making me sick all the time." Some examples of women's reporting their men's feelings include: "They (men) say a woman is no good—they keep reminding her, 'Well, you're no good . . . you can't have any more children'."[15] A woman's apprehension about losing her husband to other women can lead to postponing the hysterectomy, sometimes for six to eight years. This apprehension was most common in Mexican-American women.

Although the equating of the uterus' presence with an adequate sexual relationship is probably most common in certain ethnic and social class groups where concepts of a woman's "intactness" as a woman is related to the presence of her uterus, the concept of the uterus being important in maintaining sexual function is found in other women as well. It does exist in all socioeconomic classes, educational, and women's occupational groups. Some women verbalize a fear of losing sexual desire, responsiveness, or sexual attractiveness and the ability to gratify men. Anxiety about sexual appeal may be expressed by reaction formation in feeling "sexier" or "oversexed" after the hysterectomy. Women who express these feelings may comment that they cannot leave their husbands (men) alone. Therefore, they increase their seductive behavior toward men as one form of reassurance about their femininity.

If a woman has not married, or is divorced or widowed, she may have hoped to have a child to please her future husband. She may experience regret: "I had hoped to have a child from my second husband. He might want to have a son of his own and, if he did not, he might resent my child by my first husband." "There are certain things expected of a woman by a man. One of them is having a child for him." These statements reflect a woman's awareness of competition between men in producing children and, particularly, a man's need for a son as a symbol of masculinity.

INTIMATE PERSONAL RELATIONSHIPS. The reaction of a woman's husband or a significant other person to her hysterectomy is of paramount importance in the woman's psychological recovery from surgery. If a woman describes her significant man as distant, detached, denying concern for or interest in her feelings or thoughts, or he is of the opinion that she is less sexually attractive, she is more apt to be depressed than if he is emotionally supportive and understanding, and if he continues to find intercourse enjoyable, if not improved. Depression may occur even though the woman has many other valued aspects of her life (children, friends, and a profession). The effect of the hysterectomy upon a woman's intimate relationships is a critical factor for feelings of depression.

The husband's attitude and behavior toward his wife's hysterectomy requires further investigation. Most of the reports are anecdotes by women who state their own impressions about what they think a man will feel or do. In addition, there are a few anecdotal comments by male gynecologists, who report that men question whether having intercourse will feel different to them after a woman's hysterectomy. For some men, the uterus seems to symbolize their dependency upon the potential mother, or the power of creation and control over death through progeny. Presence of the uterus may also alleviate anxiety about coitus with a defeminized (homosexual) partner. The thought which emerges is one which implies that "if a woman does not have a womb, then she is really not a woman. Then, if she is not really a woman, what am I if I have intercourse with her?" The critical issue for some men is their own identity and its dependency upon a woman's uterus.

SURGERY AND AFTERMATH

PREOPERATIVE AND POSTOPERATIVE ANXIETY. Researchers agree that both high levels of anxiety and absence of manifest anxiety by a woman preoperatively are foreboding signs of a poor postoperative course and long-term recovery. Furthermore, a woman's behavior in the postoperative recovery room is characteristic of her typical coping patterns in a maximum stress situation and predicts the characteristics of her postoperative recovery.[7,16,17] For example, a woman who is normally controlled and who usually assumes the leadership role will become an ally of doctors and nurses, and she may direct them; a woman who uses illness to attract attention and extract sympathy may express more pain and a greater need for nursing care and general attention in the postoperative period.

PHYSIOLOGICAL SYMPTOMS. Postoperative experiences of physical weakness, increased fatigue and need for sleep, lack of appetite, excessive appetite, bowel irregularity, and inability to tolerate certain foods, have been cited as being psychosomatic in origin. The psychological origin of these almost universal symptoms is questionable. It is likely that, for most women, physical symptoms are present to some degree and reflect the normal physiological reactions to surgery and recovery from it.

PSYCHOLOGICAL SYMPTOMS. The most frequent psychopathological long-term reaction to the hysterectomy is severe depression. The depression represents the serious disruption of a woman's role and identity. It reflects a woman's inability to reintegrate herself through the mourning process and the inadequate reestablishment of significant relationships.

The potential for a serious psychological problem of readjustment occurs when malignancy of the reproductive system is found at the time of surgery. A malignancy of the reproductive system involves issues of coping with the possibility of death. Denial is difficult to maintain during chemotherapy or in a radiation treatment program. The question is then, "Why me?" The woman may believe she is to blame and is being punished for past guilt-laden activities (e.g., an abortion, extramarital relationships); conversely she may project the blame onto others (e.g., blaming her husband for stimulating the growth of cancer through intercourse, birth control pills, or pregnancy and childbirth). The issue for these women is one of survival. The fact that their reproductive organs may be the cause of their demise can uncover repressed ambivalence and anger about having been born a female rather than a male.

RELATIONSHIP BETWEEN SURGEON AND PATIENT. In view of every woman's reevaluation of her gender identity, it is interesting that no one has written about the significance of the relationship between men and women, and between gynecologists and their patients. The choice of a surgeon often depends upon referral from a trusted family physician, usually male, who vouches for the surgical competence and skill of the surgeon. In describing the qualities which they seek in surgeons, women invariably comment about the desirability of a surgeon whose behavior and attitudes reflect gentleness, kindness, thoughtfulness, understanding, and an ability to discuss details of the surgery and postsurgical reactions. Yet relatively few women (approximately one-third) seek a woman physician or surgeon, according to recent as well as older studies.[12,18] Furthermore, gynecological surgeons write about the importance of these qualities and about listening with the third ear.[19-21]

The reintegration of gender identity and the emotional relationship between the surgeon and patient can only be a matter of conjecture. Insofar as a woman is working through her feelings about the real and fantasized aspects of uterine functioning, the surgeon may be the object of flirtatious seductive behavior or excessive dependency. The latter behavior may represent regression, assumption of the stereotypic feminine passive role, and a reaction formation against anger toward the man in power who has taken away a valued part of a woman's identity. Through the former sexualized behavior, the woman seeks reassurance that she is still physically attractive; that the fantasized link between the uterus and sexual functioning does not really exist; and that she can still potentially control a man via fantasized or actual coitus. The effect of the woman's overt and covert behavior may stimulate and reinforce a complementary role in the male gynecologist.

The interaction between a woman patient and a woman surgeon has not been studied. The patient's sexualized behavior may be modified because of the possible threat of homosexual impulses. Her regression and dependency may imply a mother–daughter relationship. The potential for reworking her self-concept through identification with a woman, whose identity encompasses more than biologically based functions, is present. If the woman surgeon is married and has children, the possibility of offering a role model of a mature woman, who has integrated a many-faceted personality structure, is also present.

PSYCHOPATHOLOGIC RESPONSE TO HYSTERECTOMY

COMPARISON OF HYSTERECTOMY WITH OTHER SURGERIES. More posthysterectomy women than postcholecystectomy women require medication by their family practitioner for depression[30] or referral for psychiatric outpatient treatment.[4] The rate of depression in posthysterectomy women is reported to be 2.5 times that of postcholecystectomy women. But reports of the frequency of depression in these two groups varies markedly from seven percent[4] to 70 percent[30] in post-hysterectomy women; and from three percent to 30 percent of women with other surgeries (the majority of the last group had a cholecystectomy). Methodological limitations pose problems for comparisons and interpretation of studies. Nevertheless, the data supports the view that depression occurs at a higher rate for posthysterectomy women. Bragg has conducted the only large-scale study of psychiatrically hospitalized women, who had either a hysterectomy (1,601) or cholecystectomy (1,162). He concluded: "The rise of admission to a mental hospital following hysterectomy was greater than that following cholecystectomy, but not significantly so."[22] This risk was higher for the age group 30 to 39. There was no significant difference in the observed and expected number of admissions for psychosis for the hysterectomy and cholecystectomy groups. Diagnostic categories other than the psychoses account for the excess admissions observed in the hysterectomized group. The hysterectomy patient remains in the mental hospital on an average of almost five times as long as the mentally hospitalized patient who has had gall bladder surgery. Hysterectomized patients are likely to have a family history of mental hospitalization, whereas cholecystectomy patients are unlikely to have a family history of mental hospitalization.

The incidence of mental hospitalization or request for outpatient psychiatric care have been compared between women who have a hysterectomy versus a tubal ligation as a contraceptive procedure. Theoretically, women should be less emotionally disturbed by tubal ligation. The few studies, which have been reported, give equivocal results.[10,23-25] Definitive data to support this idea is not available.

Very few studies of hysterectomized women specify whether only the uterus was removed or the surgery included a salpingo-oophorectomy. Thus the psychological and physiological implications of the type of gynecological surgery await clarification.

A final complication in our knowledge and understanding of the relationship between psychopathology, psychiatric hospitalization, and hysterectomy is a woman's insistence upon surgery. The surgery may not be the direct cause of psychiatric care. It may instead be an indicator of the woman's decreasing ability to maintain her personality structure. For such a woman, psychiatric treatment would have occurred with or without surgery, although the surgery may hasten the woman's psychological decompensation.

DEPRESSION. Depression is the major reason for psychiatric treatment following a hysterectomy. The woman who experiences a pathological depression has been found to possess the following characteristics: special features in her personality structure,[2,17,26-28] the discovery of pelvic pathology at surgery, a history of reacting to previous stresses with depressive episodes which necessitated psychiatric intervention,[6,29,30] and current experiences of marital discord and disruption.[4,6]

Normally, the period of mourning over the loss of a valued object is abating in six to eight weeks, and the grief period is essentially completed within six months.[31] The physician's knowledge of the grieving process and an acceptance of a physical basis for the woman's depressive symptoms may account for the frequency of requests for psychiatric intervention between six months and three years after surgery.[4,6,24,27,32] Psychiatric hospitalizations have been attributed to a hysterectomy which occurred two to five years previously. There is an implied causal relationship in the histories of these women between the hysterectomy and increase in marital problems and psychiatric hospitalization.[33] Another consideration is the possibility that there is no significant relationship between the hysterectomy and the psychiatric hospitalization.[33] This surgery is only one of many surgeries and hospitalizations, which indicate the woman's inappropriate involvement with body sensations and functions.

Symptoms of depression include agitation, insomnia, crying spells, weakness, fatigue, lack of appetite, bowel irregularities, and lack of sexual interest and responsivity. Castelnuovo-Tedesco[26] has described extensively women with chronic pelvic pain or low back pain with no organic pathology. He reports these women to have the following characteristics: immaturity, alcoholism, and a childhood marked by maternal deprivation which resulted in feeling unwanted, isolated, and lonely. As adults, these women have difficulty establishing more than fleeting, casual relationships. Promiscuity is a prominent feature of heterosexual relationships. These women have even greater difficulty in forming relationships with other women. Chronically afraid of and preoccupied with thoughts of cancer and death, the symbolic expression of their separation anxiety, they long for closeness which eludes them. Their sexual and childbearing behavior is a defense mask which, when removed, reveals the basic oral dependency character structure. Lacking the fundamental early trust relationship and subsequent separation and individuation, they have assumed sex-stereotypic gender roles. Once deprived of the organs which both symbolize the role and give it authenticity, the women are a "shell," a term they frequently use to describe themselves. They have been diagnosed as having a hysterical, schizoid, or pseudoneurotic character structure.

SUMMARY

A hysterectomy does not produce significant psychopathology in a psychologically mature and healthy woman. Yet a mourning process does occur as a woman consciously and unconsciously reintegrates her gender identity. Organic pathology of sexual organs, a woman's age, socioeconomic class, marital or another significant relationship, presence of and satisfaction with children, and vocational and avocational involvement are variables affecting all women's reactions to a hysterectomy.

The unseen and untouchable position of the uterus and ovaries, which stimulate childhood fantasies about their appearance and the meaning of their function, are reawakened by the surgery. The function of the internal sexual organs is a valued part of a woman's gender role and identity. Society in turn supports and stimulates this identity. The meaning of menstruation, bearing children, and coitus are expressed in thoughts, feelings, verbalizations, and behavior. A woman's attitude toward, and decision to have, a hysterectomy is a critical issue to her and can be influenced by cultural and socioeconomic, as well as personal factors. Each woman's characteristic coping pattern in a personally threatening situation is apparent during her hospitalization and convalescent period. In the process of reorganizing her gender role and identity, other interests (vocational and avocational) and intimate interpersonal relationships will assume new significance. Intimate personal relationships are of paramount importance in determining whether the woman will experience feelings of depression and how she will handle them. The sex of the surgeon is not as important as is her or his attitude toward and explanations of the surgery and its sequelae. The gynecologist's attitude toward a woman's role will be reflected in the treatment plans, including decision about whether or not to do surgery, the type of surgery, and the surgeon's advice and behavior.

Emotional disturbance may occur when a woman has learned during childhood to equate the presence of the uterus, ovaries, and Fallopian tubes with her sense of self-worth. In a few women, sex-stereotypic role behavior may mask an underlying dependent character structure. The deficiencies in the early trust relationship and separation-individuation leave such women ill-equipped to cope with all major stress situations. Therefore, they will be likely to have had depressive episodes or other forms of serious emotional pathology subsequent to earlier stress experiences. The disruption of the marital or other significant heterosexual relationships may heighten the sense of rejection and abandonment. The woman may feel she is no longer a woman. The appearance of symptoms of depression is the most frequent reason for seeking psychiatric intervention between three months and three years after surgery.

References

1. Money J: *Man and Woman, Girl and Boy.* Johns Hopkins Press, 1973.
2. Amias AG: Sexual life after gynaecological operations-I. *British Medical Journal* 2:608–609, 1975.
3. Newton N, Baron E: Reactions to hysterectomy: fact or fiction? in *Primary care.* Philadelphia, WB Saunders, 1976, pp. 781–801.
4. Barker MG: Psychiatric illness after hysterectomy. *British Medical Journal* 2:91–95, 1968.
5. Drellich MG, Bieber I: The psychologic importance of the uterus and its functions. *Journal of Nervous and Mental Disease* 126:322–336, 1958.
6. Melody GF: Depressive reactions following hysterectomy. *American Journal of Obstetric and Gynecology* 83:410–413, 1962.
7. Menzer D, Morris T, Gates P, et al: Patterns of emotional recovery from hysterectomy. *Psychosomatic Medicine* 19:379–388, 1957.
8. Dennerstein L, Wood C, Burrows GD: Sexual response following hysterectomy and oophorectomy. *Obstetrics and Gynecology* 49:92–96, 1977.
9. Dorpat TL: Phantom sensations of internal organs. *Comprehensive Psychiatry* 12:27–35, 1971.
10. Hampton PT, Tarnasky WG: Hysterectomy and tubal ligation: a comparison of the psychological aftermath. *American Journal of Obstetrics and Gynecology* 119:949–952, 1974.
11. Rheingold JC: *The fear of being a woman.* New York, Grune & Stratton, 1964, pp 109–130.
12. Roeske NA: Unpublished data on 21 posthysterectomy women, 1975.
13. Rodgers J: Hysterectomies: a quandary for women. *Special Features, Los Angeles Times,* September 21, 1975.
14. D'Esopo DA: Hysterectomy when the uterus is grossly normal. *American Journal of Obstetrics and Gynecology* 83:113–122, 1962.
15. Williams NA: Cultural patterning of the feminine role. *Nursing Forum* 12:381–387, 1973.
16. Johnson JE, Leventhal H, Dabbs, JM Jr: Contribution of emotional and instrumental response processes in adaptation to surgery. *Journal of Personality and Social Psychology* 20:55–64, 1971.
17. Moore JT, Tolley DH: Depression following hysterectomy. *Psychosomatics* 17:86–89, 1976.
18. Haar E, Halitsky V, Stricker G: Factors related to the preference for a female gynecologist. *Medical Care* 13:782–790, 1975.
19. Good RS: After office hours. The third ear. Interviewing technics in obstetrics and gynecology. *Obstetrics and Gynecology* 40:760–762, 1972.
20. Marbach AH: Psychiatric problems in obstetrics and gynecology. *International Surgery* 48:524–532, 1967.
21. Mathis JL: Psychiatry and the obstetrician-gynecologist. *Medical Clinics of North America* 51:1735–1780, 1967.

22. Bragg RL: Risk of admission to mental hospital following hysterectomy or cholecystectomy. *American Journal of Public Health & Nations Health* 55:1403–1410, 1965.
23. Barglow P, Gunther MS, Johnson MA, et al: Hysterectomy and tubal ligation: a psychiatric comparison. *Obstetrics and Gynecology* 25:520–527, 1965.
24. Ellison RM: Psychiatric complications following sterilization of women. *Medical Journal of Australia* 2:625–628, 1964.
25. Meikle S, Brody H, Pysh F: An investigation into the psychological effects of hysterectomy. *Journal of Nervous and Mental Disease* 164:36–41, 1977.
26. Castelnuovo-Tedesco P, Krout BM: Psychosomatic aspects of chronic pelvic pain. *Psychiatry in Medicine* 1:109–126, 1970.
27. Henker FO: Female genital surgery and mental illness. *Southern Medical Journal* 57:746–749, 1964.
28. Youngs DD, Wise TN: Changing perspectives on elective hysterectomy. *Primary Care* 3(4):765–779, 1976.
29. Lindemann E: Observations on psychiatric sequelae to surgical operations in women. *American Journal of Psychiatry* 98:132–139, 1941–2.
30. Richards DH: A post-hysterectomy syndrome. *Lancet* 2:983–985, 1974.
31. Clayton P, Desmarais L, Winokur, G: A study of normal bereavement. *American Journal of Psychiatry* 125:64–74, 1968.
32. Hollender MH: A study of patients admitted to a psychiatric hospital after pelvic operations. *American Journal of Obstetrics and Gynecology* 79:498–503, 1960.
33. Patterson RM, Craig JB, Dinitz S, et al: Social and medical characteristics of hysterectomized and nonhysterectomized psychiatric patients. *Obstetrics and Gynecology* 15:209–216, 1960.

Chapter 17

Breast Disorders

SIGRID LEMLEIN TISHLER

Throughout the woman's life cycle, the breast occupies a unique role in both her physiology and psychology. Cultural and psychological forces combine to focus the woman's attention on this part of her anatomy. In addition, major physiologic evolution takes place in the normal breast during each phase of life. These changes further serve to underscore the significance of this organ at every stage. Thus, pathologic changes in the breast understandably evoke stress in the woman, and tax the emotional resources of the patient, family, and medical team alike. These stresses are most apt to occur in conjunction with those abnormal breast conditions commonly encountered in practice, and in which there is medical controversy regarding the options available to the informed patient.

ANATOMY AND PHYSIOLOGY OF THE BREAST

The breast is generally considered by the public and the medical profession alike as part of the reproductive system. Such notable texts as *Gray's Anatomy* describe the anatomy of the breast in the section on female genitalia. This is an accurate reflection of the physiologic role of the breast, but does not reflect the embryology of this organ. The mammary glands have most in common histologically with sweat glands, and are therefore most accurately considered specialized skin appendages. The primordia of mammary glands are identifiable in the sixth week of embryologic life, forming strips of special tissue called "milk lines" on both sides of the fetus from axilla to groin. Under usual conditions, only the areas closest to the axillae develop into

SIGRID LEMLEIN TISHLER, M.D. ● Assistant Professor of Medicine, Beth Israel Hospital, Harvard Medical School; Internist, Harvard Community Health Plan, Boston, Massachusetts 02215.

breasts. Primitive ducts are formed, and later, an area of pigmented skin appears to form areola and nipple. Complete absence of breasts, or presence of extra breasts, are extremely rare phenomena. Polythelia, the presence of extra nipples, is less rare, occurring in about 1 percent of the population. The accessory nipples generally can be found along the milk lines, and rarely have any clinical significance.

At birth, the normal breast consists mainly of ducts and is thus only partially developed. There may be secretion of so-called "witches' milk" from the nipples under the transplacental influence of maternal hormones. This disappears soon after birth, and true glandular development awaits the hormonal changes of puberty.

Breast development at puberty is a result of a complex interaction among several hormones. Although there is much evidence that the hypothalamus, pituitary, and ovaries all function in children prior to puberty, there is no clear agreement as to the precise hormonal mechanism that initiates the changes recognizable as pubescence. For example, prolactin levels in prepubertal boys and girls are about the same, suggesting that this hormone may have no immediate relationship to breast development at puberty. However, patterns of pituitary hormone secretion vary with sleep–wake behavior, and the entire hormonal axis is under current investigation for subtler differences than were previously appreciated. Breast development at puberty parallels the growth spurt, the maturation of genitalia, and the appearance of pubic hair. On the average, breast changes are the earliest sign of puberty, and the breast undergoes continuous modification over a period of about four years to reach adult configuration. The immediate biochemical antecedent of nipple and duct development seems to be a rise in estradiol secreted by the maturing ovary. Further rounding of the breast occurs as alveoli respond to menstrual cycles and secretion of progesterone by corpora lutea. In the absence of normal ovarian function, therapy with estrogen and progesterone results in development of breast tissue characteristic of puberty.

The adult female nonlactating breast is a protuberance from the anterior chest wall. The average weight is about two hundred grams. Asymmetry between right and left breasts is common, and may be so pronounced as to generate medical consultation. The nipple and areola are pigmented and richly innervated, containing muscle fibers which cause erection in response to stimulation. The breast is composed of glandular tissue arranged in lobes which are separated from each other by fibrous bands, some of which connect the fascia below to the skin above.

There is adipose tissue interspersed among the glands. Each lobe of glandular tissue leads into an individual lactiferous duct; about fifteen to twenty such ducts perforate the nipple. The glandular tissue is unevenly distributed in the breast, with more than half occurring in the outer quadrants. It is this inequality of distribution that accounts for the greater occurrence of tumors, benign and malignant, in the outer portions of the breast. Glandular tissue also extends superiorly out to the axillary fold, forming the tail of Spence. The glands, which develop after puberty, are composed of alveoli lined with secretory columnar epithelium. Proliferation of glandular epithelium and vascular engorgement are characteristic responses to elevated estrogen and progesterone levels in the latter part of the menstrual cycle, and during pregnancy. Bilateral breast pain, or mastodynia, may occur at these times. Although distressing, it is generally not a sign of serious disease, and can be expected to decrease with menses or delivery. Small doses of diuretics have been found to be useful in the week prior to menses for patients who experience pronounced engorgement and discomfort.

The cessation of ovarian function at menopause results ultimately in characteristic breast changes. There is marked regression of glandular tissue, and cyclic variation disappears. The breasts then consists mainly of fat, and on examination, no longer has the glandular or gritty texture of the premenopausal breast.

THE BREAST IN PREGNANCY

The most dramatic physiologic changes in the breast are those of pregnancy and lactation. Teleologically, this is the most important aspect of the life cycle of the breast, since the purpose of the structure in all mammals is the sustenance of the young. Cultural and social attitudes toward breasts emphasize their importance and attractiveness in women at every stage of life; the relationship between these social attitudes and the nutritive role of the breast in preservation of the species seems apparent.

By the second month of pregnancy, the breasts begin to enlarge, with growth of central lobules and development of new glandular tissue in the periphery. Estrogen stimulates proliferation of the ductal system, and progesterone induces alveolar growth. As pregnancy goes on, the connective tissue softens, engorged veins appear more visible on the surface, and striae—or stretch marks—may appear. The nipples and areolae become more deeply pigmented and erectile. In late pregnancy, there may be some oozing of colostrum, a forerunner of milk.

Maximal breast development takes place after delivery. In breasts prepared by the estrogen and progesterone activity of pregnancy, prolactin initiates and maintains lactation. On the third day postpartum, the breasts become hot and tense. This is not true inflammation, but marks the beginning of active milk secretion. Colostrum is exuded from the breast first. This is a watery, yellowish fluid, containing fat globules thought to be remnants of glandular epithelial cells. True milk secretion is well established by the fourth to sixth day postpartum. The regulation of lactation involves an extraordinary complex interaction among hormones. The stimulation of suckling leads to hypothalamic reflexes which result in the synthesis and release of regulatory polypeptides. These chemicals, among them prolactin releasing factor and prolactin inhibiting factor, control levels of prolactin which has a direct effect on breast tissue and is ultimately responsible for ejection of milk into the breast sinuses. Milk ejection is well-known to be sensitive to the emotional well-being of the nursing mother. The precise mechanism of the interaction between brain and endocrine tissue is only partially understood, and remains an area of intense interest and research.

Breast enlargement, or gynecomastia, and lactation, or galactorrhea, can each occur in women who are neither pregnant nor postpartum. These are abnormal conditions under such circumstances and require medical investigation. A frequent explanation is the use of a drug known to be associated with breast changes. The list of such drugs includes a number of commonly used antihypertensive medications, and a class of psychotropic agents called phenothiazines. Their mechanism of action involves a neurotransmitter, dopamine, which is in turn important in the regulation of the polypeptides prolactin releasing factor and prolactin inhibiting factor. Alpha-methyldopa (Aldomet), for example, inhibits dopamine and thereby reduces the secretion of prolactin inhibiting factor. This leads to an excess of prolactin and, in some cases, to gynecomastia and lactation. Galactorrhea can also occur as a symptom of pituitary dysfunction, often the result of a tumor. This is a rare condition, requiring special medical attention.

ABNORMALITIES OF THE BREAST

INFLAMMATORY DISEASE. Breast inflammation, or acute mastitis, is a fairly common condition most often associated with lactation. It is a bacterial infection which may be quite superficial and localized only to the skin, or may progress to deeper layers of the breast and require urgent medical care. The bacteria gain access to the normally sterile milk-producing glands through small cracks or fissures in the nipple and may evoke an intense inflammatory response. The patient becomes febrile as the breast becomes red, swollen, painful. Therapy consists of temporary cessation of nursing on the affected side, warm compresses, and antibiotics appropriate to the invading bacterial organism, usually staphylococcus or streptococcus. The inflammation generally resolves in a few days and nursing can resume. Rarely, surgical drainage of a deeper infection may be indicated.

Inflammation of the breast can occur in nonlactating women as well, but is much less common. Small abrasions in the skin are the route of entry for the bacteria. This diagnosis in nonlactating women must be made most carefully to avoid missing the occasional breast tumor which presents as an inflammatory mass. In both nursing and nonnursing women, the clinician must follow the infection to complete resolution. Any residual mass, following antibiotic therapy, deserves special attention and probable biopsy. An uncommon condition, fat necrosis, may occasionally present as an inflamed mass lesion, as may certain cancers, further underscoring the need for careful follow-up of apparently simple breast infections.

Fibrocystic Breast Disease. The most common abnormal breast condition is chronic cystic mastitis, or fibrocystic breast disease. This condition is so prevalent in premenopausal women as to be considered essentially normal by some authors. At the very least, careful definition of the syndrome is required if the diagnosis is to have any prognostic significance at all.

The frequently encountered granularity of premenopausal breasts, most common in the upper outer quadrants and often dramatically responsive to cyclic hormone variation, may best be called fibrocystic change, not fibrocystic disease. This condition occurs in over 30 percent of all women, tends to be familial, and generally disappears at menopause. It is often associated with premenstrual breast tenderness and fullness which regress after the menses. Intermittent diuretics may be helpful premenstrually.

True fibrocystic breast disease (FBD) is the presence of benign tumors in the breast. These may be cystic in nature and arise from glandular elements, or they may be solid fibroadenomas, containing connective tissue elements. True fibrocystic disease, especially with atypical ductal changes and marked dysplasia, is a predisposing lesion to breast cancer.

Women with "lumpy breasts" suffer from the physical and psychological burdens of repeated examinations, x-rays, and, often, excisional biopsies. There is no accurate way to evaluate the histology of a breast mass except by microscopic examination. For some patients with lumpy breasts, self-examination is extremely anxiety-provoking and may be virtually uninterpretable. An alternative is professional examination by nurse or physician at some regular interval, perhaps two or three times yearly. Persistent, enlarging, or solitary masses—so-called "dominant" masses—require further diagnostic study. Cystic masses may be aspirated. This is the withdrawal of fluid from the cyst with a fine needle and is virtually painless in skilled hands. The area of the cyst must then be reexamined at intervals to be certain that there is no residual mass. If there is any question of residual mass, biopsy of the area is indicated.

Patients frequently ask whether the presence of fibrocystic breast disease is a contraindication to the use of oral contraceptives. The use of female hormones has become increasingly widespread since the early 1960s. Oral contraceptives, consisting of diverse estrogens and progesterones in various combinations, have been used at some time by virtually all sexually active women under the age of thirty, and by a large percent of those currently between thirty and fifty. The physiologic effects of these steroids on breast tissue have been thoroughly studied, and can, in gross oversimplification, be summarized as promoting growth and hypertrophy of glandular and ductal elements. There has been longstanding concern that oral contraceptives might cause breast cancer, or activate a clinically dormant tumor. Multiple epidemiologic studies have shown no influence on the incidence or age distribution of breast cancer in the general oral-contraceptive-using population. In fact, there has emerged the curious statistic that there appears to be less fibrocystic breast disease among users than in a control population.[1] Although these data might reflect, in part, a bias in patient selection, their confirmation in long-term follow-up would be of great importance. Since fibrocystic disease is a risk factor for breast cancer, the incidence of malignancy might be favorably affected by a decline in incidence of fibrocystic disease. In addition, the benign condition is itself responsible for considerable morbidity as discussed above.

The story, however, is not so simple. Recent epidemiologic studies have shown that in the subpopulation of patients with fibrocystic breast disease who use oral contraceptives, there is a higher risk of breast cancer than in similar patients using no oral contraceptives.[2] Because of these data, still to be confirmed, current recommendations are the avoidance of birth control pills by patients with known fibrocystic disease, and the discontinuation of the pills by patients who develop the condition while taking them. In addition, women who have had breast cancer are advised to avoid hormones, except under very special circumstances. Some physicians advise avoidance of hormones by any woman with a high risk of developing breast cancer, because the hypertrophy of glandular tissue caused by estrogen may confuse the clinical examination and might result in either delayed detection or stimulation of a preexisting tumor.

In the postmenopausal population, use of estrogen replacement for treatment of hot flashes has apparently not resulted in any increased incidence of breast cancer.

Careful follow-up and clinical examination of the breasts should be part of any hormonal management program.

CANCER OF THE BREAST

Breast cancer is responsible for an enormous number of deaths, a tremendous amount of sickness and disability, and an overwhelming incidence of fear and anxiety in the American female population. About one woman in every fourteen will develop breast cancer some time in her life.[3] There are about 30,000 deaths per year in this country from this disease; this year, about 80,000 new cases will be discovered.[3] The overall survival rate for all patients with this disease is only about 55 percent at five years.[4] Despite the expenditure of untold amounts of research energy, the overall survival figures have changed very little over the past several decades. In this section, we will review the current understanding of the epidemiology of breast cancer, recommendations for screening and early detection, and several areas of therapeutics.

Attempts have been made over the years to define a population of women at high risk for developing breast cancer.[5] It would then be most rational to deploy medical resources among this population, aimed at early detection and treatment of the disease. The risk of cancer of the breast increases with age. Family history of the disease, especially of the bilateral form in multiple relatives at an early age, is a strong predisposing factor. Certain patterns of urinary hormone excretion correlate with risk. The often-cited protection of nursing is no longer thought valid, but is probably related to the age of the mother at the time of her first delivery. That is, the older a woman is at her first birth, the greater her risk of developing breast cancer at some time. The disease correlates with upper socioeconomic class and urban origin, and may be more prevalent in Jewish women. In some studies, the presence of fibrocystic disease, especially with marked dysplasia, is a strong risk factor. Early menopause appears protective. In summary, the hypothetical woman at greatest risk is over forty, nulliparous, well-educated, and comes from the city. She has severe fibrocystic disease, is still menstruating regularly, and has a family history which includes breast cancer in her mother and two aunts.

Why do we bother to study the epidemiology of this disease? Is there any evidence that early detection affects the outcome of therapy? Despite the gloomy statistic of the overall low survival rate in breast cancer, it is well-documented that women with small, early tumors which are totally confined to breast tissue have a much higher five-year survival rate, from 70 to 90 percent. It is also known that the best predictor of long-term survival is the presence or absence of metastases in the axillary lymph nodes. With negative nodes, the survival rate is well in excess of 70 percent, while with metastases in four or more nodes, that figure falls to 30 percent.[6] The likelihood of nodal metastases roughly correlates with the size of tumor. Therefore, it seems clear that the earliest, smallest lesions are the most likely to be cured, and the greatest impact on survival rates could be made by early detection and treatment.

Because it has been shown that early detection matters, and because we can identify a subpopulation of women at relatively high risk of developing breast cancer, current medical practice emphasizes mass screening programs for detection of the disease in susceptible populations. Screening may involve breast self-examination, regular physical exams by clinicians, and the use of thermography, xerography, or mammography as aids to diagnosis. Each of these modalities has a contribution to make, and the combination of several—physical exam plus mammography, for instance—is probably the best approach. It should be emphasized, however, that the yield of new cases of breast cancer per thousand women screened is very low, perhaps two or three at most.[7] The demand this makes on the medical system is so great as to require thoughtful deployment of resources among the populations at greatest risk, and in situations where the techniques have been proven useful. At present, most oncologists recommend self-examination once a month at the end of menses for all women over age 25, yearly or biannual exam by clinicians for all women over 25, and the yearly or biannual use of mammograms or xerograms only in women over the age of 50.[8] The routine use of mammograms in younger women is less useful, largely because the technique is not so accurate in hormonally active breasts. In addition, an increased survival rate in women screened for breast cancer has only been demonstrated in the over-fifty age group.[7] These are screening recommendations only; they are applicable to women with no complaints referable to the breasts. Clinical and x-ray techniques of examination are useful under other circumstances in women who present with lumps, pain, or other breast symptoms.

There exists some question as to the safety of breast x-rays. It is well-known that radiation can itself induce cancer, and it is possible that repeated exposure of susceptible women to the radiation of xerography or mammography may increase their risk. To date, there are no long-term data on this point, though the dose of radiation per study is very small, using modern equipment and special film. The current medical literature urges caution in the frequency of films and suggests the guidelines reviewed earlier for mass screening programs.

Most breast cancers are detected by the patient in the course of self-examination. It is critical that any breast lump be promptly examined and appropriately treated. Unfortunately, the fear of cancer, or of surgery, prevents many women from seeking medical help, and this delay may ultimately be costly. As the possibility increases for multiple approaches to treatment, and as women are given a greater role in the choice of therapy, perhaps the fear and the delay will decrease, resulting in improvement in survival. It should be emphasized that over 90 percent of all breast lumps biopsied turn out to be benign.

Whether suggested by the patient, by the doctor or nurse, or by a screening x-ray, the diagnosis of cancer is made with certainty only by tissue biopsy. Once confirmed, this diagnosis raises multiple questions concerning therapy and rehabilitation. The classical surgical approach to breast cancer has been the radical mastectomy—the removal of the breast, the muscle layer beneath, and the contents of the axilla. Over the years, this operation has evolved into a modified radical mastectomy in which the muscle layer, the pectoralis major, is left intact, with better cosmetic result. Recently, there has been undertaken a review of the success of each operation, and a comparison of these therapies with more limited surgical procedures.[9] Various approaches to surgical therapy are being investigated, ranging from radical mastectomy to such limited operative intervention as excisional biopsy, or "lumpectomy." Intermediate procedures, such as simple mastectomy, are also under study. The more limited surgical procedures are often combined with irradiation therapy in some form to gain long-term local control of the disease.

The success rate for the radical or modified radical mastectomy is well-known, and remains the standard against which all other types of management must be compared. Under certain clinical circumstances, the major operations have a limited success, and under these conditions, a more conservative surgical approach might prove as successful and more humane. The central question is whether limited surgery and radiotherapy can be considered adequate treatment for those early, well-localized tumors most often "cured" by radical surgery. The data on this point are uncertain, partly because of the difficulty in doing a controlled study of this type, and partly because the natural history of breast cancer requires a follow-up in excess of ten years.

Preliminary reports are encouraging, and suggest an important role for "lumpectomy" followed by radiation therapy as a primary treatment modality.[10] For patients with large tumors, or with very strong personal resistance to mastectomy, this combination can be offered with at least some rational belief in its success.

The traditional approach to the therapy of breast cancer has been radical surgery followed by postoperative irradiation of the chest wall and the nodal areas draining the breast, including the axillary, supraclavicular and internal mammary nodes. In the past decade, postoperative irradiation has been used less frequently, since its contribution to survival may be minimal. It is, however, an excellent tool in the management of local recurrence, and of certain distant metastases. It is still used postoperatively in selected cases where the likelihood of local recurrence is high.[11]

The use of radiation therapy as a primary treatment for breast cancer is a newer approach. This involves treatment of the breast, after surgical removal of all gross tumor, with high doses of external beam irradiation. Under some conditions, small needles containing radioactive material are implanted briefly into the tumorous area, thus delivering an even higher dose locally while sparing the rest of the body the effects of irradiation. With modern techniques, these procedures cause a minimum of discomfort and result in a cosmetically very acceptable breast. Minimal changes of induration and shrinkage of the treated breast are to be expected. Many women, especially the very young, prefer this treatment plan to radical surgery, and the preliminary data appear to justify its use in selected cases.[10]

For many years, recurrences of breast cancer have been treated with a vast array of hormonal and chemical therapies. Once the disease has recurred, it cannot be cured, although many treatments offer a good chance of comfortable survival for an indefinite period of time. The use of female hormones to suppress cancer in older women, and the removal of hormone function by oophorectomy, adrenalectomy, or hypophysectomy in premenopausal women are well-established, useful therapeutic maneuvers.[12] Their chance of inducing a remission is in the 30 to 40 percent range and, if successful, may provide one or two years of disease control. Recent studies demonstrating the presence of estrogen receptors on the surface of some tumor cells may increase the precision with which we may predict the likelihood of response of an individual patient to hormonal management.[13]

Many drugs have been developed to treat tumor recurrences in women whose disease fails to respond to hormones. Among these drugs are the alkylating agents (Cyclophosphamide, nitrogen mustard), antimetabolites (Methotrexate, Flurouracil), corticosteroids, and an assortment of others. Used in combinations, they offer great promise for remission of disease in about 50 percent of patients—providing about a year of disease control for those who respond.[14] The side effects of these drugs can be unpleasant and even dangerous. They should be used by physicians skilled in chemotherapy, and patients should be well-informed of their potential toxicity. For example, mouth ulcers, nausea, hair loss, fall in blood counts, and risk of infection generally result from chemotherapy. In well-trained hands, these risks can be managed with reasonable comfort and safety and do not outweigh the possible benefits of the drugs in most cases.

Review of survival data has revealed that women who die of breast cancer succumb not to local recurrence, but to metastatic spread to vital organs. Though apparently cured of disease, such patients must already have microscopic spread of the tumor at the time of primary management, whether surgical or radiotherapeutic. Based upon the concept of total cell kill derived from leukemia therapy, where cure by chemicals alone seems occasionally possible, an adjuvant role for chemotherapy in breast cancer is being defined. In brief, this is the preventive use of drugs in potentially cured women for about one year following primary therapy. Microscopic implants of tumor will, theoretically, be killed by the drugs at a time when the tumor burden is minimal. This may enable a greater number of women to enjoy permanent disease control than previously possible using a local approach only. Early data do suggest that in premenopausal patients fewer recurrences occur with this treatment than in control patients.[15] It is impossible at this time to determine whether long-term survival will be favorably influenced, because the follow-up time is currently well under five years. It is possible, although unlikely, that the immunologic suppression caused by these drugs could adversely affect long-term survival. The use of adjuvant chemotherapy represents an exciting potential advance, but must be considered strictly investigational until longer follow-up is available. The use of chemotherapy in patients with documented metastatic disease, however, is well-founded, and rests on theoretically very different grounds from the adjuvant use of chemotherapy in potentially already-cured patients.

REHABILITATION AFTER MASTECTOMY

In the previous section, great attention has been paid to the issue of long-term survival in breast cancer, and the success of various treatment programs related to the likelihood of survival at an arbitrary end point, five or ten years. An additional and equally important issue concerns the quality of life after therapy, and it is to this point that the next paragraphs will pertain.

Two obvious areas of concern in the rehabilitation of breast cancer patients are first, the immediate restoration of physical comfort and symmetry; and second, the long-term facilitation of psychological adjustment to the disease and to the outcome of therapy. Patients undergoing mastectomy have need for sympathetic, informed counseling in both areas. The mere choosing of a prosthesis, often simply ordered by the surgeon, takes on enormous significance to the patient. This act, of purchasing a substitute, synthetic breast, is one of the first confrontations experienced by the mastectomy patient. The loss can no longer be denied; the irrevocability of the amputation must be faced, dealt with, and integrated into a reasonable projection of future normal life. In many communities, the American Cancer Society's Reach to Recovery program may be available to counsel patients on the mechanical aspects of a prosthesis, to suggest exercises to improve the mobility of the arm, and most important of all, to provide patients the opportunity to meet other postmastectomy women. The advantages are obvious: many women feel that it is impossible for any doctor or nurse to understand their loss without having personally experienced a similar crisis. The Reach to Recovery volunteers, all of whom are postmastectomy patients themselves, can be of great help in anticipating questions patients may find difficult to ask their doctors and nurses, and can be a valuable resource to the family of the patient as well.

A certain degree of depression almost inevitably follows mastectomy. The patient has sustained a series of losses. The breast itself is gone, and with it, important pieces of a woman's self-image. Chief among these are previous assumptions about her health and her sexuality. Patients with breast cancer, whether they ultimately consent to mastectomy or not, often handle their fear of death by focusing exclusively on their feelings about the loss of their breast. They may be able to handle each of these issues more effectively if they can be helped to distinguish between them.

The role of the family is not to be minimized. A patient with breast cancer needs to feel that she has a future, and that her value to the particular elements of her emotional world is undiminished by the disease. One of the most sensitive problems is sexuality. Many women feel unattractive, unfeminine, and undesirable after breast surgery. In extreme cases, patients may be unable to undress before their mates, or even before a mirror. On another level, some women experience mastectomy as punishment for forbidden sexual fantasies or practices, and are thereby further sexually crippled. Self-help support groups may be useful for certain patients, but others will clearly need referral to professional counseling.

Occasionally, patients ask about cosmetic surgery after mastectomy. This has been tried in a variety of ways, using silicone implants, and attempting to preserve the nipple and areola at operation. When surgery is done for cancer, however, the goal is clearly to remove breast tissue as thoroughly as possible, and technical limitations often make the use of an implant inadvisable.

In this chapter, the normal anatomy and physiology of the breast have been reviewed. The complex physical and psychological processes of breast development have been emphasized as the background against which abnormal breast conditions must be understood. Multiple poorly defined factors, some endogenous and others probably environmental, may result in common abnormalities, such as inflammation, fibrocystic disease, and breast cancer. Future research will undoubtedly be concerned with better definition of these factors and clarification of their possible interaction with the continually changing normal breast. Pending eradication of breast cancer, major research efforts must be continued in the areas of early detection, and refinement of the approach to therapy and rehabilitation.

References

1. Ory H, Cole P, MacMahon B, et al: Oral contraceptives and reduced risk of benign breast diseases. *New England Journal of Medicine 294*:419, 1976.
2. Paffenbarger RS, Fasal E, Simmons ME, et al: Cancer risk as related to use of oral contraceptives during fertile years. *Cancer 39*:1887, 1977.
3. *National Vital Statistics*, U. S. Public Health Service, 1934–1971.
4. End Results Group, *National Cancer Institute: Survival Experience of Patients With Malignant Neoplasms*. Public Health Service Publication No. 789. U.S. Government Printing Office, Washington, 1960.
5. MacMahon B, Cole P, Brown J: Etiology of human breast cancer: a review. *Journal of the National Cancer Institute 50*:21,1973.
6. Fisher B, Slack N, Katrych D, et al.: Ten year follow-up results of patients with carcinoma of the breast in a cooperative clinical trial evaluating surgical adjuvant chemotherapy. *Surgery, Gynecology and Obstetrics 140*:528, 1975.
7. Shapiro S: Evidence on screening for breast cancer from a randomized trial. *Cancer 39*:2772, 1977.
8. Bailar JC: Screening for early breast cancer: pros and cons. *Cancer 39*:2783,1977.
9. Fisher B, Montague E, Redmond C, et al: Comparison of radical mastectomy with alternative treatments for primary breast cancer. *Cancer 39*:2827, 1977.
10. Levene MB, Harris JR, Hellman S: Treatment of carcinoma of the breast by radiation therapy. *Cancer 39*:2840, 1977.
11. Stjernswärd J: Adjuvant radiotherapy trials in breast cancer. *Cancer 39*:2846,1977.
12. Farrow JH: The management of metastatic breast cancer by hormone manipulation. *Bulletin of the New York Academy of Medicine 38*:151,1962.
13. McGuire WL, Pearson OH, Segaloff A: Predicting hormone responsiveness in

human breast cancer. In *Estrogen receptors in human breast cancer*. Edited by McGuire WL, Carbone PP, Vollmer EP. New York, Raven Press, 1975, pp 17–30.

14. Carbone PP, Bauer M, Band P, et al: Chemotherapy of disseminated breast cancer. *Cancer 39*:2916,1977.

15. Bonadonna G, Rossi A, Valagussa P, et al: The CMF program for operable breast cancer with positive axillary nodes. *Cancer 39*:2904,1977.

Chapter 18

A Psychological Consideration of Mastectomy

Malkah T. Notman

Breasts are important symbolically and realistically to both men and women. For a woman they represent an important component of her femininity, combining nutrient maternal potential with sexual attractiveness. Her capacity to nourish and to give is important not only in her actual functions as a nursing mother or in the role of a lover, but in creating the sense of worthwhileness and adequacy which underlies self-esteem.

Our society idealizes the breasts and their contribution to a woman's sexual desirability. Although changing styles of dress and standards of taste have affected the degree of visibility and emphasis on the breast, and the women's rights movement has criticized the focus on breasts alone, their central importance remains. Since breasts are not part of a child's body but grow in adolescence, their development symbolizes the girl's movement into adult womanhood. A girl growing up with small breasts still has to struggle with feelings of envy and, although an adult woman can learn to accept her body as it is, the adolescent with more prominent breasts is generally admired, and the breasts are integrated into her own image of her sexual attractiveness.[1] Other meanings of the breasts vary with the individual; for some women the prominence of their breasts as adults may make up for their fantasied anatomic inferiority when they were little girls comparing themselves to little boys. For other women an important meaning is the link to mother.

The significance of her breasts to a woman goes beyond realistic

Malkah T. Notman, M.D. • Psychiatrist, Beth Israel Hospital; Associate Clinical Professor of Psychiatry, Harvard Medical School, Boston, Massachusetts 02215.

considerations alone. One woman with the congenital absence of one breast made an excellent adaptation from many points of view, including marriage and successfully nursing two children with her one breast, yet she still felt a lingering sense of defectiveness which formed part of her adult personality. Psychotherapy was helpful in helping her see the source of these feelings. She also benefited from reconstructive surgery, which resulted in her feeling socially more comfortable and less conspicuous.

The symbolic importance of the breasts remains throughout life. One woman who at 48 consulted a physician with a small lump was told "your breasts are no longer functional" with the implication that she need not hesitate to have them removed. Needless to say, she was indignant.

Issues in Mastectomy

The impact of a mastectomy raises a number of issues: there are those relating to the confrontation with a life-threatening illness, those deriving from the loss of a body part, and the specific concerns related to the breast itself.

For the surgeon, the dominant aspect is usually the life-threatening illness. Appropriately, he/she is first concerned with the patient's survival, then with the morbidity associated with both the malignancy and the cure, and finally with the patient's physical and emotional response to the whole experience. Many physicians feel they protect the patient by not fully communicating this concern to her. There may be a discrepancy between what the physician knows and what he tells the patient and family, and therefore what the patient must deal with. There may also be a discrepancy between what the doctor thinks he/she is doing, namely helping the patient and treating the illness, and how the patient perceives this, which is both as a helpful procedure for her survival and cure, but also as an attack.

Even if family members are aware of the extent of illness they sometimes cannot confront the patient. Although this approach may be helpful to some people at some times, it can give rise to confusion and mistrust. The tendency to reassure and play down distress characterizes many aspects of the doctor–patient relationship. Although reassurance and cheerfulness are helpful, inappropriate reassurance may infantilize a patient who is then not best able to deal with reality. Some patients may prefer to have the surgeon take over their care, since his omnipotence in their eyes provides some control and protection against their fears and feelings of helplessness in the face of the serious illness. To some extent this wish is true of all patients who approach their physicians with trust and the expectation of being helped. However, false reassurance may create a conspiracy of avoidance and unreality. The patient can deal with feelings only indirectly or superficially and her total cure may suffer. This may also be regressive for her, encouraging dependency rather than eventual mastery of the experience.

RESPONSE OF THE PATIENT TO TRAUMA AND CRISIS

An individual's response to trauma and crisis is important in understanding her reactions to mastectomy. An emotional trauma may be defined as an experience in which a person is confronted with overwhelming stimuli, more than he or she can master, which may be disorganizing. In this case, the illness and then the surgery is perceived by a patient as a threat, as if an external event breaks the balance between internal ego adaptation and the environment.[5,6] Although consciously the patient recognizes the rational reason for the surgery, she may not be able to integrate the situation in the limited time which is available. A rare patient may externalize the illness, seeing her condition as brought on by the process of making the diagnosis or even by the physician, and become paranoid.

In any traumatic situation, although there are cultural and personality style differences, descriptions of stress reactions generally define three stages varying in intensity and duration:[4]

1. An anticipatory or threat phase in which a degree of anxiety facilitates perception of potentially dangerous situations so they can be avoided or met. Most people protect themselves with a combination of defenses which maintain an illusion of invulnerability, with enough reality perception to be able to act adaptively. Where potential stress may be planned, such as elective surgery, an individual can protect his/her integrity by strengthening those defenses and ward off feelings of helplessness.

2. An impact phase with varying degrees of reaction and disintegration.

3. A posttraumatic phase where emotional and behavioral control are gradually regained.

Most individuals perceive their own adaptive and maladaptive defenses and assess their reactions. A positive or negative view of how one has coped may effect not only this particular experience but future capacity to respond to stress as well. Janis,[4] in his study of surgical trauma patients, states that any threat which cannot be influenced by the individual's own behavior may be unconsciously perceived in the same way as childhood threats of parental punishment for bad behavior. This results in attempts to control anger and aggression to ensure that there is no provocation. Overt anger may be repressed, to appear later in nightmares, explosive outbursts, or displacement of anger which occur as the individual attempts to master the experience.

The individual who has suffered any traumatic experience tends to repeat aspects of the experience in an attempt at mastery. The repetition consists of talking about it, of reconstructing the circumstances, and of exploring alternate responses. In this process he/she takes an active role, the activity helping overcome the feelings of vulnerability related to the helplessness and passivity of the experience. To master a crisis, some emotional work is necessary. Without grief, mourning, some depression, some active consideration of the implications of the illness a resolution is not really possible. However, in an attempt to reduce discomfort, create an atmosphere of optimism, and encourage the patient to feel well, the hospital and staff may promote an environment which reduces for the patient the significance of what is happening to her. For instance, one 49-year-old woman became mildly depressed three days after surgery. She had some discomfort but no severe pain. She was given medication, quickly reassured that everything was going well, and at the same time chided for her upset. In looking back on this period she said, "It is hard to attend to what is happening when nothing seems to be happening."

Generally the model for medical care has been that of a passive patient, in this case a woman, and an active physician, generally a man. This repeats some aspects of the childhood situation in which an immature and less knowledgeable child is dependent on strong parents. Although there is considerable realistic basis for this in the relationship between patient and physician, there is generally little attempt made to develop participation by the patient where possible, on the model of a team in which both patient and doctor work together for the best care. Some women may wish to avoid this participation; however, the possibility of being more actively involved in their care is of particular importance to women with certain kinds of personality structures. A woman who relies strongly on maintaining control of her body and her life, whose self-image is one of a strong competent person, may find it especially helpful. A woman who is phobic or with a dependent personality may wish to turn the treatment over to the doctor.

FEARS OF LOSS AND MUTILATION

The acuteness of the situation has a considerable effect in the kind of trauma which a mastectomy represents. A sudden change from a state of apparent good health to one in which a major loss has occurred creates greater potential for disorganization. There are psychological advantages to allowing the patient adequate time between diagnosis and surgery, during which she can be prepared. When possible, adequate preparation of the patient and her family is critical. There are many misconceptions about cancer and mastectomy which may cause anxiety. Exploring the fears and fantasies of the patient and her family makes it possible to answer many questions and offers an opportunity to anticipate reactions. Many women feel taken in by their doctors because they were not informed of the nature of their illness or the consequences of the surgical procedure. There may be a gap between what the surgeon feels he has explained and what the patient, under conditions of great stress, hears and understands. The prestige and status of the doctor may also make her hesitate to raise questions. Here the family may be helpful. An intellectual understanding can be an important source of strength in helping a woman deal with this potential assault to her body and self.

Loss and the Grief Process. A major component of the reaction to mastectomy is a reaction to loss and the restitutive efforts made. Loss of the breast and of her bodily intactness must be dealt with, by grief and mourning, to some degree by every woman. However the loss touches on more profound and extensive concerns. The diagnosis of cancer creates a confrontation with one's own mortality. Fantasies of being immune, special, or omnipotent are destroyed. Women often say, "I never thought it would happen to me." Each individual brings her own past history and adaptive potential to this task of acknowledging mortality and losing a part of oneself. Some individuals have more internal resources for confronting difficult reality than others. The physician may be particularly helpful here by being open to questions and encouraging the expression of fears. Sometimes the physician's reluctance to confront these questions produces further denial by the patient, making it difficult for her to be realistic, and may then lead to depression. The reaction to the loss of a breast may also represent a response to earlier losses which have not been worked through. For instance, excessive grief at the loss of a breast may represent an unresolved reaction to the loss of a mother many years before. A severe reaction to the loss of a breast may really reflect the patient's concern about dying.

Loss as a Threat to Sexuality. The loss of sexual attractiveness is a concern of many women. This is generally assumed to be most prominent for younger women. Certainly younger women are anxious about the reaction of husbands and lovers. It is tremendously reassuring for a woman to feel that her partner is really not repulsed by her body and does not consider her disfigured or undesirable. However, this alone may not be enough to restore her self-esteem until her changed body image has been reintegrated. The significance of the loss to a particular individual is very important. For a woman whose self-definition rests on her attractiveness, it may be particularly meaningful to have support and reassurance about this from the people close to her. For such a woman the loss of the breast and the concern with attractiveness and desirability may be more critical than for a woman who has other sources of self-definition.

Older women may be just as concerned with their sexual desirability as younger women. A menopausal woman who is worried about the effects of aging on her physical attractiveness may be particularly vulnerable to the effects of a mastectomy which further intensify the feeling that she is losing her sexual identity. In the last few years, in the climate of increased acceptance and openness about sexuality, women have become more outspoken about their sexual feelings and needs. There has been a tendency to minimize the active sexual interest of older women, and to assume that they do not share the concerns of younger women. The physician's support for the legitimacy of these needs can help the woman through this stressful period.

MUTILATION. The feeling of being mutilated and damaged can result from minor body injury. Even the loss of a tooth can create a change in one's self-image. The loss of any body part revives childhood fears of being hurt and damaged and also fears of being abandoned because one is defective. The feeling of defectiveness is usually greater than the actual realistic change in the body. The sense of disfigurement from the loss of a breast may be considerable, even though the absence of the breast may be hidden under clothing. It is manifested in a variety of ways. One woman found her awareness of her ribs along the upper chest wall to be startling and repulsive. It concretized the missing breast.

The disfigurement from the lymphedema and the muscular limitations sometimes resulting from radical surgery, when this is performed, can result in intense feelings of awkwardness and cause social and occupational restriction, severely limiting rehabilitation. The embarrassment may be further restricting. It makes public the diagnosis of cancer and intensifies the feeling of defectiveness. Some depression is normal in response to this crisis. Women respond also with denial, displacement, fear, anger, anxiety, and even guilt, depending on their personality style and defenses available to them. For some women the denial may be helpful and keeps them from becoming depressed or feeling more helpless. For instance, one woman in her fifties had bilateral mastectomies for separate primary tumors. She spoke freely and publicly about this, taking the position that what mattered to her was being attractive when clothed. However, denial may break down, revealing deeper, more distressed feelings.

The removal of one breast leaves the woman with only one breast remaining, which is then regarded with ambivalence. Much may be made of the remaining breast. However the possibility of recurrence creates anxiety. The contrast with the mastectomy scar and the bodily asymmetry also may heighten feelings of disfigurement.[3]

LOSS AND RECONSTRUCTIVE SURGERY. Reconstructive surgery following simple mastectomy in suitable patients may create a positive emotional reaction.[2] It also conveys the physician's belief in her recovery since someone thinks it worthwhile to invest in reconstruction. Sometimes the possibility of reconstruction mobilizes the patient's awareness of the degree of her upset. One woman read about reconstructive breast surgery in a magazine article five months after her own mastectomy. She was then also considering preventive surgery in the other breast. When she saw the article she became furious at the surgeon for not having suggested reconstruction, and then realized that behind the anger at the surgeon was previously unexpressed anger at the whole experience—the cancer, the loss of the breast, and the disfigurement. She reproached the surgeon for not having helped her recreate her undamaged body.

There seem to be mixed medical attitudes about reconstruction even for suitable patients. Some physicians stress the patient's good fortune to be alive and convey to the patient some sense of the "frivolousness" of this wish, as if to imply that one must pay for survival by suffering. The patient may project her own anxiety and conflict onto the doctor and feel criticized and punished. Perhaps this also relates to the sexuality which is implicitly associated with the patient's wish to be whole and attractive, and this sexuality is viewed ambivalently.

FAMILY FACTORS IN THE RESPONSE TO MASTECTOMY

Family factors are extremely important in the reaction to mastectomy. The stability of a marriage, sexual reassurance, the capacity of family members to tolerate the truth, and the anxiety of uncertainty about the future are pivotal in the amount of support the patient has in regaining her emotional balance.[5] The capacity to offer support of course varies with the personal experience of each individual member as well as the family pattern of response to crises and loss. The role of the ill member in the family will also determine the reaction of the other family members. For instance, a woman who is the stabilizing and most dependable member of a family described her husband's decline from a chronic disease as originating at the time she had a mastectomy. Physical absence of the mother in a family and her depression, if it is significantly long or severe, are major life crises for young children, accentuated if there is no other family member able to be supportive. The physician may need to assess the family situation, its resources and vulnerabilities, in planning for the rehabilitation of the patient. Preparation of the family means making decisions about what to tell them, including what to tell young children. A husband's anxiety as to how to treat his wife and his own conflicting feelings may lead to his withdrawal which she interprets as rejection.

One woman described contrasting reactions in two daughters, both in their twenties. One was flat chested. In her adolescence she had fantasied large breasts but had come to terms with her body. She was able to talk realistically with her mother following the surgery, to look at the scars, and offer reassurance by her acceptance. The other, for whom her own fullbreasted figure was a source of great pride, found it difficult to acknowledge what had happened to her mother, and perhaps to deal with the competitive feelings aroused by this as well. She could not face this unthinkable possibility, avoided talking about the illness, and also withdrew from her mother, depriving her of a potential source of support.

In rehabilitation of the postmastectomy patient, the family may thus help or hinder in her acceptance of the loss of the breast and in her reintegration of her self-image as that of a person whose body has changed but who feels worthy of love. The family as well as the patient must face the possibility of a recurrence. To do this and keep a balance between reality and optimism may be difficult.[3] Sometimes help for a family member should be considered.

Discrimination against cancer patients socially or in the job market provides a barrier to successful rehabilitation. Hiding the illness may lead to guilt, anxiety, depression or further reinforce denial. The follow-up visits can confront the patient with the reality of the illness which she encounters nowhere else. She may overreact to innocuous procedures because of residual feelings from the initial surgery. Sometimes the reactions are displaced into other settings. Agitation may be expressed in other groups at work or at home. A woman may find herself irritable and diffuse with children.

In summary, mastectomy constitutes a potential major life crisis for a woman and her family. In any case the patient must deal with losses, changes in her body image, anxieties about the future, her own femininity, and her relationships with people. In helping her, the physician should be able to understand the significance of the loss of the breast to this particular woman and assess her capacity to handle stress. He should also be aware of the resources available to her from family and community. Preparation, encouragement of questions, and participation of the woman in her care where possible are helpful. The patient needs help in facing the reality of the illness and also in planning. For some people, despite the stress and losses, there is still something positive to be gained from the experience, from confrontation with feelings, the changes in relationships, which sometimes become closer, and the mastery of a major life experience.

REFERENCES

1. Asken MJ: Psychoemotional aspects of mastectomy: a review of recent literature. *American Journal of Psychiatry* 132:56–59, 1975.
2. Gifford S: Emotional attitudes toward cosmetic breast surgery: loss and restitution of the 'ideal self,' in *Plastic and reconstructive surgery of the breast*. Edited by Goldwyn RM. Boston, Little, Brown, 1976, pp 103–122.
3. Healey JE, Jr: Role of the rehabilitation medicine in the care of the patient with breast cancer. *Cancer* 28:1666–1671, 1971.
4. Janis I: *Psychological stress*. New York, John Wiley & Sons, 1958.
5. Klein R: A crisis to grow on. *Cancer* 28:1660, 1971.
6. Notman M, Nadelson C: The rape victim: psychodynamic considerations. *American Journal of Psychiatry* 133(4):408–413, 1976.

Chapter 19

The "Difficult" Patient: Observations on the Staff– Patient Interaction

Eileen B. Kahan and Elizabeth B. Gaskill

Breast cancer is the most common form of cancer in women in the United States. It is the leading cause of death among women age 40–44 and 6 percent or 1 out of 17 women are expected to develop breast cancer at some time in their lives.[1] These facts have resulted in a significant effort in the scientific community to treat this disease effectively, both physically and emotionally.

In this chapter we describe our observations concerning the emotional impact of breast cancer on a group of women who illustrate a range of responses to their disease. In addition, they illustrate an often overlooked aspect of medical care: the interaction between patients and those caring for them.[2] What characterizes this group is that they are viewed as "difficult" management problems by their caretakers.

The "Difficult" Patient

One of our observations has been that those patients who are considered "difficult" are likely to reflect difficulties in the staff–patient interaction. By "difficult" we mean the label often applied by medical staff to patients who ask many questions, repeatedly, requesting explanations that take up more time than the staff is accustomed to giv-

Eileen B. Kahan, M.D. • Department of Psychiatry, Peter Bent Brigham Hospital; Harvard Medical School, Boston, Massachusetts. Currently engaged in private practice of psychiatry, 44 Hancock Street, Lexington, Massachusetts 02173. Elizabeth B. Gaskill, M.S.W. • Department of Social Service, Peter Bent Brigham Hospital, Boston, Massachusetts 02115.

ing. This may be an indication that the patient is having difficulty coping with the illness as well as possessing a generally noncompliant style. However, often the staff person feels his/her competence is being questioned. This may produce considerable discomfort (i.e., anxiety) in the staff, who may then, out of anger at feeling anxious, respond by labeling the patient as "difficult." This "difficult" patient is often more readily referred to the psychiatrist or social worker.

Review of the Literature

We shall present, briefly, the contributions of some investigators whose work has clinical relevance in describing and understanding the range of emotional reactions seen in women with breast cancer and those close to them.

The treatment of breast cancer depends on its stage. In simplified terms, early stage disease is localized to the breast and later stage disease extends to other parts of the body. Early stage disease can be treated by mastectomy of various types and radiotherapy. Treatment of later stage disease often involves chemotherapy, adrenalectomy, and oophorectomy to control the body's hormonal milieu. Thus, the literature examining the psychological effects of surgical removal of breasts, ovaries, and adrenal glands are useful today.

An early study in 1941 by Lindemann[3] reveals that women undergoing pelvic operations had a higher frequency of postoperative psychiatric sequelae (i.e. restlessness, sleeplessness, agitation, and preoccupation with depressive thought content) when compared to women undergoing removal of the gall bladder. In 1960, Hollender[4] found that of women admitted to psychiatric hospitals following surgical operations, the group admitted following pelvic operation was almost twice as large as the group admitted for operations of all other types. These studies seem to address an underlying question which is still being asked, "Does removal of a woman's sexual organ result in emotional sequelae?" The validity of scientific, psychological research directed at this issue is beyond the scope of this chapter. However, it should be noted that this is a currently debated issue. Though there are methodological problems with much psychological research, we answer this question affirmatively for many women, fully recognizing that increasingly sophisticated methods for measurement are yet required.

Others who have built on this early work have attempted to examine several related areas: the emotional impact of having cancer of any type,[5,6] the impact of mastectomy and/or breast cancer specifically,[7-10] the sexual sequelae of breast cancer surgery, [11-15] and the sexual sequelae of pelvic surgery.[16-21] To date, there are no long-term descriptive studies detailing the natural history of the emotional impact of breast cancer. Nor are there any controlled outcome studies regarding the effectiveness of psychological intervention with this population.

We shall review some of the clinical impressions discussed in the literature, keeping in mind that one usually observes a shifting pattern of reactions to a life stress [5,22] in an attempt to master it.[15]

Hearing that one has a diagnosed cancer has been likened to "a heavy blow on the head. . . . The person characteristically feels stunned or dazed."[5] Despite vast improvements in treatment, the word cancer still connotes a death sentence[7] "and in one sudden moment, we learn we are really mortal, after all."[10] Other fears emerge, in addition to death anxiety, such as fear of physical pain, body mutilation, and changes in social and family structure. In fact, some patients reveal that they "could handle the progression of their disease, but they could not handle the pain as a constant reminder that death was inevitable."[23]

Denial and avoidance are often the first line of defense in response to this anxiety. Use of these defenses has been particularly studied because they may result in delay in seeking treatment.[6,8,21,24,25]

When a person can no longer deny or avoid the existence of the cancer, other feelings may be experienced:

> intense anxiety and fear, shame and guilt, rage, despair, helplessness and/or hopelessness, and feelings of giving up or having given up. The victim feels helpless in a world not of his own making. One may feel shame or guilt about some current or past event seeing the traumatic loss as a punishment for real or imagined "crimes." All traumas instill the feeling of something being lost—not only the possibility of life itself, but also power and control over one's destiny.[11]

In this context, it is of more than historical interest to note that mastectomy is mentioned in the Code of Hammurabi as a form of actual punishment.[26]

Given this panoply of emotions, the in-hospital experience may reinforce feelings of helplessness and dependency. Caretakers, particularly physicians, may then be imbued with the traits of omniscience and omnipotence which the patient perceives as lacking in himself/herself.[6] Others who need to maintain a strong sense of independence may have difficulty in asking for assistance at all when it may be very necessary[23] out of fear of acknowledging any dependency needs.

Emotional reactions to loss of specific organs, such as breast, ovaries, and uterus have been described because of their special meanings. "Any organ with special symbolic meaning becomes more highly prized and more catastrophically injured by cancer."[11] For many the breast represents at least a dual nature—symbolizing motherhood and nurturing functions as well as female sexuality.[7,8] Other studies have revealed that to many women the "removal of the uterus and ovaries meant the end of all sexual life at least in a feeling way."[4] Others cited

> concern for loss of childbearing ability . . . regret that menstruation would cease. It was seen as a valued and necessary function for the maintenance of health and well-being . . . some expressed fear of losing their sexual desire, fear that they would be unable to respond to their partner, fear of the loss of sexual attractiveness . . . fear that their partners might not receive satisfaction from them because the operation had damaged their sexual equipment. Some even thought they would not be able to carry out their everyday activities at home or at work . . .[21]

When one's body is altered, one loses a sense of intactness.[19] It is as though one's relationship with one's self is altered and that affects interpersonal relationships. There is widespread acknowledgment, then, that the loss or change of a body part in one sexual partner affects the other partner.[7-10,12,13,17,27-29] Perhaps emanating from the notion that fantasied fears are worse than the reality of mastectomy, some suggest confrontation by the sexual partner of the operative site[9,13] in the hope that early acceptance of this reality will lead to early resumption of usual sexual activity. It has been pointed out that "successful sexual functioning in this group can provide an important means of tension reduction at a time when it is most useful and necessary."[19] "Sexual success . . . is particularly reassuring . . . that with its defects, the body can give both pleasure and a sense of mastery."[17]

One study has demonstrated that patients usually will not raise the issue of sexual concerns until the physician does.[20] Thus, a discussion of the patient's sexual concerns should be part of standard care. This will provide an opportunity to educate the woman and her partner as to normal anatomy and physiology, and what changes will and will not occur as a result of treatment. Instituting this dialogue invites questioning by the patient and her partner with the further chance of dispelling personal misconceptions.[16]

Recently, women who have experienced being treated for breast cancer have added a dimension to our understanding with their firsthand reports.[30,31] They clearly describe the emotional impact of the process of diagnosis and treatment and their personal attempts at their mastery of this stress. They demonstrate the necessity for the patient's exercising some control in the decision-making process regarding treatment modalities. It was through personal accounts such as these that many were sensitized to the need for a two-stage procedure for diagnosis and treatment as opposed to a one-stage procedure (i.e., one-stage: breast biopsy, to be followed by immediate mastectomy if a malignant tumor were found). The one-stage procedure resulted in considerable psychological trauma as the woman was unable to prepare herself adequately for a mastectomy. This need is being incorporated into surgical practice more commonly with outpatient breast biopsy for diagnosis preceding the inpatient hospitalization for mastectomy.[32] It also demonstrates that patients can affect the type of care they receive.

As women begin to take a more active role in influencing the type of care they receive, they ask questions. Sometimes the caretaker perceives these questions and the emotions behind them as challenging his/her competence and authority when, in fact, the patient is requesting information. This distortion or misperception reverberates within the relationship sometimes resulting in the caretaker's labeling the patient as "difficult."

CLINICAL ILLUSTRATIONS

The clinical illustrations we discuss demonstrate difficulties in patient-caretaker interaction. We attempt to understand what behaviors generated the labeling process. As a group, the women described as "difficult" were characterized as highly anxious with a strong need to be in control, especially in decision-making situations. These patient characteristics may be particularly difficult for physicians to deal with because the physician is, in part, characterized as a decision-maker who is in control of life-death situations. Patient and physician needs may then conflict, resulting in a situation in which all the participants feel helpless and angry. How the anger generated by this situation is recognized and handled will affect the doctor-patient relationship and the outcome of treatment. Those involved in the care of patients need to understand the patient's behavior as an expression of her inner emotional experience and characteristic coping style. If the patient's anger is met by an accepting rather than angry, distancing response by treatment personnel, a smoother course will usually follow. The following case histories are illustrations of some of these observations.

Case 1
A 30 year old woman discovered a breast lump. She promptly sought medical attention, had a biopsy, and was advised to have a mastectomy. She was intelligent, achievement-oriented, and when first seen was in process of completing her masters degree in a highly competitive field. Given her style of making a decision only after carefully researching known data,

she began to read extensively and intensively on the major treatment modalities for breast cancer. She discovered conflicting opinions and began to consult experts in the field locally. During this two-week period, she experienced considerable anxiety. She was referred for consultation as someone who was "shopping around for a doctor," "asking a lot of questions," and "might be getting out of control." The pejorative flavor of these phrases seems to reflect certain attitudes. For example, the person who is "shopping around for a doctor" implies a lack of trust in any one doctor's opinion. The issue of the doctor's competence is raised, and often this results in a defensive attitude on the doctor's part. This may then cause him/her to react defensively and become hostile. This hostility may have been reflected in the view that her anxiety was unproductive and negative, rather than as constructive and necessary to her decision-making process. Some of this attitude may reflect the still unusual aspect of the patient taking part in the decision-making aspect of treatment, of choosing one among several doctors, and assuming the role of consumer rather than patient. This direct confrontation of the traditional role of doctor as ultimate decision-maker may further engender anxiety and anger in the doctor.

The psychiatric discussion of this patient raised concerns about her assertiveness. The implications of it varied, depending on the sex of the observer. The two women who interviewed her saw her anxiety as related to the decision-making process, and likely to be relieved once her conflict regarding treatment was resolved. She was seen as trying to gain increasing control but certainly not "out of control." They felt it unlikely that the patient would have any continuing emotional difficulties unless her disease worsened.

Female radiotherapy technicians complied with the patient's requirement that treatment sessions be rescheduled when her classes conflicted with appointments. She consistently acted as though she had no time to devote to having cancer and emphasized her strong desire to continue with her new career plans. She would not allow this cancer to achieve a role of primacy. This behavior appeared to be an adaptive form of denial as it permitted her to comply with treatment and continue with her work.

A male staff member, in contrast, regarded her high energy level and controlling style as indicating psychopathology that would likely result in a severe emotional impairment at some point. Part of this opinion was also based on the patient's history of losing her father at an early age, and her changing careers in order to better her mother's life-style. These facts were interpreted as resulting in rage at an early loss and as overdependence on her mother. He saw her present high energy level as "excessive" and as an outlet for her rage at having cancer. Her wish to manipulate and control was viewed as a maladaptive attempt to deny her illness.

Follow-up at 6 months revealed that she was pleased with the job she had obtained following graduation. She was resettled in a new community. Although she reported feeling lonely occasionally, she had made friends and was "keeping busy" (her characteristic style), and she was complying with her treatment plan.

What seems important to emphasize are the expressed attitudes about the patient's assertiveness and denial. The female staff may have overidentified with her, and underplayed certain aspects of her history and behavior, while the male staff reacted mainly to confrontation with an assertive woman. By denying her illness, she remained the assertive, achievement-oriented individual she had been prior to her illness. Those traits were unchanged. If assertiveness is difficult for people to accept in healthy women perhaps it is even less acceptable in a woman who is ill. There may be an underlying assumption that in illness, one becomes passive and compliant, as experience often confirms. This then becomes the anticipated reaction. When that anticipated reaction is not forthcoming, hostility may be generated. This may then be expressed toward the patient in viewing her emotional responses as "maladaptive" and "pathological." It is likely that this negative view emanated from their hostility toward an assertive woman. This is an issue of utmost concern to women (and health consumers) as they express their need to influence the type of care they receive.

Case 2

The following case illustration involves the attitudes expressed toward a woman in an acute crisis. The patient was an elderly woman with late-stage breast cancer who was brought to the emergency room by her family, with whom she had been living since an adrenalectomy 5 months earlier. There was a history of early morning awakening, some minor physical combativeness toward her niece, and monetary gifts to her relatives which were out of character with her previous parsimonious behavior. Her admitting diagnosis was "psychosis" and the issue first raised was, "Can she be committed to a mental hospital?" When interviewed shortly after admission, she did not have an overt disorder of thinking but showed signs of denying her illness. She had poor judgment and was hostile when she discussed emotion-laden issues. An incipient mania was also possible given the history of her gift-giving. She remained in the medical setting to allow evalution of the possibility of organic etiology for her symptoms. However, no organic pathology was found to be contributing to her emotional symptoms. During her evaluation, further history revealed that she had become increasingly combative coincident with the anniversary of her mother's death one year previously. Over the next few days, she was able to accept the fact that her family would not take her back, and that she could not live alone. She cursed them and cried. None of her family would care for her as she had cared for her mother. Once she experienced staff support and intervention to help her deal with the crisis, she was then able to mobilize her strengths. Prior to going to a rest home, the patient dressed herself in street clothes, went out to dinner with a friend, and began doing needlepoint.

Symptoms suggesting mental illness often frighten professionals who do not have specific training in this area. In her state of panic, she appeared irrational and frightened. This frightened her family and then she was labeled "crazy." Her helplessness instilled a sense of helplessness in those initially evaluating her, so that the first impulse was to send her away, despite the fact that her physical disease could have produced her emotional symptoms. Her symptoms cleared when her caretakers took the time to listen to her, to obtain the relevant history, to allow her to ventilate her own anger in a safe environment, and to assist her in making plans.

Case 3

Professionals, families, and patients often have difficulty coping with stress. Because the case of Mrs. N illustrates this so clearly, it is presented in some detail. Mrs. N was a woman in her 40s with late-stage metastatic breast cancer who had undergone a unilateral modified radical mastectomy 4 years previously, oophorectomy 2 years previously, and adrenalectomy 4 months previously. She had a history of marital difficulties. She requested consultation with a psychiatrist after she and her husband returned from a difficult vacation together. It was a disappointing experience for Mrs. N because she had been expecting that her husband, a physician, would alter his "rigid" schedule to comply with her own. He was unable to do this and had to interrupt their vacation for a professional meeting. Following their return, Mrs. N "talked at" her husband for 3 hours during which time "he said nothing." This she recognized as "his style when he feels attacked." She cried, could not sleep, and called her local physician who advised, "Double all your medications." (These included antidepressants, tranquilizers, and barbiturates.) At this point she was labeled a "difficult" patient. In retrospect, it would appear that her physician may have been responding to her implied request, "Please do something." Unfortunately, medications are often prescribed to treat the physician's helplessness.

During her consultation, she described a fantasy imagining her husband and his next wife spending all the money Mrs. N and he had worked so hard to save. She felt intensely lonely and then became furious. She continued in intermittent therapy where she dealt with loneliness and anticipated separation. Most of the meetings were at times of crisis, usually before a scheduled return visit to the local cancer treatment center. At these times she experienced increasing feelings of rage toward her husband, coincident with the anticipatory dread of her visit with the oncologist. Between visits she cared for her children, continued decorating their home, volunteered at a thrift shop, and played tennis vigorously, often despite bone pain. When she talks about her tennis, she says, "That is the one time that I feel really healthy . . . and I tell God, 'You're not going to get me today.' " For her this activity is a coping mechanism that effectively channels her energy.

Under the stress of her recent hospitalization for an adrenalectomy, her fears of loneliness and separation surfaced. Ultimately, she was able to say she feared dying all alone. Her rage was directed not only toward her husband, but toward hospital personnel. When she was given a bed on an open ward, she immediately called her surgeon and oncologist, demanding, "Let's see how much pull you've got around here to get me a private room." She later threatened to write letters complaining of the food and the housekeeping. She focused most of her anger on her husband when he arrived later than the beginning of visiting hours, or on any separation during visiting hours.

Often this kind of behavior is described as "entitlement." The patient feels entitled to something more or better and often overwhelms others with her or his expressed neediness. Mrs. N. felt out of control as she saw her disease progress and attempted to restore some sense of control by engaging in behavior with predictable results. She recognized the effects on her husband of her late night calls to various physicians. He became overtly angry and they could then predictably spend many hours in heated debate. She grinned with delight one day as she imagined how angry her husband would be to discover that all her long distance calls were billed to his office. Conflict was one way Mrs. N could remain in control of something. As she became more helpless, epitomized by the in-hospital experience, she acted so as to make everyone else feel helpless also. The staff did not respond with angry, distancing behavior but by helping her deal with her fear of loneliness and her rage at not getting what she is entitled to (i.e., a long life, great wealth), her fears diminished.

Additional sessions enabled her to see that her husband had his own coping mechanisms, just as she had her tennis. He may have used these when confronted with the reality of her disease. His "rigidity" about his schedule was an example. She understood that these mechanisms helped him stay in control and made him feel more comfortable. She was able to give up her wish for "the perfect husband" and deal with the reality, "the good enough husband." In that context, instead of focusing on her fear that he might not be there when she would need him, she has been able to acknowledge that he has been there when she has needed him.

Case 4

The next case is an example of how people deal with ambivalence and how it leads to anxiety in both patients and caretakers. The response of the caretaker will affect the patient's resolution of the anxiety. Mrs. B was a 45-year-old married mother of 3 who was seen postbiopsy, at the time she was beginning to consult oncology specialists to select mastectomy or primary irradiation as the treatment of choice for her breast cancer.

Mrs. B's initial anxiety began the previous summer when she first noted nipple discharge which was examined by a physician and discounted. Six months later a mammogram was obtained which showed a lesion in the left breast. She was advised that surgery, radiation, or a combination of the two should be considered. During the next two weeks, she consulted with radiotherapists, an oncologist, and a surgeon.

She was a highly educated, well-read woman, and initially physicians responded to her in a sensitive, individualized manner, trying to help her sort out what would be the best treatment for her particular tumor. The more information she obtained from different specialists, the more she sensed the lack of definitive guidelines in the treatment of breast cancer. Views of treatment changed with the perspective of each specialist. Her anxiety escalated and her questions became obsessional and repetitive. Her physicians became wary and perceived her questions as a test of their competence and skill. Their guarded answers served to increase her anxiety, anger, and mistrust of physicians. At one point, she indicated that she probably would choose surgery and one of her radiotherapists expressed relief because she had become such a taxing individual. A note in the medical chart at the time of her lumpectomy stated that she had "Extensive consultation with many individuals regarding her choice. . . . Tonight she has finally decided to proceed with radiotherapy as the primary mode." Tolerating her ambivalence had been difficult for both patient and doctor.

In understanding the mutual interaction between Mrs. B and her caretakers, it should be recognized that from the very beginning, Mrs. B was suspicious of her doctors. She had found something in her breast six months before and the physician she consulted had not taken it seriously.

When the diagnosis was confirmed, she was terrified that her disease had metastasized and that she was going to die. She was looking for definitive treatment. When she was not able to find this, she became increasingly indecisive and obsessional. Rather than getting the advice and support she needed from the physicians, her confrontational style pushed them away.

An essential element in understanding the problem this patient struggled with was her difficulty tolerating the need to make a decision based on incomplete data and the physicians' inability to tolerate her ambivalence. In Mrs. B's case, additional factual information compounded her problem. She discovered the conflicts in the medical community regarding treatment. Her continued efforts were attempts to find someone who could assimilate all the conflicting information and tell her what to do. This person was not to be found.

Some clinicians have expressed the opinion, after hearing of such spiraling anxiety in the face of conflicting information, "It's a pity these women have so much information today. It just stirs them up." To us this reflects the notion, "Doctors know best. . . . Don't bother your pretty head with all that. . . . Let us decide what's best for you." It seems far more honest, in our opinion, to acknowledge that conflicts as to treatment recommendations exist and then help our patients bear the considerable anxiety that this uncertainty may engender in order for them to make choices about their care.

Case 5

Some patients arouse strong feelings in all who come in contact with them. These feelings are often difficult for the staff to deal with because of their strong identification with the patient and her situation. Mrs. W, a 29-year-old woman with metastatic breast cancer who was admitted to the hospital with severe headaches, presents this problem. One-and-a-half years before she was diagnosed as having carcinoma of the left breast. She underwent a modified radical mastectomy. There were no positive nodes, but because of extensive lymphatic invasion, she was placed on chemotherapy. At this time she began raising questions about the effects of chemotherapy on her ability to become pregnant and have a healthy child. Her oncologist researched her questions and talked with her. Her ambivalence about therapy was tipped negatively when the oncology resident left, and the new resident was less attentive. She decided, at that point, to end her chemotherapy. Six months later, she became pregnant. She was 32 weeks pregnant at the time she was admitted to the hospital for severe headaches. A CAT scan revealed a large lesion in the right parietal area of her brain, for which she underwent radiation therapy. A month later she delivered a healthy baby girl. Two months later, she began to have seizures. Chemotherapy was started again. The seizures recurred 4 months later and tests revealed liver metastases. In spite of her metastases and the debilitating effects of chemotherapy, she remained organized and able to meet her responsibilities. Both she and her husband, a graduate student with considerable teaching responsibility, described their relationship as "mutually supportive." He felt it was very important for her to make her own decisions regarding treatment.

All the staff were acutely aware of her rapidly progressive course and the utter ineffectiveness of any treatment modality in limiting the growth of the tumor. They felt helpless and impotent especially since it was very easy to identify with her situation and her social role as mother of an infant with an earnest, hard-working husband.

The feelings she engendered in the staff were difficult to reconcile with her cheerful, optimistic manner. One psychiatrist, in fact, described her as "comforting." At times she described feeling sad or angry but it was always in relation to a past event, never in the present. One encounter she did describe involved a radiotherapist who said, "I'm not sure how much time there is the way your tumor is progressing . . . but these are my recommendations." She became incensed at how "coldly and rudely" he relayed his opinion to her. Although she felt she had been assaulted, she recovered quickly.

Staff members expressed many kinds of feelings regarding Mrs. W. There was anger that she had been "irresponsible" in discontinuing her chemotherapy and having a child. Some were uncertain as to how to respond to her optimism when they felt so pessimistic. One physician shared how nonplused he felt when she greeted him smilingly on the elevator saying, "My cancer has spread to my liver." Most interpreted her attitude as denial. Some even felt it to be of psychotic proportion.

As her disease progressed, her husband became busier and more involved in his work. Meetings with staff members were less frequent. This helped him avoid and deny the impact of her rapidly progressive illness. Unlike many staff members, he appeared to be less conflicted about supporting her denial. His support of this style probably made it possible for her to cope as well as she did.

This particular woman did not conform to staff expectations in that she genuinely seemed to be happy most of the time. When staff were able to gain some distance through discussion of their own feelings, they could accept the patient's coping style as legitimate for her. In this case her denial was maladaptive in a medical sense since it resulted in her not completing treatment early in her disease. However, it was adaptive when one considers her strong need to have a child—as she accomplished this goal though sacrificing her life.

CONCLUSION

It is hoped that the case studies discussed have revealed the importance of staff-patient interaction, especially when conflict arises in that interaction. The traditional nature of this relationship is caricatured by the mythical doctor-patient relationship in which the doctor is omniscient and all-powerful and the patient is passive and compliant. Though this is generally acknowledged to be a myth, there is evidence that at times both patients and staff behave as though their expectations of each other developed from this myth. When these long-held expectations are unmet, anxiety and hostility may be generated which then seek expression, usually directed at the frustrating object. Case histories were presented to illustrate this type of interaction. Emphasis was given to that particular form of hostility expressed by

268 EILEEN B. KAHAN AND ELIZABETH B. GASKILL

labeling the patient as "difficult." We believe an awareness of the issues underlying this labeling process will result in a more empathic staff–patient interaction.

REFERENCES

1. Wilson RE: The breast, in *Davis-Christopher textbook of surgery: the biological basis of modern surgical practice*. Tenth edition. Edited by Sabiston, DC Jr. Philadelphia, WB Saunders, 1972, pp. 580–586.
2. Artiss KL, Levine AS: Doctor-patient relation in severe illness: a seminar for oncology fellows. *New England Journal of Medicine 288*(23):1210–1213, June 7, 1973.
3. Lindemann E: Observations on psychiatric sequelae to surgical operations in women. *American Journal of Psychiatry 98*:132–139, 1941.
4. Hollender MH: A study of patients admitted to a psychiatric hospital after pelvic operations. *American Journal of Obstetrics and Gynecology 79*:498–503, March 1960.
5. Shands HC et al.: Psychological mechanisms in patients with cancer. *Cancer 4*:1159–1170, 1951.
6. Mastrovito RC: Cancer: awareness and denial. *Clinical Bulletin 4*(4):142–146, 1974.
7. Renneker R, Cutler M: Psychological problems of adjustment to cancer of the breast. *Journal of the American Medical Association 148*:833–838, 1952.
8. Bard M, Sutherland A: Psychological impact of cancer and its treatment. IV. Adaptation to radical mastectomy. *Cancer 8*:656–672, 1955.
9. Ervin CV, Jr: Psychological adjustment to mastectomy. *Medical Aspects of Human Sexuality 7*(2):42–65, February 1973.
10. Klein R: A crisis to grow on. *Cancer 28*:1660–1665, 1971.
11. Grinker RR, Jr.: Sex and cancer. *Medical Aspects of Human Sexuality 10*(2):130–139, February 1976.
12. Kent S: Coping with sexual identity crises after mastectomy. *Geriatrics 30*(10):145–146, October 1975.
13. Witkin MH: Sex therapy and mastectomy. *Journal of Sex and Marital Therapy 1*(4):290–304, Summer 1975.
14. Byrd BF: Sex after mastectomy. *Medical Aspects of Human Sexuality 9*(4):53–54, April 1975.
15. Notman MT: A psychological consideration of mastectomy, in *The woman patient*, Vol I. Edited by Nadelson CC, Notman MT. New York, Plenum Press, 1978.
16. Huffman JW: Sexual reactions after gynecologic surgery. *Medical Aspects of Human Sexuality 3*(11):48–57, November 1969.
17. Ford AB, Orfirer AP: Sexual behavior and the chronically ill patient. *Medical Aspects of Human Sexuality 1*(10):56–60, October 1967.
18. Waxenberg SE, Drellich MG, Sutherland AM: The role of hormones in human behavior. I. Changes in female sexuality after adrenalectomy. *Journal of Clinical Endocrinology 19*:193–202, 1959.
19. Labby DH: Sexual concomitants of disease and illness. *Postgraduate Medicine 58*(1):103–111, July 1975.
20. Vincent CE, et al: Some marital-sexual concomitants of carcinoma of the cervix. *Southern Medical Journal 68*(5):552–558, May 1975.
21. Drellich, MG, et al: The psychological impact of cancer and cancer surgery. VI. Adaptation to hysterectomy. *Cancer 9*:1120–1126, November–December 1956.
22. Vaillant, GE: Natural history of male psychological health: the relation of choice of

ego mechanisms of defense to adult adjustment. *Archives of General Psychiatry* 33:535–545, May 1976.

23. McCorkle MR: Coping with physical symptoms in metastatic breast cancer. *American Journal of Nursing* 73(6):1034–1038, 1973.
24. Gold MA: Causes of patients' delay in diseases of the breast. *Cancer* 17:564–577, 1964.
25. Eardley A: Triggers to action. A study of what makes women seek advice for breast conditions. *International Journal of Health Education* 17:256–265, 1974.
26. Degenshein GA, Ceccarelli F: The history of breast cancer surgery, Part I: early beginnings to Halsted. *Breast, Diseases of the Breast* 3(2):28–36, April–July 1977.
27. Lobsenz NM: What will our marriage be like now? *McCall's*: August 1973.
28. Daly MJ: Psychological impact of surgical procedures on women. *Comprehensive textbook of psychiatry*, Vol II, 2nd ed. Edited by Freedman AM, Kaplan HI, Sadock BJ. Baltimore, Williams & Wilkins, 1975, pp. 1477–1480.
29. Roth P: *The professor of desire*. New York, Farrar, Straus, and Giroux, 1977, pp. 107–110.
30. Kushner R: Breast cancer: a personal history and an investigative report. New York, Harcourt Brace Jovanovich, 1975.
31. Rollins B: First, you cry. Philadelphia, JB Lippincott, 1976.
32. Baker RR: Out-patient breast biopsies. *Annals of Surgery* 185(5):543–547, May 1977.

Chapter 20

The Woman and Esthetic Surgery

ROBERT M. GOLDWYN

Most patients seeking esthetic surgery are female. Most surgeons performing it are male. These facts reflect the present status and attitudes of women and, conversely, of men in our society.[2,19] Our culture places a higher value on the attractive appearance of the female than on the male; and the female, deprived of the many sources of gratification available to the male, has learned to use and value her body, consciously and unconsciously, to please herself and/or others. This behavior is rewarded and is perpetuated and reinforced throughout her life by such acts as using makeup, adopting hair and clothing styles, and keeping "young and trim."

Inculcated with the desideratum of attractiveness and bombarded by measures and stratagems for acquiring it, many women feel obliged to change or maintain their body to promote pleasure for themselves and others.[9,15] To aid her in the battle for beauty is the plastic surgeon who, as noted, is generally a man and does not think it is unusual for a woman to enhance her appearance through surgery.[1]

This chapter will consider the principal kinds of cosmetic surgery as well as a specific type of reconstruction (breast replacement after mastectomy) sought by women. I have not included operations deemed noncosmetic or essential, for example, the repair of a cleft lip or the revision of scars, even though they obviously have cosmetic significance.

ROBERT M. GOLDWYN, M.D. ● Associate Clinical Professor of Surgery, Harvard Medical School; Head of Plastic Surgery, Beth Israel Hospital; Surgeon, Peter Bent Brigham Hospital, Boston, Massachusetts 02215.

THE NOSE

The most common esthetic procedure in the adolescent girl is rhinoplasty. Generally, she has initiated the idea of modifying the shape of her nose, but occasionally, her mother is the instigator. In the latter instance, the mother herself may have had the procedure or may have wanted it, but was denied it because of "circumstances." Usually, the father is the last to concur with his daughter's wishes since he sees "nothing really wrong with the nose." It is important to emphasize that the adolescent girl rarely says she wishes a beautiful nose; rather she wants to get rid of the "ugly nose." She wants to blend with her peers and not be singled out negatively because of an inherited feature.[14,16]

Following the operation, most female adolescent patients are very pleased with the result. They ignore imperfections which might bother the mother and the surgeon. This is in marked contrast to the older male who frequently is dissatisfied postoperatively. A possible explanation is that the patient may have a conflict in sexual identification and is uncertain whether he wants a "masculine" or a "feminine" nose.

In conjunction with rhinoplasty, a frequent procedure is chin augmentation: correcting a recessed chin, usually by an implant, generally of silicone, inserted through the inside of the mouth or a small incision under the chin. Not every patient is prepared for changing both her nose and chin at the same time. The surgeon should be careful not to overwhelm an individual with anatomic inadequacies. Sometimes it is better to delay the chin operation until after the rhinoplasty, if, indeed, the patient still desires it.

EARS

Psychologically, prominent ears can be an unpleasant reality for a child or an adult. The female has the advantage of hiding the problem with her long hair. Today, when even males tend to wear their hair long, the frequency of correcting prominent ears has decreased. If undertaken, surgery should wait until the child expresses a desire for it. Although the average age for operation is around five, it is not unusual for a woman in her thirties to have this procedure. Frequently, the patient will say, "Now that I have raised my family I think I can do something for myself." Even though plastic surgeons may spend hours talking to one another about the "best technique" to reduplicate each contour and crevice of the normal ear, patients are almost always pleased if the ears no longer project.

As in rhinoplasty, occasionally the mother may wish the procedure done soon after her daughter's. In these situations, the father and
mother may have a poor marriage and the joint surgical undertaking
by the mother and daughter is an aggressive act on the part of the
mother to exclude him.

THE BREAST

Breast development is the hallmark of puberty, and in some, it
goes awry: breasts may become too large, asymmetrical, or may fail to
develop. Small breasts are generally not treated in adolescence unless
there is some degree of agenesis or significant asymmetry. Excessively
large breasts may constitute not only cosmetic but functional difficulties: back and shoulder pain, poor posture, intertrigo, and difficulty in
buying clothes. The young woman may avoid summer sports and may
actually become obese in her frustration. The oversized breasts become the unwanted focus of her relationships with boys. Unlike the
adolescent male with enlarged breasts (gynecomastia), the female is
not confused in her sexual identity; she is excessively aware of it.[7,8]

Many male physicians are insensitive to the emotional and physical burden of this condition and like the girl's father, are reluctant to
recommend any reduction in the size of the breasts. If the girl has a
good relationship with her mother, particularly if the mother is similarly affected, she will be aided in her quest for relief and will also
have less anxiety about the operation; furthermore, she will have a
better convalescence. After years of feeling encased by custom-made
bras, the teenager may yearn to go braless. Yet, she will still wish to
retain a good figure and consequently frequently instructs the surgeon:
"Don't take too much off." The older girl, who may have an intimate
relationship with a male, may bring him to the office. He should enter
into the decision about the surgery. Usually, but not always, the boyfriend or husband are supportive if their relationship is one of mutual
care and respect. Generally, she has told him of her feelings of being
"grotesque" or being misshapen, but he has liked her with the breasts
that she now has. It is not unusual for many women who are large
breasted to have sex only with their bras on and only in the dark.
After reduction mammaplasty, although there will be scars and may
be decreased sensation in the areola and nipple, and even though
nursing may not be possible, patients are almost always very pleased
because they have been relieved of a "deformity." Their self-image
improves. They may begin a strict weight reduction program and may
enter into other areas of activity with zest and confidence. They also

report feeling more at ease in sexual situations and state that their sensuality is increased.

The surgeon should be very clear about the patient's expectations regarding size and shape. Some women, married or not, in the 18–30 age range, may postpone the surgery if they cannot be guaranteed that they can nurse. Naturally the patient should determine the timing of this elective operation and should not be talked out of the desire to breastfeed. Aside from the psychological benefit to mother and child, the act of nursing may confer a protection against the subsequent development of breast cancer. This last point is controversial, however.

BREAST ENLARGEMENT

Augmentation mammaplasty is usually done in the older female, 20–45 years of age, for small breast size and for mild degrees of sagging. From a personal series of patients undergoing augmentation mammaplasty, Gifford[8] concluded that many had

> unhappy childhoods, experiences of loss of maternal deprivation, and conflicts in identification with parents. They tended to make early marriages, in which they played a submissive or frankly masochistic role. . . . Many described longstanding feelings of inferiority or low self esteem, and several described periods of clinical depression. The "typical" breast augmentation patient seemed to have reached an emotional turning point in her life, when she had decided against having more children and was seeking a new direction, increased self-assertiveness, some kind of personality change. In these women the breasts had come to represent something more than sexual attractiveness, because their breast was their representation of an ideal self, real or imagined. This was an image of themselves as they were at some former time or as they had hoped to be, an ideal self which they had been deprived of or lost through hardship, childbearing or the vicissitudes of life. The operation represented the restitution of this loss, the restoration of an ideal or former self. . . .[8]

Many patients for augmentation mammaplasty are in transition—between marriages, affairs, or careers. It is important to assess what the patient expects the operation to do for her life at this time.[3,6,12,13,18]

Breast enlargement can be performed on an outpatient basis under local anesthesia supplemented by intravenous medication. The return to work is rapid (about a week) and the relative ease with which this procedure can generally be done may lead some women not to consider it "surgery." The surgeon has the obligation to make the patient understand that she is indeed having a surgical procedure which has associated morbidity and mortality, albeit extremely low. Also, because of the unpredictability of wound healing, a thickened capsule might form around the implant, causing the breast to become abnormally firm. Scars are usually well hidden, particularly if the incision is made within the areola. Although the procedure of augmentation itself and the insertion of the implant cannot be indicted as causes of cancer, the breast, of course, could still develop cancer. Periodic breast self-examination and visits to the doctor are required. The patient, once so preoccupied by her breasts, may now refuse to think about them in terms of their cancer potential once her "ideal self" has been restored or achieved.

Despite the fact that after augmentation some patients have breasts which lack normal softness and contour, almost all are happy with their result.[4,5] In two weeks or so, they consider the implant as part of their own body—an attitude different from that which they had while wearing a padded bra. To them, the padded bra was indeed a "falsie," but the implanted breast is their real breast.

BREAST RECONSTRUCTION FOLLOWING MASTECTOMY

Increasingly, the plastic surgeon is asked to reconstruct the breast following operations either for premalignant or malignant disease. Although the technical aspects are not within the scope of this chapter, certain points deserve emphasis. The female who has had a simple, or radical, or modified radical mastectomy, probably felt coerced into that surgery because of the threat to her life. The act of later inquiring about breast reconstruction may be a sign of emotional recovery. Whether or not she eventually has the procedure, she now feels that she is in control over her body and over her life course. Hopefully, now, surgeons who remove breasts are more sympathetic to the feelings of women who must bear this loss. It is not sufficient that a patient should be told: "You should be glad that you are alive." Many women no longer feel truly feminine.[1] They consider themselves deformed and they refrain from physical intimacy. The reconstruction of the breast is, in many ways, like the restitution of the self, noted earlier in patients with micromastia who had augmentation. Here again, the mastectomized female does not wish to become a super female, but simply to be like every other female, with two normal breasts. Ideally, the surgeon who must do the mastectomy should confer preoperatively with the plastic surgeon about rebuilding the breast. The patient, of course, should be part of this discussion. In some instances, the procedure may not be in the best interests of that patient, but she should at least have that information and know the alternatives.

If cancer detection programs prove successful, then women with a marked potential for developing malignancy will be identified and their breast tissue can be removed prophylactically (subcutaneous mastectomy).[11] Breast reconstruction, by implants, can then be done. The fear of deformity after mastectomy has kept many women away from periodic breast examination and early cancer detection. As reconstruction becomes more available and better esthetically, more cancers will be prevented since patients will be seen earlier and treated sooner.

Insurance companies, which are controlled by men, have been slow to provide financial support to their subscribers for breast reconstruction, which they consider cosmetic. Admittedly, what is cosmetic may be difficult to define but certainly breast rebuilding seems as worthy of insurance coverage as is remaking the nose after amputation because of cancer. Although the male may view the breast as an adornment or a secondary object of sexual attentions, to the female, it is integral to the self. Its restoration is not to capture beauty but to be acceptable to herself.

For some patients, to recommend psychotherapy in order to have them adjust to their mastectomy may be unrealistic and unhelpful; breast reconstruction can prevent a great deal of anguish not only for the woman but for her family and friends.

EYELIDPLASTY AND FACE LIFT

The patient desiring surgery for the aging face is most likely a white, middle- or upper-class married female between the ages of 40 and 58, generally around 45. Characteristically, she is energetic and active both socially and professionally. She is by no means one of the "idle rich." She tends to be narcissistic, and having been considered attractive throughout her life, she fears losing what has been such an important asset to her. Most patients who wish an eyelidplasty and face lift do not do so to dissimulate their age, but rather to reaffirm to themselves that they are still youthful, optimistic, and effective in thought and action.[10] Many say they do not wish to look young, but really wish to look their age and not "older." Many still think of themselves as younger than they are chronologically. For some, a sagging face is symbolic of life's inexorable downhill course. They do not wish to see their life contracting coffin-like around them; they want to rid themselves of the daily reminders of decay.[7]

Surgery for the aging face is frequently sought after a recent loss, such as a separation, a divorce, a death, or termination of psychotherapy.[9,10,17] The 45-year-old female is either in the menopause or facing it. Losses start overcoming gains, the body ages; loved ones leave; a husband's attentions may flag; at work she may feel excluded by those younger; there is less sand in the hourglass than at 25.

The process of aging is generally imperceptible and proceeds slowly, but cumulative changes go beyond the subliminal level and then become noted. This particularly is true if there has been an emotional trauma. A patient may say, "Suddenly, I look so old. I don't mind getting older, but not this fast." Some patients have familial tendency to premature facial aging. One patient remarked: "Why should I go on looking like this when every other part of me feels young?" Some express their resentment at being the bearer of this inherited trait, especially if an older sibling has escaped it.

Many women wish to appear younger for professional reasons, as in the performing arts, or because of a liaison with someone younger. It is not unusual for a patient to feel guilty about wanting the surgery. Some are disappointed that, despite their college or postgraduate education, they have capitulated to a quirk of our culture, the glorification of the younger-looking woman. Their feelings of guilt have been increased by pronouncements of women's groups, which tell them to accept themselves as they are.

The individual wanting to look younger often must wage her battle alone. It is, after all, a losing battle since inevitably aging and decline supervene. Friends may consider her foolish; her husband may call her "crazy." One patient said that the entire process of obtaining a face lift was a lonely vigil. In a world where the haves are reminded of the have-nots, she may feel more guilty because she is spending money—often her husband's, since cosmetic surgery and the associated hospitalization are generally not covered by insurance. Many apologize for taking the doctor's "valuable time" and for occupying a hospital bed "meant for sick people."

An eyelidplasty or face lift can be done on an outpatient basis or during a brief hospitalization. Recovery time is rapid in terms of general well-being. Most patients seeking this kind of surgery do not wish to be passive or dependent in their life style. In fact, they usually do not want anyone to know that they have had an operation and they push to resume their social and professional activities as quickly as possible.

The operation of improving the aging face is generally viewed by the patient as an enhancement and such patients easily accommodate to the "new look" since it is really the old look—"the way they were." However, it should not be assumed that all patients having eyelidplasty and rhytidectomy are satisfied. Many are, but others feel disappointed because there are "still some wrinkles." Those individuals who had the operation not just to look younger, but actually to recapture youth, will be disappointed. Their lease on life has not been extended. The plastic surgeon who carefully questions his patient following this procedure will detect more depression than has commonly been reported. This is true in many patients having surgery, especially esthetic operations. In the instance of the patient with large breasts, the reaction in the immediate postoperative phase may be one of depression over loss of a permanent feature in the body image. However, with time, things get better for the patient emotionally. This is not always true for the patient who has had surgery for her aging face. With time, things can get ultimately only worse.

Abdomen and Thighs

Patients for abdominoplasty and thigh lift are almost always female and may desire these procedures after weight loss or pregnancy. They may remark that they wish to wear a bikini or jeans. One patient, recently divorced, said that she wanted "to start a new life. I wish that I were a snake so that I could get new skin." Many have "always hated" their bulky thighs, which may be a familial trait and cannot be slimmed by exercise and massage. The idea for the surgery is almost always the patient's. A husband or boyfriend may occasionally support her, but more frequently acquiesces, thinking that it is "unnecessary" or "absurd." Despite the inevitable scars, most patients, if properly selected, are extremely happy with the outcome. They have been relieved of a disturbing feature in their self-image.

Patient Selection

Not everyone who wishes plastic surgery should have it. Certain patients should be refused because they will not be satisfied with the outcome. Potential problem patients include the following:

1. The perfectionistic patient. This is the individual who wishes the result to be "perfect"—every wrinkle gone, or "the nose just so." It is usually impossible to satisfy that individual because surgery and wound healing are not that precise or controllable. The skin is not marble.

2. The indecisive or vague patient. This person may schedule surgery and then cancel it. Her vacillation is an indication that she is not prepared to undertake the operation.

3. The patient with minimal deformity. Surgery is potentially hazardous no matter how slight it may seem, and if the object of the surgery is only a minimal deformity, the risks may outweigh the gains.

4. The plasti-surgiholic patient. This individual may wish multiple procedures: rhinoplasty, correction of breast ptosis, abdominoplasty. The surgeon may be successful in one of those procedures, but luck for both the patient and the surgeon may run out. That individual has a generalized low self-esteem and may actually be in the midst of a depression. She (most of them are female) would be best treated by a psychiatrist.

5. The acquiescing patient. This is a form of masochism in which no surgeon should get involved. The willingness of some women to expose themselves to possible harm, to undergo pain, and to go through another operation to correct the results of a previous one is truly astounding, and the willingness of surgeons to operate on these individuals without benefit of psychotherapy is equally amazing.

6. The patient with a recent loss. The stimulus to plastic surgery, as mentioned, may follow a recent loss. Although this does not necessarily preclude an individual's having an operation, it should make the surgeon sufficiently wary of an underlying depression which might worsen precipitously after surgery. Psychiatric advice preoperatively can be very helpful.

7. The paranoid or depressed patient. Elective surgery of a cosmetic nature, in general, is best not done in these individuals. With psychotherapy, that person eventually may be suitable for operation, but its timing must be carefully chosen.

8. The complaining and disagreeable patient. This is a difficult category to define, but there are persons who, if presented with a dozen roses, would note only the thorns. Their bitterness about life, their insatiability, and their hostility, will focus on the postoperative result no matter how technically acceptable it is.

In these few pages, it has been impossible to detail all aspects of the woman as a plastic surgical patient. The surgery of appearance has been emphasized, since it gives some insight into the attitudes and behavior of women within our society. Admittedly, society is changing, although it is impossible to predict what direction women's values and value will take. Will the woman of tomorrow, given more opportunity than today, rely less upon her appearance to find happiness? Will she become less passive and not submit her body to surgery so easily and so enthusiastically? While theoretically it might be a better society if less emphasis were placed on appearance, the probability is that physical beauty, particularly for women, will still be pursued, at least for the next few decades. The needs of these women should be answered with maximum care and understanding, but without exploitation.

REFERENCES

1. Asken MJ: Psychoemotional aspects of mastectomy: a review of recent literature. *American Journal of Psychiatry* 132:56, 1975.
2. Bettman AG: The psychology of appearances. *Northwest Medicine* 28:182, 1929.
3. Druss RG: Changes in body image following augmentation breast surgery. *International Journal of Psychoanalysis and Psychotherapy* 2:248, 1973.
4. Edgerton MT, McClary AR: Augmentation mammaplasty: psychiatric implications and surgical indications. *Plastic and Reconstructive Surgery* 21:279, 1958.
5. Edgerton MT, Meyer E, Jacobson WE: Augmentation mammaplasty: II. further surgical and psychiatric evaluation. *Plastic and Reconstructive Surgery* 27:279, 1961.
6. Edgerton MT, Knorr NJ: Motivational patterns of patients seeking cosmetic (esthetic) surgery. *Plastic and Reconstructive Surgery* 48:551, 1971.
7. Gifford S: Cosmetic surgery and personality change: a review of some clinical observations, in *The unfavorable result in plastic surgery*. Edited by Goldwyn, RM. Boston, Little, Brown, 1972, pp 11–33.
8. Gifford S: Emotional attitudes toward cosmetic breast surgery: loss and restitution of the "ideal self.", in *Plastic and reconstructive surgery of the breast*. Edited by Goldwyn RM. Boston, Little, Brown, 1976, pp 103–122.
9. Goldstein DL: Psychology of the prospective plastic surgery patient. *Journal of the Medical Society of New Jersey* 66:647, 1969.
10. Goldwyn RM: Operating for the aging face. *Psychology in Medicine* 3:187, 1972.
11. Goldwyn RM: Reconstruction after mastectomy. *Archives of Surgery* 110:246, 1975.
12. Hoopes JE, Knorr NJ: Psychology of the flat-chested woman. *Aesthetic surgery of the face, eyelid and breast*. Vol 4. Edited by Masters FW, and Lewis JR. St. Louis, Mosby, 1972, pp 145–148.
13. Kolin IS, Baker JL, Bartlett ES: Psychosexual aspects of mammary augmentation. *Medical Aspects of Human Sexuality* 8:88, 1974.
14. Linn L, Goldman IB: Psychiatric observations concerning rhinoplasty. *Psychosomatic Medicine* 11:307, 1949.
15. MacGregor FC, Schaffner B: Screening patients for nasal plastic operations: some sociologic and psychiatric considerations. *Psychosomatic Medicine* 12:277, 1960.
16. Meyer E, Jacobson WE, Edgerton MT, et al: Motivational patterns in patients seeking elective plastic surgery: 1. women who seek rhinoplasty. *Psychosomatic Medicine* 22:193, 1960.
17. Reich J: The surgery of appearance: psychological and related aspects. *Medical Journal of Austria* 2:5, 1969.
18. Stern K, Doyom D, Racine R: Preoccupation with the shape of the breast as a psychiatric symptom in women. *Canadian Psychiatric Association Journal* 4:243, 1959.
19. Sontag S: The double standard of aging. *Saturday Review* Sept. 23, 1972.

Chapter 21

An Overview of Problems in Sexual Functioning

Carol C. Nadelson

Complaints about problems with sexual functioning in heterosexuals as well as homosexuals are seen more frequently now than they were in the past. This is related to the social acceptability of acknowledging sexual difficulties as well as to the knowledge about the causes and treatment of these disorders.

Sexual complaints may be at the level of desire, performance, or gratification. However, "sexual dysfunctions" are specific disorders of coital performance which are caused by physical and/or psychogenic factors. Those symptoms which are based on the lack of interest in sexuality are more related to intrapsychic or interpersonal problems and thus they are not specifically dysfunctions.

Sexual dysfunctions may be classified as primary or secondary. An individual with a primary dysfunction has never, under any circumstances, successfully completed a specific sexual act. Thus, the man with primary impotence has never been able to maintain an erection long enough to have successful intercourse, and the woman who suffers from primary anorgasmia has never had an orgasm under any circumstance. Those individuals with secondary dysfunctions report previously successful attempts. The problem may be situational or it may be related to a chronic progressive problem, for example, impotence in the diabetic man.

CAROL C. NADELSON, M.D. • Psychiatrist, Beth Israel Hospital; Associate Professor of Psychiatry, Harvard Medical School; Director, Medical Student Education, Department of Psychiatry, Beth Israel Hospital, Boston, Massachusetts 02215.

SEXUAL RESPONSE CYCLE

In order to discuss sexual dysfunctions a brief review of the sexual cycle is necessary.

The cycles of both female and male can be divided into four phases.[1] Evidence from studies of the male cycle indicates that there is a biphasic response. Erection is primarily mediated by one component of the autonomic nervous system (the parasympathetic nervous system), and the emission phase of ejaculation by another (the sympathetic nervous system), as well as by somatic nerves.[2] Clinical evidence from dysfunctional syndromes in females suggest that similar mediation exists.[3]

1. The excitement phase is characterized by increasing blood flow into the pelvic and penile vessels. This produces erection in the male, and vaginal lubrication and genital swelling in the female. In addition, there are changes in the position of pelvic organs and an increased size of the vagina.

2. The plateau phase occurs when there is maximal enlargement and vascular engorgement of pelvic organs with shifting positions of organs, including elevation of the uterus. Immediately prior to ejaculation in the male is the period called ejaculatory inevitability. This is a time when it is no longer possible to voluntarily inhibit ejaculation. There is no comparable period in the female cycle. Thus the female cycle can be interrupted by internal or external stimuli at any time while, after a certain point, the male cycle cannot be interrupted.

3. Physiologically the orgasmic phase in the male occurs with ejaculation. It consists in the male of involuntary contractions of the muscles surrounding the base of the penis and of the penile urethra. The female response is similar. It is important to note that while the emotional components of orgasm may vary from individual to individual and may be affected by the partner, the time, and the situation, the physiological process remains the same.

4. The resolution phase results in an abatement of the vascular congestion and a return to the previously unexcited state. For the male there is a refractory period, during which time the excitement phase cannot recur. This period of time varies primarily with age. It may last for a few seconds in adolescents, or it may take several days in a man who is over 70. There is considerable individual variation, and no specific "normal" time. For the female, the absence of this phase means that multiple orgasms can occur in rapid succession. The pattern of multiple orgasms, however, does not occur in all women. In fact, those women who are multiorgasmic may not be all of the time. There are a number of women who do not reach orgasm at all, or who only reach

orgasm by masturbation and not by intercourse. There is no reason to believe that this is a pathological situation, but it appears to be a variant of functioning, within the "normal" range.[2]

SEXUAL DYSFUNCTIONS IN WOMEN

There is considerable confusion in the conceptualization and classification of female sexual dysfunctions. The term frigidity is a catch-all term which has meant many things, including failure to be erotically stimulated, and/or inability to achieve orgasm. Kaplan's[2] classification scheme is based on the same sexual response cycle as exists in the male.

1. *Sexual unresponsiveness*[3] most closely approximates the more common usage of the term *frigidity*, and refers to inhibition of sexual arousal. The woman experiences a lack, or inhibition, of sexual feelings. Physiologically, she suffers from an impairment of the early or vasocongestive part of the cycle, so that she does not have sufficient vaginal lubrication or change in vaginal size. The etiology of this problem includes negative attitudes about sexuality, psychological problems, or difficulties in a particular interaction with a partner. This symptom rarely has an organic etiology.

2. *Orgasmic dysfunction* occurs in sexually responsive women who do not reach orgasm when aroused and it rarely has an organic basis. It occurs most often in women with fear or anxiety about loss of control or unrealistic expectations about sexual performance, that is, if the woman believes that orgasm should occur only via coitus she may feel that she or her partner is inadequate. Anxiety appears to be mobilized at the moment of impending orgasm with the resultant involuntary inhibition of the reflex.

3. *Vaginismus* is defined as the involuntary spastic contraction of the outer one-third of the vagina, and it thus interferes with sexual intercourse. It is also rarely organic in etiology. It can be considered a conditioned response often to a previously traumatic sexual experience. It may or may not be related to psychological problems.

This symptom may account for many of the cases which were called "imperforate hymen" in the past. Severe vaginismus may entirely prevent intercourse. Women with this symptom often avoid coitus because they experience severe pain, thus pain may be the presenting problem. A definitive diagnosis can only be made on physical examination.

4. *Dyspareunia* or *painful intercourse* is perhaps the most common disorder causing sexual difficulties in women. Since the pain is frequently organic in etiology, a careful medical evaluation is essen-

tial. Pain may result from disorders involving the vaginal opening, clitoris, vagina, uterus, Fallopian tubes, and/or ovaries so that each area must be carefully examined. Another cause of dyspareunia may be related to insufficient lubrication, because sexual excitation is minimal. Since some couples do not engage in foreplay sufficiently stimulating to cause excitation and lubrication, they often need to change or modify their technique or their attitudes toward sexuality. Another cause may be related to changes in the vagina following menopause, resulting in insufficient lubrication.

ETIOLOGY OF SEXUAL DYSFUNCTION

The symptoms of sexual dysfunction are generally nonspecific. A particular physical disorder or psychological characteristic is not necessarily responsible for a particular symptom. The same sexual problem in one person may well have a different, even opposite, cause in another. In order to eliminate any potential organic causes, or to assess the relevance of factors like age, pregnancy, cardiac disease, radical surgery, etc., an adequate sexual history and physical examination is necessary. Since sexual dysfunctions exist within relationships, both partners and the relationship should be evaluated. The factors which must be considered before specific treatment can be recommended include motivation for therapy and the coping mechanisms and ability of each partner to adapt, as well as physical or psychological disorders.

While sexual dysfunction symptoms are often multifactorial, they can be divided into three basic groups, depending on whether the etiology is primarily physical (3–20 percent of sexual dysfunction, depending on the specific population studied), primarily psychological, or combined. In this latter group, an existing organic problem can result in psychologically based symptoms. For example, a person with cardiac disease may lose interest in sex because of anxiety about possible cardiac damage. Or, a person who has had radical surgery may have serious problems with body image resulting in sexual symptomatology.

PHYSICAL CAUSES OF SEXUAL DYSFUNCTION.[1,2] The physical causes of sexual dysfunction can be grouped according to the mechanism of action:

1. Dysfunction related to biochemical-physiological factors producing systemic effects. These include disorders of major organs, i.e., heart, kidneys, etc. as well as infections and malignancies. The effect on sexual functioning is generally related to decreased libido and thus sexual arousal or potency is impaired. General debilitation, pain, or

depression are the major problems. Specific effects can also result from tumor, infection, or hormonal changes, related to the disease process or to the treatment changes.

2. Dysfunctions caused by anatomic or mechanical interference primarily with local genital or adjacent structures. These include disorders producing pain, local damage, or irritability such as infection, vaginitis, or allergic reactions. Approximately three-fourths of women treated with radiation for cervical cancer have sexual dysfunction following therapy.[4] At times intercourse in advanced pregnancy may be uncomfortable.

3. Dysfunctions occuring following surgical procedures. These occur because of damage to genitals directly or indirectly by interfering with nerve supply or hormone production. Women may have dysfunctions if they have had severe obstetrical trauma or as a complication of hysterectomy.

4. Neurologically related dysfunctions. These include disorders where there is damage to the brain [tumor, trauma, cerebrovascular accident (stroke)], or when spinal cord damage occurs (multiple sclerosis, surgery, or trauma). In the case of brain damage the primary effect is a change in libido or motor ability. With spinal damage libido is generally not affected, but the ability to have orgasm changes.

5. Drugs and Medications. Drugs or medications can affect sexual responses directly or indirectly by changing sexual responsiveness, by interferring with the nervous system, or by altering the blood flow to an organ. The effects of drugs are difficult to assess because mood, personality, and perception are variable, especially with drugs like LSD and marijuana. Drugs that are most frequently used and do alter sexual performance in women include alcohol and barbiturates. Although these are usually considered depressants, in small amounts they reduce anxiety and inhibition, and thus can increase sexual responsiveness. Psychotropic medications for anxiety or depression appear to have a similar effect. They may improve sexual behavior because of reduction of anxiety or depression, but they also have been reported to decrease sexual interest.

Psychological Aspects of Sexual Dysfunction. The psychological factors in sexual dysfunctions may be related to past and/or current issues. Recent therapeutic approaches, originating with Masters and Johnson,[1] have attempted to modify the immediate antecedents of sexual problems and to treat problems using behavior modification techniques. These may, however, ignore the more remote causes. Kaplan[2] has utilized a multicausal and integrated approach with more limited goals than those of traditional psychotherapy or psychoanalysis. The attempt is to relieve the sexual dysfunction symptom where possible, rather than affect personality change or marital harmony. Often people who are seen for sexual therapy have had previous psychotherapy or seek it afterward. This is probably related to the complexity of the symptomatology, and to the issues that are uncovered during the therapy.[1,2,5,6]

Kaplan[2] considers the dysfunctions to be the physiological concomitants of anxiety, rather than defenses against the emergence of anxiety which result from the reactivating of early feelings and fantasies. This concept implies that stress may result in symptoms like sexual dysfunction. Thus, illness, life-threatening situations, anger, or even lack of attraction to a partner may produce a symptom.

Since sexual responsiveness is complex, and since aspects of the physiological component are reflexive once they are initiated, sexual function is successful when a person is relaxed, undistracted, and not consciously monitoring performance or involved in obsessive ruminations. The psychogenic factors which are etiologic in the symptoms reported are related to early sexual attitudes and experiences that include (1) lack of information because of ignorance, fear (of pregnancy, venereal disease, etc.), unrealistic expectations (bells ringing or supreme ecstasy), or persistence of myths (simultaneous orgasm is necessary or men are always interested in having sex, but women are not); (2) negative family or societal attitudes which may produce guilt, anxiety, or dislike of sexual practices; (3) past history of a traumatic sexual experience such as rape or incest; or (4) homosexual experiences which may produce anxiety about sexual identity or partner choice.

Situational factors may include family or work stress, marital communication problems, infidelity, or boredom. Differences in life stage and interests between partners are often important factors.

Problems related to deeper intrapsychic and interpersonal issues range widely from simple performance anxiety when there has been a previous history of failure in sexual functioning to serious depressions. Sexual symptoms may serve as an entree into psychotherapy for some people. The major psychological problems producing sexual symptoms are related to:

1. *Low self-esteem.* This may be manifested by fear of failure or rejection, performance anxiety, or concern about sexual identity.

2. *Dependency.* For the individual who is dependent the desire for a sexual relationship may be secondary to the need to be taken care of.

3. *Depression.* There are multiple etiologies for depression and it is important for these to be clarified before treatment is recommended. One must distinguish between a depression caused by a sexual dysfunction, which can be treated by behaviorally oriented and other specific techniques, and a depression which causes sexual problems

and must be treated primarily as a depression, using psychotherapy and/or drugs.

4. *Control issues.* When erotic feelings and orgasm are perceived as a dangerous loss of control, the individual may respond defensively. People with problems in this area often report that they go through the motions of sexual involvement but are unable to experience sexual feelings. They become "spectators" or they develop obsessional and unrelated thoughts which diminish their sexual pleasure.

5. *Communication problems.* If these are limited to the physical and sexual aspects of the relationship, they may be amenable to a behavioral approach therapeutically. They may, however, be an indication of more extensive difficulty in the relationship, requiring another type of therapeutic approach. At times couples insist on direct sexual therapy (behavioral approach) when it is not appropriate. In such cases it may well be ineffective because it produces pressure for communication and arouses the anxiety which had been masked by the symptom.

6. *Symptoms related to earlier unresolved conflicts.* Early life conflicts involving parents or siblings may be related to the development of sexual symptoms. Thus, during pregnancy, when a wife becomes a mother or a husband becomes a father, the partners may begin to experience changes in sexual feelings related more to conflicts in their relationships with their parents than to the reality of their current relationship.

THERAPEUTIC PRINCIPLES

While there are a number of methods of treating sexual dysfunctions, we will consider the developments of the past decade beginning with the pioneer work of Masters and Johnson,[1] since their method has yielded better treatment results for problems, where the indications are appropriate, than have other treatment techniques. Their work has also provided the impetus for further study, and for the development of therapeutic modifications. We will not consider more traditional forms of individual, couple, and group therapy, since treatment of sexual dysfunctions by those techniques does not differ substantively from the treatment of other disorders by those techniques.

The "new" sex therapies involve treatment procedures for specific dysfunctional syndromes, not for sexual orientation or gender identity problems. The most successful model of treatment involves a synthesis of theory and procedure from several perspectives, with a focus on psychological understanding of the partners. An attempt is made to modify the immediate antecedents of sexual difficulties, recognizing that deeper roots exist, but assuming that resolution of many symptoms can occur at a more superficial level.

When viewed from a transactional systems perspective, the relationship itself, rather than the individuals, are considered together and an attempt is made to clarify and resolve the reciprocal dynamics which lead to the disorder. Learning theory principles are utilized in the process of identifying the mechanisms by which problematic transactions occur, in order to provide appropriate behavioral modifications. The symptom, then, is seen as the disorder, rather than as the symptom of an underlying disorder. This is not inconsistent with, but can expand, a psychodynamic understanding. In addition, some understanding of how roles are established and maintained is useful in working with couples with sexual problems.

In order to succeed in their sexual functioning a couple must be able to develop mutual trust and avoid being judgmental, overcritical, or needing to maintain control. Since guilt and performance anxiety also impair function, and treatment may intensify anxiety, the couple must also be prepared to tolerate this. Resistance to progress in therapy arises because the discussion and the specific exercises do increase anxiety. Most often resistance appears first in excuses about not having had time to do the assigned exercises. Occasionally there may be anger, attempts at sabotage, or complaints that the exercises are too mechanical. The firm support of the therapist is most critical in facilitating progress despite these negative feelings. However, because of the sensitivity of the situation, the therapist must be cautious and have a good understanding of each partner before proceeding.

There are several general operational principles in the approach to the therapy of sexual dysfunctions:

1. *Shared responsibility of the couple.* It is assumed that regardless of the specifics of the etiology of a symptom, the treatment is a shared responsibility. It is not acceptable to place blame or to focus specifically on one partner as the one with "the problem."

2. *Permission for sexual enjoyment.* Sexuality is seen as a way of communicating, sharing, and relaxing. Partners are encouraged to be spontaneous and less rigid in their definitions of acceptable sexual behaviors, or in the times and places they choose for sexual enjoyment.

3. *Decreased pressure to perform coitus.* There is more emphasis on enjoyment of sensuality without requiring orgasm each time.

4. *Communication is emphasized.* Partners are encouraged to understand and accept each other's values, preferences, and differences as "normal."

5. A *time limit* keeps the pressure to progress at optimal levels, prevents the couple from falling into prolonged patterns of resistance,

and prevents involvement in more complex psychodynamic issues which can be counterproductive for some couples. On the other hand, periodic reevaluations are important so that if the therapeutic approach is not effective it can be modified or changed. The use of modification of techniques and interventions such as more psychodynamically or system-oriented work may be helpful.

6. *Conjoint or cotherapy with a male/female therapy team.* The validity of this principle has been debated. Masters and Johnson[1] feel that it is critical, since it provides the support of a partner of the same sex, and also decreases the intensity of the transference response to the individual therapist. Others, including Kaplan,[2] feel that an experienced therapist of either gender, provided that person is well-trained in traditional therapies as well as sexual therapy, is suitable. The author's experience indicates that it is important to have therapists of each gender when one of the partners demonstrates more extensive psychopathology and/or when the modification of treatment may take the form of individual meetings interwoven with couples meetings.[6]

Treatment of Sexual Dysfunctions

The basic therapy format proposed by Masters and Johnson involves two weeks away from home and work, devoted totally to the treatment. While this has been reported to be extremely successful, it is not easily adaptable. The financial and time commitments for both patients and therapists may be prohibitive. In addition, their approach may not be applicable in all situations. It is often the case that those people who are ready to consider going to the Masters and Johnson clinic may already be on their way to successful treatment by that time.[6]

Sex therapy clinics have arisen in all parts of the country, adapted to meet the specific problems and characteristics of the populations involved, as well as the motivation and resistances of specific patients. Currently there is no one method that is applicable to all problems. Cultural and individual differences are important considerations. Techniques range from those oriented around individuals who are involved in relationships to those that provide surrogate partners when an individual does not have a partner or when the partner cannot, for whatever reason, cooperate. This latter method raises many moral and ethical questions, as well as questions relating specifically to its psychological impact.

There are certain principles and methods used by most therapists who treat people with sexual dysfunctions. These include (1) an initial period of coital abstinence to reduce performance anxiety and facilitate communication; (2) the use of systematic tactile stimulation and exploration to focus on the substitution of giving and receiving pleasure for the exclusive goal of orgasm; and (3) specific technical suggestions and directions including sequences and variations in those techniques which facilitate and reinforce success.

FEMALE DYSFUNCTIONS

What follows here is a summary of some specific aspects of the treatment involved in dealing with female sexual dysfunctions. These will be considered briefly in this chapter and discussed in greater detail in the next chapter.

SEXUAL UNRESPONSIVENESS (FRIGIDITY). The goal of therapy is to create an undemanding and relaxed environment for sexual interaction to occur. Women with this symptom often defend themselves against erotic feelings because of guilt or fear of rejection. They need support for sensual expression. The treatment principles include:

1. Sensate focus experiences which emphasize pleasuring without demand for the first four to eight sessions. Coitus and ejaculation are generally prohibited and the couple explores a variety of nongenital, and later, genital, kinds of stimulation. The emphasis is on enjoyment. The sensate focus exercise is a critical component in the treatment of unresponsiveness as well as many other sexual problems. The permission for and encouragement of sexuality produces dramatic effects particularly if no specific sexual demands are made. It is important that the woman experiences her own sexual feelings rather than perform according to expectations or rules. She is encouraged to be more active in her participation.

2. Dispelling obsessive thoughts. "Spectatoring" is actively discouraged. Overconcern with the feelings or judgments of the partner prevents relaxation. Permission for focusing on oneself is necessary.

3. Resumption of coitus. Generally after four to ten sessions enough confidence is restored so that the couple can resume coitus. Coitus is introduced slowly and under the woman's control. Negative reactions about the experience, including disbelief that there will be any positive effect, and/or obsessive thoughts are not uncommon and may take time to work out.

ORGASTIC DYSFUNCTION. The basic goal for this treatment is to enable the patient to give up her need for controlling the orgastic response. This involves maximizing stimulation and preventing those factors which trigger the response from being activated. This is a complex task and requires a thorough understanding of the dynamics of the inhibition and/or the environmental interference. It may initially involve removing the partner. The woman can be taught to bring herself to orgasm through masturbation manually or with a vibrator, providing that she is ready to accept this practice. Fantasies are encouraged and she may need to be reassured that they are not "sick," regardless of the content. Spectatoring is discouraged.

Approximately 8 percent of the female population has been reported to be anorgastic by any means.[2] A larger percentage achieve orgasm by means other than coitus. For the woman who is primarily anorgastic the major objective is to achieve the first orgasm. This dispels her fear that she is incapable of orgasm and facilitates further progress. Treatment proceeds on the premise that the reflex has been inhibited, not destroyed, in such a woman. If the inhibition is related to unconscious determinants, then referral for psychotherapy may be necessary. Barbach has reported good results using group treatment techniques.[7] Of 83 women in her program 92 percent achieved orgasm after five weeks via masturbation, and were able to transfer this success to coitus with a partner within eight months.

Vaginismus. Treatment of this disorder involves progressive deconditioning of the involuntary spasm of the vaginal muscles. Before this can be done, the woman's phobic avoidance of vaginal entry must be alleviated. Frequently this can be initiated in the gynecologist's office with a gentle pelvic examination and the use of a series of dilators that are graduated in size. The presence or involvement of the partner may facilitate treatment. Encouragement and support are of primary importance. This is in contrast to the usual situation, where the partner may be angry and feel rejected, often not understanding the unconscious nature of the symptom, but interpreting it as willful. Psychotherapy in conjunction with this direct approach is sometimes indicated.

Treatment Results

Since the treatment modality discussed here is relatively new, and the patient populations are so variable, long-term follow-up data has been difficult to obtain. Treatment failures seem to occur when motivation is not evaluated prior to beginning therapy. It is clear that the therapist must have an understanding of physical and psychological processes in order to properly evaluate and treat sexual dysfunctions.

References

1. Masters W, Johnson V: *Human sexual inadequacy*. Boston, Little, Brown, 1970.
2. Kaplan HS: *The new sex therapy*. New York, Brunner/Mazel, 1974.

3. Kaplan HS: The classification of the female sexual dysfunctions. *Journal of Sex and Marital Therapy* 1(2):124–138, 1974.
4. Weinberg J: Dyspareunia. *Journal of Sex and Marital Therapy* 1(2):1974.
5. Meyer JK.: Psychodynamic treatment of the individual with a sexual disorder. *Clinical management of sexual disorders.* Edited by Meyer JK. Baltimore, Williams & Wilkins, 1976.
6. Nadelson C: Unpublished data, Sexual Dysfunction section of Psychiatric Out-Patient Division, Beth Israel Hospital, Boston, 1977.
7. Barbach LG: Group treatment of preorgasmic women. *Journal of Sex and Marital Therapy,* 1(2):139–145, 1974

Chapter 22

Female Sexual Dysfunctions: A Clinical Approach

Maj-Britt Rosenbaum

Female sexuality has long been seen from the male perspective. Sex was something men did to women. Women were expected to adapt to the sexual force emanating from men. *He* played the active part, she was the passive participant. This attitude is expressed by the term: frigidity, a pejorative label. It is the description of a frozen state that does not respond to the ardent flame of male sexuality. It is also a term too vague, too all-inclusive to tell us anything more than that sexuality was not freely expressed and enjoyed.[1]

Since the already classic groundbreaking work of Masters and Johnson[2,3] women have come into focus as subjects, not objects, in sexual behavior, as active participants, not passive recipients, of the sexuality of their partner. The terminology used in describing the various sexual dysfunctions, male as well as female, does not have a cohesive diagnostic framework. The author will present a clinical approach to the problems of women using a diagnostic organization which reflects current approaches in the field of sexual dysfunction therapy.

Sexuality from the Female Perspective

Before describing specific dysfunctions, it is important to focus briefly on some of the obvious differences between male and female behavior because these differences are mirrored in the way women experience sexual difficulties.

Maj-Britt Rosenbaum, M.D. ● Director, Human Sexuality Center, Long Island Jewish-Hillside Medical Center; Associate Clinical Professor of Psychiatry, Albert Einstein College of Medicine, New York 10461.

The fact that female sexuality has for so long been suppressed, culturally and individually, results in women tending to struggle under the burden of more inhibitions in the expression of their sexuality. They have been brought up to subordinate their sexual needs and to see sexuality as something to respond to, not act upon. This conditioning has at times worked so effectively that women have been able to go through a lifetime of taking part in sexual intercourse, bearing and rearing children, and never experience their sexuality in orgasm. This attitude toward the sexual lives of women is reflected in the current lack of sexual knowledge and information about female physiology, including the character of the female orgasm. Also, little has been written about the feelings women experience during sexual excitement.[4] No wonder there is many a Sleeping Beauty still waiting behind the thorny hedge of inhibitions, repressions, and defenses against sexuality.

Girls have been said to masturbate considerably less than boys. They have tended to be introduced to erotic sexual sensations in the context of petting.[5] First coital experiences are only rarely sexually satisfying to the young woman. It is unusual for a woman to experience orgasm during her first experience of intercourse, in contrast to the experience of the young man. Thus it has tended to take women longer to become familiar with and comfortable with their sexuality, to learn how their bodies feel and react when sexually aroused.[6]

Another important aspect of female sexuality is the ability of women, because of their anatomy, to take part in a full range of sexual interaction without necessarily being aroused, whereas men need some level of sexual excitement in order to proceed to intercourse. This has implications in terms of sexual control, and is also reflected in the form of many of the problems women have.

The fact that women have the capacity to become pregnant is a further important dimension in their sexual interaction. The fear or wish for pregnancy, the fear of intrusion, not only by the penis, but by the potential baby, is a crucial factor in many women's sexual behavior.

DIAGNOSTIC CLASSIFICATION

The diagnostic categories presented here are based on the sexual response cycle as set forth by Masters and Johnson.[2] They describe the phase of the physiological sexual response that has been interfered with and that will be discussed in greater detail as the chapter proceeds.

1. Problems related to lack of sexual interest, lowered libido
2. Excitement phase disorder
   a. Primary
   b. Secondary
3. Orgasmic phase disorder
   a. Primary
   b. Secondary
4. Vaginismus (Intromission disorder)
5. Dyspareunia (Pain)
   a. Organic
   b. Psychogenic
6. Relationship problems

Clinical Approach

Women's concerns tend to cluster around three main themes. The first complaint is: "I don't have orgasms," or, "I don't think I have the 'right kind' of orgasm or the right number, in the right locations, with the right partner." The second theme sounds: "It hurts when I have sex." Intercourse may be uncomfortable, there may be pain before penetration or after coitus. The third group of women state: "I don't like to have sex—I am not interested, not turned on." Among them are also the women who find sexuality disgusting, and seek to avoid it.

Let's take a closer look at these women—applying the next magnification in our diagnostic microscope.

No Orgasm. Women with this problem make up the largest group of those who seek help with sexual complaints.

It is important to ascertain whether the woman has ever had an orgasm by any means—intercourse, petting, masturbation, or fantasy. If not, she is a primary nonorgastic woman. Estimates vary as to the frequency of this disorder. Kinsey reported that about 30 percent of newly married women are anorgastic, although after ten years of marriage the figure dropped to 10 percent.[7] Kaplan estimates that 8 to 10 percent of women do not experience orgasm.[8] Among women who complain of not experiencing orgasm there are many different personal descriptions of the problem. Some women experience very intense levels of arousal, they lubricate freely, experience full and pleasurable sexual sensations in their genital area, but they are not able to achieve orgasm. Among these women are those who "spectator," who anxiously monitor their own sexual responses, who feel anxious and tense about their capacity to reach orgasm or about being adequate sexual partners; but there are also women who have not received enough sexual stimulation to trigger the orgastic reflex. These women may have partners who do not or cannot stimulate them. This, coupled with their inability to ask for or actively participate in the sexual interaction, may prevent receipt of adequate stimulation. Some women are fearful of losing control of their impulses. They fear the disruptive quality of what they imagine orgasm to be, or they fear their partners' response to their loss of control, so they hold back for fear of being ashamed or embarrassed.

Some women have actually been experiencing sexual arousal as well as physiological orgasms, but have not defined them as such. They have often expected something much more intense, earthshaking, and dramatic. They may be disappointed to learn that this is "all" there is to it. Usually they report, however, that after labeling their subjective experiences as orgasm, they relax, and often start experiencing orgasms that are increasingly more intense and pleasurable. Some women report very little sensation in their bodies when sexually stimulated. They may describe vaginal anesthesia or aversion. Some of these women have encountered traumatic sexual experiences early in life, e.g., rape. Others may have grown up in very repressive environments which precluded sexual learning, or introduced severe taboos against all sexual feelings and experiences. Vaginal anesthesia is probably best conceptualized as a conversion symptom.

The majority of nonorgastic women can be considered to have secondary orgastic dysfunction. In this group are the women who have previously experienced orgasm, but who are now no longer orgastic coitally. This may result from disturbances in the couple's relationship, or there may be organic causes, e.g., diabetes, medications, neurological disorders, or surgical conditions; or it may represent a psychological reaction to illness, surgery, pregnancy, or traumatic bodily events, such as abortion, mastectomy, or hysterectomy.

Most women report that they are able to achieve orgasm by direct clitoral stimulation, either through self-manipulation manually or with the help of mechanical devices such as vibrators, streams of water, etc., or through direct clitoral stimulation by their partner, manually, orally, or mechanically; but that they are unable to reach orgasm solely through the stimulation they receive during coitus. There is considerable controversy as to whether these women should be considered dysfunctional at all, or whether they simply represent one form of normal female sexual expression.[8] They may need more direct clitoral stimulation than they receive through coital activity. Many of these women can be helped to "bridge" the clitorally induced orgasm into a vaginally elicited orgasm; others will be reassured that an orgasm is an orgasm is an orgasm, whatever the primary mode of stimulation. An orgasm is, in the final analysis, in the mind and body of the beholder, and not in the physiology laboratory, nor in the statistical tables.

There has been too much of a tendency to focus on the purely physiological aspects of orgasm. Orgasm is a complex psychophysiological reaction, with many components, only one of which is the climactically integrated reflex activity that constitutes the physiologically measurable orgastic contractions. Another aspect is the proprioception of these phenomena, and proprioceptive capacity varies from individual to individual. Other components are the external perceptions of skin against skin, of total body contact and pressure. Most important, there is the input from the higher nervous system, the expectations, thoughts, memories, and fantasies that accompany the experience, and to such a large degree color it with pleasure, satisfaction or frustration.

PAINFUL SEX. Women who complain of pain or discomfort when they engage in sexual activity fall roughly into three categories: those with vaginismus, dyspareunia, and excitement phase disorders. *Vaginismus* in its milder forms, with some degree of tension of the muscles guarding the opening to the vagina, is not uncommon among young sexually inexperienced women. In its more severe forms, the spasm of the circumvaginal muscles is so great that nothing can be admitted into the vagina. This is often accompanied by considerable pain on attempted entry. There may be a history of having experienced one or several instances of uncomfortable or painful intercourse. Vaginismus can be conceptualized as a conditioned reflex, which may guard a phobic woman, who is fearful of painful intrusion, fearful of pregnancy, or fearful of anything entering her body and "getting lost in there." Some of these women may also experience cramplike closures of other orifices and body openings, such as difficulty in releasing the anal sphincter or a constriction of the throat.

The condition is usually relatively simple to treat by using progressive dilation, either with dilators or fingers. Vaginismus may not interfere with sexual feelings. Many women with it become very aroused during sexual activity and can attain orgasm through other means of stimulation.

Another group of women who complain of painful intercourse can be considered to have *dyspareunia*—painful intercourse. There is a tendency to ascribe the cause to psychological reasons before an adequate assessment is made. It is of paramount importance to fully investigate the possibility of an organic cause for pain, because it has a high likelihood of having an organic etiology. A careful history should be aimed at eliciting when the pain occurs; is it at the moment of penile entry? during penetration? is it vaginal or deep pain? is the pain felt genitally or in the pelvis or abdomen? does the pain subside after coitus? does it intensify after intercourse is completed? The history can give important clues to the etiology. Are we dealing with a vulvar or a vaginal infection or laceration? Is there endometriosis or ovarian pathology? Are there adhesions or torn uterine ligaments? A careful physical examination is essential before one even considers the possibility of a functional cause for the dyspareunia. I have not been impressed, in my own clinical work, with the presence of functional dyspareunia in those who are sexually aroused, although it certainly does occur. It is probably best conceptualized as a psychosomatic symptom, a compromise solution developed when a conflict exists in the sexual area, and the wish for sex struggles for supremacy with the prohibitions against it.

Pain on intercourse as the presenting symptom, should however, lead us to consider *lack of arousal*. The vagina in its nonexcited state is not adequately prepared for the entry of the penis, resulting in discomfort and irritation.

DISLIKE OF COITUS. *"I don't like sex"* is the problem of another group of women. Complaints may range from: "I don't like to have sex as often as my partner—although I enjoy it when we engage in it . . ." to, "I would give anything to be able to avoid having sex for the rest of my life!" Between these poles fall the women who enjoy sexual activity on certain occasions, or with one partner but not with another, as well as women who have come to see sex as a necessary duty and a marital chore, those who could take it or leave it. In approaching these problems the history is important. It is necessary to find out when the problem started, within what setting, and with what partner and what was the nature of the relationship? The first step for the clinician is to rule out any of the dysfunctions discussed above, all of which can lead to an avoidance of sexual activity, as it becomes decreasingly less pleasurable.

The other area to be considered is the woman's level of sexual interest. The best tool is the clinical history: Has there been a recent change in interest, perhaps related to significant life events, illness, separations, losses? Is there the possibility for an underlying depression that would lessen the sexual appetite? Is there any possibility of an endocrinological disturbance that affects libido, for example, functional lowering of the testosterone level (which "sets the thermostat" for sexual interest in men and women alike)?

On rare occasions the use of the contraceptive pill has been implicated. Although the data are not clear, it has been reported to lower libido in some women.[8] Another important factor are the changes in interest that many women experience during their menstrual cycles.

Most women report heightened interest immediately premenstrually and midcycle.[9] Although we still have a rather poor understanding of the individual variations and fluctuations in libido, we postulate a wide range of normal "appetites" in the sexual area as well as in other biological aspects of life. Although there certainly are temporal variations in sexual drive, with fluctuations depending on life circumstances, illness, etc., each individual appears to have a rather constant quantity of erotic drive that finds different expressions throughout life.[7] It is important, but often difficult, to differentiate between a low level of erotic drive activity, and a quantitatively "normal" drive, that has been suppressed, inhibited, or distorted. Acute changes in libido are often amenable to therapeutic intervention. However, some very thorny situations can arise when a man and a woman have very different levels of sexual interest. It may be hard to find a compromise and the conflict can easily deteriorate into frustration or anger. Clinically, these are among the most difficult and recalcitrant problems to deal with.

Of considerable clinical interest (and difficulty) are women who develop an increasing disinterest and, even in some cases, an aversion to sexual activity. Sexual aversion tends to be partner specific, so when it occurs, it is important to look very closely at the relationship. The woman may have unfilled expectations, hostility, and resentment. She may fear dependency or commitment or have other negative emotional reactions to her partner.

Whether determined mainly by biology or biography, women still tend to view sexuality as one aspect of a larger emotional commitment. Although there is a shift in this attitude, most women continue to be unable to derive full sexual satisfaction from a relationship that has deteriorated in its other parameters. It is of interest to point out that women often complain about not being satisfied sexually, or not finding sex pleasurable or gratifying, whereas men tend to more readily complain of performance disturbances. There are women who, in emotionally shattered relationships, may report that they still experience orgasms, but that the enjoyment has gone out of the sexual activity.

ETIOLOGY

The etiology of sexual dysfunction can have two main sources: psychological and physiological. These often have considerable overlap. It is always important to keep the physiological underpinnings in mind and to ascertain that there is no organic impediment to adequate sexual functioning. Organic difficulties tend to play a relatively smaller part in female than in male sexual dysfunction, since female sexual physiology is less vulnerable to organic problems than male sexual physiology.

Intercurrent illnesses, trauma, infection, and surgical, malignant, or degenerative changes in the genital apparatus, e.g., neurological disease, diabetes, neuropathy, as well as many medications and drugs may inhibit sexual functioning, either centrally or peripherally,[8,10,11]

Ignorance and misinformation, faulty conditioning, lack of both intellectual and experiential learning, and inadequate role models play a significant part in faulty female sexual functioning. We have alluded to the role played by cultural repressions, by the stereotypes in our society that have contributed to a double standard in sexual morality, and to the inhibiting influence of religion on the development of female sexual expression.

Other causes for sexual dysfunction which seem to play an increasingly larger role are: performance anxiety, anxious self-observation, the fear of failure, the excessive need to please the partner, and the overemphasis on genital sexual activity.[3,8] Interpersonal conflicts come to the forefront in female sexual function and dysfunction as do the quality and quantity of communication between a couple, the level of trust and intimacy, and the relative absence of rivalry and hostile destructive interaction.

In some cases the leading role is played by intrapsychic conflicts. Early development, early patterning within the original family, may have caused neurotic conflicts. When these have not been resolved, guilt, anxieties, shame, and hostilities may have to be worked out in a more traditional psychotherapeutic format rather than in a briefer therapy.

TREATMENT

Whenever the area of sexuality is discussed, it is important to provide a supportive atmosphere where the person can feel free to air difficult material. We are all, patients and professionals alike, struggling with what has for so long been a taboo area for open communication. It often takes considerable time to reverse this cultural conditioning. It is also important that professionals be aware of their own anxieties so that they are not acted out in the therapy. Premature advice, hasty judgmental comments, or rapid reassurance may hinder progress since it may serve to minimize rather than take the problem seriously.

The sexual area offers an opportunity for prevention. A considerable amount of education and information can be transmitted during contacts related more specifically to other issues. Myths can be dispelled and attitudes and behaviors can be supported. Especially critical phases of a woman's life—menarche, pregnancy, postpartum, menopause, and old age—offer excellent opportunities for an educational approach which may help avoid potential difficulties. There are many other opportunities, for example, when discussing contraception, especially in relation to an abortion or VD, where there is discussion of genital surgery, hysterectomy, mastectomy, as well as nonspecific illnesses. Sexuality is an everpresent accompaniment to the totality of a woman's life.

Many women need more specific therapy to correct or reverse a sexual symptom. These individuals may benefit from the many techniques that are being developed for the rapid treatment of sexual dysfunction. Most of them follow the basic format introduced by Masters and Johnson, whose already classic themes in these telescoped times have many new variations. In addition to the couple-oriented techniques developed by Masters and Johnson[3] conducted by a dual sex therapy team, there is an increasing amount of work being done by single therapists.[8,10,11,12]

Largely based on the assumption that many women have not had the opportunity for adequate experiential learning in the sexual area, many programs have also been developed that are aimed specifically at women, either individually or in groups. These are practical programs that in a progressively steplike fashion teach or—more correctly—allow women to freely experience the sexuality inherent in their normal bodily functions.[13,14,15,16] The time-limited direct and directive techniques developed to treat sexual dysfunction in a matter of weeks or months should be very seriously considered when a woman presents with a specific sexual dysfunction. The experience so far has been that two-thirds of the women with specific dysfunctions, e.g., excitement phase or orgasmic phase disorders, show marked improvement or reversal of their symptoms. The results in vaginismus are even more gratifying.[3,17] Work is currently under way at several centers to systematically evaluate the results of "sex therapy."[18] Further data should enable us to more precisely delineate the kind of problems that can be alleviated by short-term techniques, separating them from those that would respond better to a different treatment modality, such as individual or relationship psychotherapy.

The challenge in the field today is to effectively integrate the newer therapeutic techniques to sexual dysfunctions with other forms of medical and psychological treatment.

REFERENCES

1. Faulk M: Frigidity: a critical review. *Archives of Sexual Behavior* 2(3):257–266, 1973.
2. Masters W, Johnson V: *Human sexual response.* Boston, Little, Brown, 1966.

3. Masters W, Johnson V: *Human sexual inadequacy*. Boston, Little, Brown, 1970.
4. Hite S: *The Hite report*. New York, Macmillan, 1976.
5. Gagnon J, Simon W: *Sexual conduct*. Chicago, Aldine, 1973.
6. Rosenbaum M-B: Female sexuality or why can't a woman be more like a woman? in *Sex and the life-cycle*. Edited by Oaks WW, Melchiode A, Ficher I. Grune & Stratton, 1976.
7. Kinsey AC, Pomeroy WH, Martin CE, Gebhard PH: *Sexual behavior in the human female*. Philadelphia, W B Saunders, 1953.
8. Kaplan H: *The new sex therapy*. New York, Brunner/Mazel. 1974.
9. O'Connor J: *Behavioral rhythms related to the menstrual cycle in biorhythms and human reproduction*. New York, Wiley & Sons, 1974.
10. Meyer JK: *Clinical management of sexual disorders*. Baltimore, Williams and Wilkins Co., 1976.
11. Lief HI et al: Normal and abnormal human sexuality, in *Comprehensive textbook of psychiatry*. Vol 2. Edited by Freedman AM, Kaplan HI, Sadock BJ. Baltimore, Williams & Wilkins, 1975, pp 1349–1608.
12. Kaplan HS: *The illustrated manual of sex therapy*. New York, Quadrangle, 1975.
13. LoPiccolo J, Lobitz WC: The role of masturbation in the treatment of orgasmic dysfunction. *Archives Sexual Behavior* 2(2):163–172, 1972.
14. Kline-Graber G, Graber B: *Woman's orgasm*. Indianapolis, Bobbs-Merrill Co., 1975.
15. Kohlenberg RJ: 1974. Directed masturbation and the treatment of primary orgasmic dysfunction. *Archives of Sexual Behavior* 3(4):349–356, 1974.
16. Barbach LG: *For yourself. The fulfillment of female sexuality*. New York, Doubleday, 1975.
17. Schumacher S: Preliminary report as presented at Masters and Johnson seminar on future trends in sex therapy. New York, 1974.
18. Kuriansky JB, Sharpe L: Guidelines for evaluating sex therapy. *Journal of Sex and Marital Therapy* 2(4):303–308, 1976.

Chapter 23

The Impact of Rape

Elaine Hilberman

Any really useful discussion of rape must begin with an exploration of the meaning of rape, because empathic treatment of rape victims is contingent on one's comprehension of the meaning of the crime. The profound impact of the rape stress must be understood in the context of a crime against the person and not against the hymen. Bard and Ellison[1] remind us that victims of violent crimes in general frequently experience a life crisis which goes unrecognized. Burglary, for example, is experienced as a violation of the self in that one's home and possessions are symbolic extensions of the self. Armed robbery intensifies the stress by the added dimension of an encounter between victim and criminal. The self-violation is thus compounded by a forced deprivation of independence and autonomy, in which the victim surrenders his/her controls under the threat of violence. An actual physical assault in addition to the robbery further stresses the victim for whom the injury to the body (or envelope of the self) serves as concrete evidence of the coercive surrender of autonomy. Rape, then, becomes the "ultimate violation of the self"[1] short of homicide, with invasion of one's inner and most private space, as well as the loss of autonomy and control. In this schema, it becomes irrelevant to differentiate vaginal from oral or anal violation; it is the self and not an orifice that has been invaded. Thus, for the virgin, the prostitute, the housewife, and the lesbian, the core meaning of rape is the same.

The problems of victims of sexual assault who are courageous enough to identify themselves as such are well known. The act of reporting a rape initiates a most complex process. The victim is confronted with the usual institutional patterns of the hospital and the

Elaine Hilberman, M.D. ● Assistant Professor, Department of Psychiatry, University of North Carolina School of Medicine, Chapel Hill, North Carolina 27514.

criminal justice system, which are confusing and alien. She presents herself to these authorities at a time of crisis—one which differs from other crises in that her usual support system is more likely to be disrupted. In addition, the crisis is never limited to one's person since the victim, by the act of reporting, involves herself in a public process, so that she is at the mercy of the hospital, police, courts, media, and community opinion. Rape is an act of violence and humiliation in which the victim experiences overwhelming fear for her very existence and a profound sense of powerlessness and helplessness which few other events in one's life can parallel. The victim's needs, then, are for empathy and safety, and for a sense of control over herself, including what will happen to her in her dealings with hospitals and with the law. Without sensitivity to these needs, the experience of reporting becomes another assault.

RAPE DEFINED

Rape is defined legally as carnal knowledge of a person by force and against her will.[2,3] While male rape and statutory rape occur and present added dilemmas, the majority of victims are female. This chapter will address itself only to the female victim of forcible rape. Two elements are necessary to constitute rape: (1) sexual intercourse and (2) commission of the act forcibly and without consent. The slightest penetration by the male organ constitutes carnal knowledge; neither complete penetration nor emission is required. The concept of force includes the use of actual physical force to overcome the victim's resistance, or the use of threats which result in acquiescence because of fear of death or grave bodily harm. Rape experiences encompass a wide spectrum, ranging from a surprise attack with threats of death or mutilation to an insistence on sexual intercourse in a social encounter where sexual contact was unexpected or not agreed upon. In instances where assailant and victim have a prior relationship, nonconsent is often misinterpreted by assuming that certain social situations imply willingness for a sexual relationship.[4]

SOCIOCULTURAL CONTEXT: THE MYTHOLOGY

Until recently, the mobilization of rape crisis facilities was initiated only after a victim had been extraordinarily abused by medical and/or criminal justice institutions. The following example illustrates this:

> In the fall of 1973, a child was brought to the emergency room of a major teaching and referral hospital by a distraught mother who gave the

history that the youngster had been raped. The hospital, which had only vague procedural guidelines for the treatment of rape victims, informed the mother that her daughter would not be examined unless she had a warrant for the assailant's arrest. The parent was driven some twenty miles away to the Sheriff's office where she was told that a warrant could not be issued unless the child was first examined, and medical evidence of rape confirmed. Back at the emergency room, a physician reluctantly examined the child, but refused to tell the mother the results of the examination.[5]

In order to develop more effective services to victims of rape, it is first necessary to understand how a group of ordinarily well-meaning and empathetic individuals representing both hospital and law enforcement could have unwittingly collaborated in such inappropriate behavior. A review of the medical literature on rape through 1973 is enlightening. Most striking is the absence of any significant literature about the victim, other than that relevant to medico-legal concerns, although there were a number of articles dealing with the need to understand and rehabilitate the rapist. The reader is provided with a mass of instruction designed for medico-legal protection of the examining physician rather than the care of the victim. Further, the assumption permeates many articles that the victim was not an innocent party to the rape. Rather, she was seen as seductive, sexually promiscuous, drunk, willing, or violating some other societal norm. The burden of proof of innocence has been the responsibility of the victim. As a spokesperson for a hospital noted, "If she doesn't want to report it, she probably wasn't really raped."[6] While no such remark was made by either hospital or law enforcement in the previous case report, the existence of differing guidelines for treating the victim who does or does not wish to report or prosecute and the combined behaviors of those personnel in connection with the child victim suggest the identical attitude.

In March of 1974 a bill that would have temporarily prevented the publication or broadcast of a rape victim's name was defeated by the House Judiciary Committee of the North Carolina General Assembly. A member of that committee warned that delayed publication of the victim's name for ten days would result in the filing of capricious charges: "So many women would scream rape if they knew they could hide behind the bill. . . . I'm sitting in jail for ten days because some floozy has charged me with rape."[7] Similar attitudes are reflected in the criminal justice system, in which rape has been the only violent crime requiring corroboration. Corroboration is defined[8,9] as support of a fact by evidence independent of the mere assertion of the fact. It is not considered "supporting evidence that can be used to strengthen the prosecutor's case, it is evidence that is required to prove that rape occurred."[9] The victim's testimony, then, is insufficient grounds for conviction even if her testimony is probable and consistent.

One of the consequences of the corroboration requirement is that it is the victim who stands trial. The assumption that women will make false accusations against men "makes the victim's testimony the central object of inquiry and not the rape incident itself."[9] In the case of Coltrane v. United States in 1969, the need for corroboration was supported because "we know from the lessons of the past that all too frequently such complainants have an urge to fantasize or even a motive to fabricate. . . ."[3] This view has been given legitimacy by professionals, as in the following illustration:

> Women frequently have fantasies of being raped. Dr. Karl A. Menninger has said that such fantasies might almost be said to be universal. And in a hysterical female, these fantasies are all too easily translated into actual belief and memory falsification. It is fairly certain that many innocent men have gone to jail on the plausible tale of some innocent looking girl because the orthodox rules of evidence (and the chivalry of judges unversed in psychiatry) did not permit adequate probing of her veracity.[10]

The theme of woman as "fabricator" or liar pervades all of our attitudes about rape victims. The report of the District of Columbia Task Force on Rape concludes:

> Victorian anachronisms appear to underlie many judicial decisions as well as the verdicts of even the most representative juries. These include the suspicion that a "proper" person should have absorbed substantial physical brutality to evidence lack of consent; that prior sexual experience of any kind is reasonable evidence of possible misconduct or "provocation" on the part of an unmarried victim; that "nice girls don't get raped and bad girls shouldn't complain."[3]

This image of women as liars is likely the explanation for the assumption that women often make false charges of rape against men, even men they don't know. Law enforcement personnel are aware that false charges of crime do occur, but only in rape is it assumed that the usual safeguards in the system are inadequate to protect the innocent from a lying witness. The report of the Center for Women Policy Studies comments that

> the credibility of the rape victim is questioned more than that of any other victim of crime. This extraordinary concern for the authenticity of rape complaints is manifested in the Federal Bureau of Investigation's Uniform Crime Reports—forcible rape is the only crime for which an "unfounded" rate is calculated.[11(a)]*

---

*Unfounded refers to a complaint which is determined by the police to be unsubstantiated by the evidence or by admission of the complainant or by evidence contradicting her complaint. Within individual law enforcement agencies, however, the "unfounded" label may be used when an officer simply disbelieves the victim or when it is desirable to reduce the number of open cases.

Contrast a charge of rape with that of robbery, where it is understood that property is taken from the victim without his/her consent, and there is no need to prove that fear of death or grave bodily harm was at issue. Thus, the law grants more protection to property than to the person, especially if the person is female. The inconsistency inherent in trivializing the victim's complaint while exacting severe penalties of convicted rapists probably stems from the perception of rape as a violation of male property rather than as a violation of the victim herself.

Medical institutions, law enforcement agencies, and the prosecutory system all reflect the same mythology which society at large perpetuates about rape. Myths about rape are myriad and include the following:

1. The rapist is a sexually unfulfilled man carried away by a sudden uncontrollable urge.
2. Rapists are sick and therefore not really responsible for their behavior.
3. Rapists are always strangers.
4. Rape occurs on the street, so women can protect themselves by remaining at home.
5. Most rapes involve black men raping white women.
6. Women are raped because they ask for it by seductive dress and provocative behavior.
7. Only women with "bad" reputations are raped.
8. Women can't be raped unless they want to be, the corollary being that women actually enjoy rape.

Underlying much of this mythology is the notion that the victim is unreliable and her testimony is likely to be malicious and deceitful. The victim, then, is considered responsible for the crime. Recent changes in these attitudes which are now reflected in new legislation will be discussed later in this chapter.

Sociocultural Context: The Reality

A variety of studies serve to document the distortions implicit in culturally determined attitudes about rape. The reality, as summarized by Griffin, stands in sharp contrast to the mythology:

> Rape is an act of aggression in which the victim is denied her self-determination. It is an act of violence which, if not actually followed by beatings or murder, nevertheless always carries with it the threat of death. And finally, rape is a form of mass terrorism, for the victims of rape are chosen indiscriminately but the propagandists for male supremacy broadcast that

it is women who cause rape by being unchaste or in the wrong place at the
wrong time—in essence, by behaving as though they were free.[12]

In 1971, Amir reported on 646 victims and 1292 offenders.[13] In his
sample, the age of the victim varied from infancy to old age, although
most victims tended to be young women in the age group 15–24, and
most assailants were under the age of 30. The majority of reported
rapes were intraracial, with rapist and victim of the same race.

Three-quarters of the rapes involved one or two assailants (single
rape, 57%; pair rape, 16%), with group rape (three or more assailants)
the pattern in 27% of cases. Of the total number of incidents, 71%
were planned in advance, and only 16% could be considered explosive. Group rapes were planned in 90% of cases and single rapes in
58% of cases. These data challenge the "uncontrollable urge" theory of
rape. While the mythology of rape suggests that staying at home is
safe, 56% of rapes occurred in the victim's residence. In only half of
the cases was the rapist a stranger to the victim; the remainder included casual acquaintances, neighbors, boyfriends, family friends,
and relatives. Husbands are not included in these statistics because a
sexual act between husband and wife is not usually considered rape,
although many women would challenge this view.

In Amir's sample, physical force was present in 86% of cases, the
remainder involving various kinds of nonphysical force, such as coercion and intimidation, with or without weapons. Amir characterized
physical force in the following way:

Roughness (holding, pushing around) · · · · · · · · · · · · · · · · 29%
Nonbrutal beating (slapping) · 25%
Brutal beating (slugging, kicking,
    beating by fists repeatedly) · 20%
Choking and gagging · 12%

Thus, in one-third of the cases in which physical force occurred, extreme brutality was evident. When group rape occurred, there was
higher frequency of both alcohol intake and prior criminal records
among the assailants, especially of sexual offenses. The assault was
usually planned and was more brutal, with the victim subjected to
sexually humiliating practices in addition to the rape. These statistics
do not include rape which ends in death because these are usually reported in the homicide statistics rather than in rape statistics.

Victim behavior was described by Amir as submissive in 55%,
with some degree of resistance in the remainder. At the time of the as-

sault, the victim must decide whether she has a greater fear of the rape
itself or of the potential for physical injury. Her actions will reflect her
decision. Thus she is faced with a dilemma; resistance increases her
chance of escape, but also increases the likelihood of violence toward
her should she not escape. Victim-coping strategies before and during
the rape itself have been described by Burgess and Holmstrom.[14]

The most significant finding in studies of rape is that rape is a
crime of violence rather than passion, with the purpose of rape to hu-
miliate and debase the victim.[13,15,16] Groth and Burgess, reporting on
their work with victims and offenders, conclude that rape is a pseudo-
sexual act in which sexuality may play an important role but is not the
primary objective of the offender.[16] In their group of 133 offenders,
most were either involved in a consensual sexual relationship or had
access to nonforcible sexual outlets, and in no case was it necessary for
the man to rape for the purpose of sexual gratification. The assailants
made no attempts to negotiate a consenting relationship with their
victims, but used intimidation and assault immediately. Fifty-three
percent had a prior conviction for rape and 63% demonstrated an
escalation of force and aggression during their assaults over time
while none evidenced a decrease in brutality. Motivation for the assault was judged to be anger and/or power. The angry assailant used
more force than was necessary to overpower the victim, and the rape
was viewed as an expression of hatred and revenge against women.
The focus for the assailant motivated by power was domination and
conquest rather than savage brutality, with gratification and strength
achieved by putting the victim in a helpless position.

Amir suggests that rapists are a danger to the community because
they are violent and aggressive. While they often appear psychiatrically normal, they tend to have criminal records of offenses against
the person, these offenses usually committed with brutality and violence. In his series, rapists tend to be young members of lower class
subcultures in which masculinity is expressed by displays of aggressiveness, which include sexual exploitation of women. This is most
evident in group rape, in which aggressive behavior is not the result
of deviant sexuality, but of participation in a group which condones
the use of force in attaining goals. Brownmiller summarizes this
theory of the "subculture of violence" as follows:

> Within the dominant value system of our culture there exists a subcul-
> ture formed of those from the lower classes, the poor, the disenfranchised,
> the black, whose values often run counter to those of the dominant culture,
> the people in charge. The dominant culture can operate within the laws of
> civility because it has little need to resort to violence to get what it wants.
> The subculture, thwarted, inarticulate and angry, is quick to resort to vio-

lence; indeed, violence and physical aggression become a common way of life. Particularly for young males.[17]

One might extend this hypothesis to suggest that the rape phenomenon serves to reflect an aspect of the prevailing relationship between the sexes. Rape can be seen as an acting out of cultural norms, in which the rapist is not a deviant, but an extremist, whose behavior is an overt manifestation of culturally approved activities in which one segment of society dominates another.[18] Rape as a ritual of power has been the focus of considerable scrutiny by feminists, among whom Brownmiller emerges as a most articulate spokesperson. She suggests that rape has the same meaning for women as did lynching for blacks:

> A world without rapists would be a world in which women moved freely without fear of men. That *some* men rape provides a sufficient threat to keep all women in a constant of intimidation forever conscious of the knowledge that the biological tool must be held in awe for it may turn to weapon with sudden swiftness born of harmful intent. . . . Men who commit rape have served in effect as frontline masculine shock troops, terrorist guerrillas in the longest sustained battle the world has ever known.[17]

VICTIM SILENCE

Judge Hale's often quoted remark that rape "is an accusation easily to be made and hard to be proved, and harder to be defended by the party accused, tho never so innocent" is a remarkable distortion of the victim's experiences in the criminal justice system. Not only is rape the fastest growing of the Index crimes against the person,* but among these it has the lowest proportion of cases closed by reason of arrest.[11(a)] In 1974, only half of the reported rapes led to an arrest, and 40% of men arrested were never prosecuted. Of the remaining 60% who were prosecuted, half were acquitted or had cases dismissed.[19] In Denver, for example, 950 cases were reported to the police in 1971–72, and only 41 cases were brought to trial.[20]

According to the Uniform Crime Reports released by the Federal Bureau of Investigation, 46,430 women were victims of rape in 1972.[19] This volume represents an 11% increase over 1971, and a 70% increase over 1967. In 1974, there was an estimated total of 55,210 forcible

*The *Uniform Crime Reports* released annually by the Federal Bureau of Investigation defines the Crime Index offenses as murder, forcible rape, robbery, aggravated assault, burglary, larceny-theft, and motor vehicle theft. These were selected because of their seriousness, frequency in occurrence, and likelihood of being reported to law enforcement. Index crimes against the person (violent crime category) include murder, forcible rape, aggravated assault, and robbery, while the remaining Index crimes comprise the property crime category. "Unfounded" complaints are not reported in the *Uniform Crime Reports*.

rapes, an 8% increase over the preceding year, and a 49% increase over 1969. Federal Bureau of Investigation comparative statistics confirm that rape is the fastest growing of the violent crimes. While better reporting may account for part of the increase, it is felt that these statistics do not reflect the actual incidence of rape. It is estimated that between 50 to 90% of rape cases go unreported. The Federal Bureau of Investigation attributes underreporting to "fear and/or embarrassment on the part of the victims."[19] The victim anticipates public accusation of provocation or active participation in the rape. She is fearful of the reactions of those close to her, even her husband, boyfriend, parents, or friends. In the case of a young victim, the parents may wish to protect the child from the publicity and the trauma of the legal process. If the assailant is a close friend, relative, or employer, there are additional pressures not to report.

While the natural channels for reporting are hospitals and law enforcement agencies, many women trust neither of these institutions to deal with rape. Hospitals suffer from lack of personnel trained to work with victims both in the crisis period and in follow-up, and from lack of consistent and clear procedures for evidence collection. In the absence of formal policies for the treatment of victims in crisis, personal attitudes and fears prevail on the part of the staff, both with regard to the victim and the criminal justice system. A clinician, then, might choose to disbelieve the victim rather than to face the prospect of a court appearance. Similarly, law enforcement agencies also suffer from lack of personnel identified and trained to work with rape victims. The victim who reports the crime does not receive consistent treatment because of high rates of police turnover, rotating shifts, and personal attitudes. The woman may equate reporting with prosecution, or she may be fearful of harrassment by law enforcement officials if she reports and does not want to prosecute. Finally, both reporting and prosecution entail some exploration of the victim's life and past; if she prosecutes, these become public record.

Unfortunately, there is considerable reality to these fears, since jurors represent a microcosm of society in which we see:

> two different facets of the female stereotype in the mythology of male supremacy. On the one hand, the female is viewed as a pure delicate and vulnerable creature who must be protected from exposure to immoral influences; and on the other, as a brazen temptress, from whose seductive blandishments the innocent male must be protected. Every woman is either Eve or Little Eva—and either way, she loses.[21]

Gates cites a 1966 study of jury trials where the factors which influence judges and juries were explored.[22] In rape cases in which there was no extrinsic violence, one assailant, and no prior acquaintance of the victim and the assailant, the judge and jury would have reached the same conclusion in only 40% of cases. In the remaining 60%, the judge would have convicted where the jury acquitted. The judges concluded that in the absence of external evidence of violence, jurors ascribe to the complainant some contributory or precipitant behavior.

There are three major elements of the legal defense in a rape case, as delineated by Hibey[8] and Connell:[9]

1. Identification. The man accused was the perpetrator of the crime.
2. Penetration. A sexual act took place.
3. Lack of consent. Intercourse was not a voluntary act on the part of the woman.

Consent is usually the issue on which court cases hinge. Most laws demand a high degree of resistance from the victim, based on the belief that a healthy woman cannot be forcibly raped. A growing number of statutes appear to recognize that the amount of resistance depends on the circumstances of the attack and the implications of continued resistance so that victim compliance is not a sign of consent, but of futility. The report of the Center for Women Policy Studies comments on this issue:

> When and how a woman should resist a rapist are under hot debate. . . . The few published studies of convicted rapists indicate that there are three or four different categories of offenders whose motives, methods, and reactions to resistance differ. Since rapists do not wear identifying labels, a woman cannot know which type she is confronting. . . .
>
> An important element of any program on defense against rape should be emphasis of the right of the woman to submit. Although some people successfully resist robbery, others are killed in the attempt, so no one is counseled to fight a robber. Although there are different values at stake, the choice should still be the victim's. Even a person who wants to resist and is trained to fight may be unable to do so when confronted with a situation which she or he perceives as dangerous.[11(d)]

Consent is considered an affirmative defense in which the occurrence of the event is not disputed, but legitimized or excused.[8] Since the success of the consent defense depends on which version of the facts the jury will believe, the defense must not only make their case believable, but must also make the other side unbelievable. This is done largely through evidence of the complainant's general character or reputation for unchastity, the implication being that prior consensual intercourse whether with the defendant or someone else denies the woman the right to choose her sexual partner.

In addition to the complex social forces deterring reports of rape, the victim has a set of internalized beliefs stemming from her own socialization, which decrease the likelihood of reporting. She often accepts the view that the rapist is a sex-starved monster or pervert who is hiding behind some bush and hates his mother. When the reality of the rape does not coincide with this view, as it rarely does (half of the assailants are acquaintances if not trusted friends), she too is left to wonder about her own complicity in the event. She also "knows" that nice girls don't get raped and that it is not possible to rape a woman against her will, and this further contributes to her silence.

Thus, there are multiple forces which act as deterrents to reporting. One can assume that it will be necessary to create a sympathetic climate which allows the victim to identify herself to the hospital, law enforcement, and judicial systems. In 1975, the House of Delegates of the American Bar Association adopted a resolution[23] which would protect the victim from unnecessary invasion of privacy and the consequent psychological trauma. The proposed changes included the elimination of corroboration requirements which exceed those applicable to other assaults, revision of the rules of evidence relating to cross-examination of the complaining witness, development of new procedures for police and prosecution in processing rape cases, and establishment of rape treatment and study centers to aid both the victim and the offender. A number of states have redefined rape to apply to both sexes, to include oral and anal contact, and to differentiate degrees of rape contingent on the extent to which force or violence is used. Degrees of criminal conduct not requiring penetration have also been established. In Michigan and Wisconsin, for example, "sexual contact" denotes the intentional touching of the person's intimate parts or the clothing covering such areas, if the touching is construed as being for the purpose of sexual gratification. These revisions will facilitate convictions in sexual assaults where the victim shows no evidence of serious physical injury, a situation previously ignored by the criminal justice system. Resistance standards have also been revised to be dependent on "reasonable fear," that is, whether victim resistance was reasonable to expect under the circumstances of the assault. Reduced penalties for rape, in line with comparable violent crimes, should increase the likelihood of jury convictions. The impact of such changes will hopefully eliminate the distinction between victims of rape and victims of other crimes.[11(d), 22, 24]

REACTIONS TO RAPE

Rape is a personal crisis in the sense that the victim must deal with the impact and meaning of the event for herself. Rape is also a social crisis since family and friends will be strongly affected by the event. There is a possibility that there will be negative consequences in the relationship between the victim and husband or boyfriend, or in the case of child victims, parents and schoolmates.

Bard and Ellison define a crisis as a subjective reaction to a stressful life experience, one so affecting the stability of the individual that the ability to cope or function can become seriously compromised.[1] Characteristics of stressful situations which result in crisis reactions include suddenness, with no preparation time; arbitrariness, in that the event is perceived as unfair and capricious; and unpredictability, in contrast to the normal developmental or anticipated life crisis. Although reactions in crisis vary according to prior adaptive capacity, coping style, and social support, there are a set of fairly predictable responses which include disruption of normal patterns of adaptation with disturbances in eating and sleeping, diminished function, attention, and concentration span; regression to a more helpless and dependent state in which support and nurturance are sought outside the self; and increased openness and accessibility to outside intervention, which present a unique opportunity to affect the long-term outcome of the crisis. The disruption associated with a crisis may appear acutely or may come as a delayed reaction.

The first significant clinical study of rape victims was reported in 1970 by Sutherland and Scherl.[25] Their sample consisted of thirteen young social workers, all of whom were victims of rape which occurred in the context of their work setting. The authors describe a similar pattern of responses for all victims which they conceptualize as a three-phase process. Phase one, or the acute reaction, was characterized by signs of acute distress which included shock, disbelief, emotional breakdown, and disruption of normal patterns of behavior and function. The victim was unable to talk about what had happened, and was uncertain about telling those close to her, much less reporting to the hospital or police. Guilt was prominent, with fears that poor judgment precipitated the event. During this phase of overt disruption, there were many concrete concerns which demanded immediate attention: Should she tell her family, husband, lover, friends, children what had happened? What were the implications of not telling significant others? Would there be newspaper publicity? Would friends and neighbors find out? What was the likelihood of pregnancy and venereal disease? Should she have reported to law enforcement? Should she have prosecuted? Would she be able to identify the rapist? Was she in danger of another assault by the rapist? Phase two, that of outward adjustment, followed within several days to weeks after the rape with temporary resolution of the immediate anxiety-provoking issues. In an attempt to overcome her anxiety and to regain control, the victim returned to her normal life patterns. She behaved as though the crisis was resolved, thus reassuring both herself and those close to her. Sutherland and Scherl[25] comment that "this period of pseudo-adjustment does not represent a final resolution of the traumatic event and the feelings it has aroused. Instead, it seems to contain a heavy measure of denial or suppression. The personal impact of what has happened is ignored in the interest of protecting self and others." Phase three, that of integration and resolution, often went unrecognized. Depression was prominent along with the need to talk about what had happened. Emerging issues included the need to integrate the event with her view of herself and to resolve her feelings about the assailant. "Her earlier attitude of 'understanding the man's problems' gives way to anger toward him for having 'used her' and anger toward herself for in some way having permitted or tolerated this 'use.' "

Burgess and Holmstrom also reported on the crisis associated with the rape stress.[14, 26–28] On the basis of their work with 146 victims, they defined a specific "rape trauma syndrome" as a two-stage process: the immediate response in which the victim's life style is completely disrupted, and a long-term reorganization process. The syndrome includes the physical, emotional, and behavioral reactions which occur as a result of the encounter with a life-threatening event.

Immediately following the rape, there are a wide range of acute impact reactions. Emotional responses fell into two major categories, an expressed style and a controlled style. The expressed style was manifested by visible evidence of a massive affective response. In contrast, the controlled victim appeared calm and collected with little external evidence of distress, the apparent calmness reflecting shock, disbelief, and exhaustion. The primary reaction was related to the fear of physical injury, mutilation, and death, that is, the awareness that they could have been murdered. Victims learned in a profound experiential way that rape is a crime of violence and not of passion. Thus, one woman, who was the victim of repeated forced fellatio, expressed the wish to kill herself by putting a gun in her mouth and pulling the trigger.[29] Mood swings were common and included feelings of humiliation, degradation, guilt, shame, embarrassment, self-blame, anger, and fear of another assault. The primary defense was to block the thoughts from her mind as typified in the following statement: "All I want to do is put this out of my mind. I want to forget that it ever happened." Attempts to undo the event were reflected in fantasies of how she might have handled the situation differently, thereby avoiding the assault.

The wide variety of physical and physiological reactions which occurred during this time period were dependent in part on the location and extent of the injury. Complaints may refer to general feelings of soreness or to more localized pain. Specific symptoms occurred which related to the area of the body which had been assaulted. Insomnia and wakefulness were universal. Victims who were attacked in bed awoke in terror at the precise time that the rape had occurred. Appetite disturbances included anorexia, nausea, and vomiting, which must be differentiated from similar symptoms induced by the administration of hormones for pregnancy prevention.

This acute phase lasted from a few days to weeks with gradual merging into the long-term reorganization process. The manifestations of this second stage varied with the victim's age, personality style, available support system, and treatment she encountered from others. Changes in life style were prominent, with impaired level of function at work, home, and school. Many women acted on the need to get away and moved to another residence or city, while others were afraid to leave their homes, or gave up autonomy by returning to their families. Similarly, children wished to change schools or developed frank school phobias. Sleep disruptions continued, with vivid dreams and nightmares reflecting concerns about violence. Phobias appeared which seemed specifically determined by the nature of the rape experience, with fears of crowds or of being at home or outside depending on the location of the assault. An accidental physical contact on the street or the appearance of someone resembling the assailant often precipitated a panic reaction. Sexual fears were common, with a decline of interest as well as withdrawal from one's partner.

If this represents the normal reaction to rape then one can assume a more intense and complex reaction will occur in certain circumstances. The victim who is raped by a trusted friend or relative is faced with a greater burden of resolution than would be the case if the assailant is a stranger. The assailant treats the victim as an object, and if she also perceives herself as an object, she can isolate and depersonify the event in a way that is not possible with a friend. The existence of psychological problems and/or maladaptive behavior patterns prior to the rape increases the potential for pathological coping strategies following the rape. Serious medical problems either prior to or as the result of the rape may affect the outcome. Most rape counseling programs have seen victims who have been raped more than once, suggesting that some women are especially vulnerable to rape. The fact of a previous rape and its sequelae will certainly have a powerful impact on the present crisis. Other coincident life crises involving the victim's family, social network, academic or work status compound the stress. There is some preliminary evidence to suggest that a major personal crisis increases the possibility of rape occurring, in that one's energy is focused on the crisis at hand, with insufficient attention to whether or not one places oneself in a vulnerable situation.[30] The rape, then, may be followed by disabling depression, suicidal behavior, alcoholism, drug abuse, frank psychosis, or a marked increase in somatic and conversion symptoms.

In addition to the stresses already enumerated, there are also age-specific issues for the victim which vary with the developmental phase. These life stage considerations have been described by Notman and Nadelson[4] and Burgess and Holmstrom.[28] The single young woman may be sexually inexperienced, with encounters with men limited to the trusting, caring figures of her childhood, or to high-school dates. If the rape is her first sexual experience, she is likely to be quite confused about the relationship between sexuality, violence, and humiliation. If she is engaged in the process of separating from her family and in the establishment of an independent identity, her sense of adequacy may be challenged by her feeling that she really cannot take care of herself. A college student living away from home may decide not to tell her parents because of their possible insistence that she leave school and return home. The integrity of her body is also at issue, and is reflected in concerns about the pelvic examination which may be a new experience and can be perceived as being like the rape itself. The woman who has an ongoing sexual relationship may choose not to tell her partner that the rape has occurred for fear of disrupting the relationship. Her silence may realistically protect the relationship but leave her feeling anxious and guilty, and without support. The divorced or separated woman is in a difficult position because her life style, morality, and character are even more frequently questioned. The rape experience may confirm her fears of inadequacy about independence and autonomy. The woman with children must deal with the problem of what, how, and when to tell them. This becomes especially important since the event may be known in the community and at school. The middle-aged or older woman will have concerns about independence. She may already be in a crisis phase about her life role, with changes in her relationship to husband and children, role loss, and absent family members. The misconception that an older woman has less to lose by a rape than does a younger woman may seriously impede her ability to resolve the crisis.

Little information is available about the long-term consequences of rape because our awareness of rape as a crisis is recent. Clinical evidence of a silent rape reaction is documented by therapists and counselors who unexpectedly uncover the history of a previous rape in the context of ongoing psychotherapy, and find that the event is still unresolved. While it is difficult to predict all of the long-term sequelae, some of the issues which seem to reemerge at a later time are mistrust and avoidance of men, sexual disturbances, passivity in relationships, phobic reactions, and anxiety and depression often precipitated by seemingly trivial events which symbolize the original trauma.

Some general remarks about the dynamics of the victim's response to rape seem appropriate, particularly with regard to aggression. Notman and Nadelson note that the universality of rape fantasies hardly makes every woman a willing victim and every man a rapist.[4] Fantasies do not usually picture the actual violence of the experience, and while all individuals have aggressive as well as sexual fantasies, most people keep thought and action separate. The victim has had an overwhelming confrontation with the assailant's loss of control of sadistic and aggressive impulses, which serves to challenge the woman's confidence in her own defenses and controls. Further, women usually relate ambivalently to men, perceiving them as both protectors and potential aggressors. The confrontation with this violent potential has as a result a marked decrease in the woman's ability to trust men and, what is perhaps even more important, diminished trust in her capacity to control her own aggression.

Thus, it may not be surprising that there is little clinical evidence of rage in rape victims, compared with the outrage stimulated in others hearing of the rape. The anger, when it does occur, is likely to be a delayed experience. The absence of anger may be determined by a variety of issues including sex-role socialization norms in which women are discouraged from showing outward aggression, as well as environmental reinforcement for the idea that rape is a justifiable retaliatory act because the victim was provocative. It seems, however, that the encounter with the assailant's loss of control of violent impulses has a primary role in the suppression of anger by the victim. Victims themselves seem to recognize this. One victim described the impact of rape by stating, "I have become a very passive person," while another sought psychiatric help two years after an assault with the chief complaint, "Help me to get angry."[29]

Katan addresses this issue in a description of her analytic work with six adult women who were raped in childhood. The common theme for all six women was "unbelievably low self-esteem" which Katan attributes to a severe disturbance in the fusion of sexual and aggressive drives:

> My patients had no criminal or delinquent tendencies. Their aggression was turned against the self in a savage form . . . they were fragmented, they could never feel that they were whole persons. They regarded their own aggression as dangerous and raw, whether it was turned against the self or against the outside world. They felt keenly that the traumas had caused irreparable damage.[31]

Metzger, in a fictional account of her own rape, describes the violence which defines the rape encounter:

> An invasion. A tree opening to fire. And a black hollow from which no twig can emerge again. Perhaps it is a gun penetrating me and orgasm will be a round of bullets. Pain is a relief. I cherish it as a distraction from knowing. I am an enemy country. Destroy me with fire. But there is no distraction. The cloth rubs against my legs. There is a gun resting on my shoulder. I do not forget that death is the voyeur at this encounter.[32]

THERAPEUTIC INTERVENTION

It should be apparent from the elaboration of the rape trauma syndrome that it is not possible to provide a simplistic approach to the rape victim and her family. Nevertheless, it will be useful to indicate those areas in which intervention is necessary.

In the aftermath of rape, a complex sequence of events leads to rapid involvement of the victim with medical and law enforcement personnel. Issues of personal safety and control emerge as primary concerns. The victim has just had an experience in which her very existence has been threatened, with total loss of control over her fate. Her immediate needs are for a sense of physical safety as well as for assistance in assuming some control over what has happened to her and what will happen to her in her dealings with both individuals and institutions. The presence of an empathic and supportive individual, who may be a counselor, clinician, or friend, will enhance her sense of safety and her ability to deal with the crisis. She must be allowed to talk and to ventilate her feelings, with reassurance and validation of her responses. Whether this occurs in the police station, the physician's office, or the hospital emergency room, the issues are the same. She is dealing with new personnel, institutions, and procedures, and the availability of accurate information about medical and legal procedures allows her to regain control by making choices based on informed consent. The victim may or may not wish to report to the hospital or law enforcement, and this is her right. For obvious reasons, coercion has no place in the management of the rape victim.

Medical treatment usually takes place in a hospital emergency setting and has the following goals:[33, 34] (1) immediate care of physical injuries; (2) prevention of venereal disease; (3) prevention of pregnancy; (4) proper medico-legal examination with documentation by evidence collection for law enforcement; and (5) prevention or alleviation of permanent psychological damage. It is not the function of the clinician to decide whether the victim has "really" been raped. Rape is a legal and not a medical term. The fact that the victim perceives herself as having been violated remains the essential fact. Hospital treatment is facilitated by a team treatment model, the team consisting of a physician, nurse, and counselor/advocate, all of whom have clearly defined roles and a collaborative relationship with each other. Because victim treatment involves an interface between medicine and the law, programs designed by medical facilities should optimally be part of a community-oriented approach, in which there is a cooperative effort by hospitals, citizen groups, and criminal justice agencies.[5,11(b),35] Interagency collaboration must not, however, jeopardize the victim's right to confidentiality.

All recent reports stress the need for immediate availability of crisis counseling for victims with some indications that continued counseling, either formal or informal, may be necessary for as long as twelve months.[1,4,11(d),26–28,35–37] There appear to be three assumptions regarding counseling about which there is a consensus: (1) crisis intervention will facilitate working through of the trauma and diminish the likelihood of long-term psychopathological consequences; (2) the victim needs emotional support from whomever she comes in contact with during the crisis period; and (3) rape is a crisis for family members and friends and they also need emotional support.

The goal of counseling is to restore the victim to her previous level of functioning as quickly as possible. The victim is assumed to be an individual who was managing her life adequately prior to the crisis. Since the rape stress disrupts the victim's life in physical, emotional, social, and sexual areas, all of these issues are appropriate areas for scrutiny. The following are important foci for intervention in the immediate phase: the assault and the victim's relationship to the assailant; medical concerns; criminal justice implications and the decision to report or prosecute; anticipated responses of both the victim and those significant to her; and physical safety when she returns home.[5,28]

Special mention is made of the victim's social support system because her fear that the rape may affect or change her relationship with those who are important to her is invariably an issue in the immediate crisis period. In contrast to most personal crises in which the importance of sharing the crisis with loved ones is reinforced, there exists for rape victims a very real possibility that the revelation may disrupt the relationship. A husband may perceive the rape as an infidelity while parents may accuse an adolescent victim of irresponsible behavior. When the victim chooses to share the information, family counseling becomes important in sensitizing the victim's social network to the meaning of rape so that they are able both to work through the crisis themselves and to provide honest support to the victim.

Lest we think we really know how to treat victims, here is a victim who speaks directly and poignantly about her needs:[18]

> there is no treatment for rape other than community. Therapy or [consciousness-raising] can be helpful as long as no "cure" for a "condition" or "disease" is implied. Rape is loss. Like death, it is best treated with a period of mourning and grief. We should develop social ceremonies, rituals, for rape which like funerals and wakes allow the mourners to recover the spirits which the dead and rapists steal.

In a historical context, it has been women themselves who first identified rape as a traumatic event and a sexist act. As a result, the last decade has witnessed the spontaneous appearance of a nationwide anti-rape movement which currently involves both citizen groups and professionals. The eradication of rape is contingent on educating and sensitizing our society to the meaning of the crime and the context in which it occurs. Innovative and empathetic services to victims will serve as a deterrent to the crime by facilitating reporting and, thereby, apprehension and prosecution of assailants. Ultimately, however, the elimination of rape will require a reconsideration and restructuring of social values as well as a reordering of the relations between the sexes. When the sex roles of both men and women are defined by individual needs and talents, rather than by stereotypic expectations based on sex and power motives, there will be an end to rape.

REFERENCES

1. Bard M, Ellison K: Crisis intervention and investigation of forcible rape. *The Police Chief* 41(5):68–73, May 1974.
2. Evrard J: Rape: the medical, social and legal implications. *American Journal of Obstetrics and Gynecology* 111(2):197–199, September 1971.
3. *Report of the public safety committee task force on rape.* Subcommittee of the District of Columbia City Council. City Hall, 14th and E Streets, N.W., Room 507, Washington, D.C., July 1973.
4. Notman MT, Nadelson CC: The rape victim: psychodynamic considerations. *American Journal of Psychiatry* 133(4):409–413, April 1976.
5. Hilberman E: *The rape victim.* New York, American Psychiatric Association Basic Books, 1976.
6. Largen MA: A report on rape in the suburbs. Northern Virginia Chapter of National Organization for Women, 1973.
7. Raleigh News and Observer. March 22, 1974.
8. Hibey RA: The trial of a rape case: an advocate's analysis of corroboration, consent, and character, in *Rape victimology.* Edited by Schultz LG. Springfield, Ill., Charles C Thomas, 1975.
9. Connell N, Wilson C (eds.): *Rape: the first sourcebook for women.* New York, New American Library, 1974.
10. Guttmacher M, Weinhofen H: *Psychiatry and the law.* New York, Norton, 1952.
11. *Rape and its victims:* a report for citizens, health facilities, and criminal justice agencies. Prepared by Center for Women Policy Studies, Washington, D.C., April, 1975.

The report consists of four separate handbooks: (a) *The police response,* (b) *The response of medical facilities,* (c) *The response of prosecutor's offices,* and (d) *The response of citizen's action groups.* Copies are available from Law Enforcement Assistance Administration, 666 Indiana Avenue, N.W., Washington, D.C. 20531.

12. Griffin S: Rape: the all-American crime. *Ramparts, 10*:26–35, September 1971.

13. Amir M: *Patterns of forcible rape.* Chicago, University of Chicago Press, 1971.

14. Burgess AW, Holmstrom LL: Coping behavior of the rape victim. *American Journal of Psychiatry 133*(4):413–418, April 1976.

15. Sheppard DI, Farmer DJ: *Operation rape reduction: summary and recommendations of the national rape reduction workshop.* Denver Anti-Crime Council, 1313 Tremont Place, Suite #5, Denver, Colorado 80204, 1973.

16. Groth AN, Burgess AW: Rape: a sexual deviation. *American Journal of Orthopsychiatry 47*(3):400–406, July 1977.

17. Brownmiller S: *Against our will: men, women and rape.* New York, Simon & Schuster, 1975.

18. Metzger D: It is always the woman who is raped. *American Journal of Psychiatry 133*(4)405–408, April 1976.

19. Uniform Crime Reports for the United States. Prepared by the Federal Bureau of Investigation, Washington, D.C., 1972 and 1974.

20. Giacinti TA, Tjaden C: *The crime of rape in Denver.* Prepared for the Denver High Impact Anti-Crime Program. Denver Anti-Crime Council, 1313 Tremont Place, Suite #5, Denver, Colorado 80204, 1973.

21. Johnston JD Jr, Knapp CL: Sex discrimination by law: a study in judicial perspective. *New York University Law Review 46*(4):704–705, October 1971.

22. Gates MJ: *The rape victim on trial.* Presented at Special Session on Rape, American Psychiatric Association, Anaheim, California, 1975.

23. *American Bar Association Journal 61*:464–65, April 1975.

24. Wood PL: The victim in a forcible rape case: a feminist view, in *Rape victimology.* Edited by Schultz LG. Springfield, Ill., Charles C Thomas, 1975.

25. Sutherland S, Scherl D: Patterns of response among victims of rape. *American Journal of Orthopsychiatry 40*(3):503–11, April 1970.

26. Burgess AW, Holmstrom LL: The rape victim in the emergency ward. *American Journal of Nursing 73*(10):1740–1745, October 1973.

27. Burgess AW, Holmstrom LL: Rape trauma syndrome. *American Journal of Psychiatry 131*(9):981–86 September 1974.

28. Burgess AW, Homstrom LL: Rape: victims of crisis. Bowie, Maryland, Robert J Brady, 1974.

29. Hilberman E: Unpublished case reports.

30. Nadelson CC, Hilberman E: Personal communication.

31. Katan A: Children who were raped, in *Psychoanalytic study of the child,* Vol 28. Edited by Eissler R, Ford A, Kris M, Solnit AJ. Yale University Press, 1973, p 208.

32. Metzger D: *Skin: shadows-silence.* West Coast Poetry Review, Reno, Nevada, 1976.

33. Massey JB, Garcia CR, Emich JP: Management of sexually assaulted females. *Obstetrics and Gynecology 38*(1):29–36, July 1971.

34. *Suspected rape.* ACOG Technical Bulletin Number 14, July, 1970 (revised, April 1972).

35. McCombie SL, Bassuck E, Savitz R, Pell S: Development of a medical center rape crisis intervention program. *American Journal of Psychiatry 133*(4):418–421, April 1976.

36. Hayman CR, Lanza C: Sexual assault on women and girls. *American Journal of Obstetrics and Gynecology 109*(3):480–486, February 1971.

37. Wasserman M: Rape: breaking the silence. *The Progressive 37*:19–23, November 1973.

Chapter 24

A Gynecological Approach to Menopause

Johanna F. Perlmutter

Menopause is a very specific period of time in which the cessation of menses occurs. It is a diagnosis that can only be made retrospectively after one year has elapsed. The term "menopausal years" is actually a misnomer. What one usually means is the perimenopausal years which includes premenopause (that period of time leading up to the menopause), the menopause itself, and postmenopause (those years which follow the cessation of menses).[7]

In the United States, the average age of menopause is 49 years.[1] Approximately 80 percent of women will be symptomatic to some extent. Most complaints are of a minor nature and not bothersome, but may persist over prolonged periods of time. Less than a third of women are sufficiently uncomfortable to seek and pursue medical attention. Onset of symptoms, severity of complaints, and their duration cannot be predicted.

There are multiple disorders that have been ascribed to the changing hormonal balance and are equated with menopause. In reality, not all the changes that are noted are secondary to hormonal imbalances. The normal aging process is occurring concomitantly and is responsible for some of the symptoms that the patient may experience. In addition, we are living in a society which is oriented toward the young and does not revere and honor old age. Thus, the real changes caused by aging and hormones are compounded by societal pressures, fears, diminishing job security, and the degenerating integrity of the family unit.

JOHANNA F. PERLMUTTER, M.D., M.P.H. • Assistant Professor, Department of Obstetrics and Gynecology, Beth Israel Hospital, Harvard Medical School, Boston, Massachusetts 02215.

To date, there has been minimal research done on the endocrinologic alterations that occur during the perimenopausal era and their specific effects on the body. The result is that the available information is sparse and there is minimal concrete knowledge. Most reports are based on small samples, subjective findings, and bear the influence of the emotional status of the patient, clouding the issues even further. Even when factual material has become available, its relationship to symptomatology is not always clear-cut or evident.

ENDOCRINE CHANGES

The hormonal pathways for ovulation and the menstrual cycle have been worked out and are fairly well understood. Even in this area, knowledge is not complete and new hormones, pathways, releasing factors, and more intricate knowledge of what we thought we already knew have broadened our scope, clarifying issues in some instances, and causing further confusion in others. In addition to the ovarian-hypothalamic-pituitary axis, one must not forget the role of the adrenal gland in the production and synthesis of steroid hormones, particularly at the time of menopause and postmenopausally. The adrenal gland is probably responsible for most of the steroid hormones produced during the postmenopausal years and supplies small amounts of androgen, some of which is converted peripherally to estrogen.

In its simplest form, menopause can be described as a decrease in estrogen levels, accompanied by increasing gonadotrophin levels (FSH and LH). The organ systems that are involved are the hypothalamus which apparently has a regulatory effect on the pituitary, producing releasing factors which influence the pituitary to produce and release the gonadotrophic hormones. These, in turn, stimulate the ovaries to produce their hormones. The ovarian hormones that are secreted have a negative feedback effect on the hypothalamus, reducing the amount of releasing hormone being produced, thus preventing the gonadotrophins from being produced. When the ovarian hormonal level falls to a low enough level, the releasing factor and gonadotrophins are again produced in quantity. This continues on a cyclic basis until the menopausal years approach. The ovary no longer responds and estrogen levels begin to wane. The hypothalamus continues to secrete releasing factors in large quantities in an attempt to elevate the circulating estrogens. This leads to excessive production of LH and FSH (the gonadotrophins). This is an overall view and an individual look at each hormone is necessary.

ESTROGEN. During the reproductive years, the granulosa cells in the ovaries produce estrogens (estradiol, estrone). As the ovary begins to fail, the production of active estrogen begins to decline. Following menopause, the estradiol blood levels decline by over 90 percent. The levels of estrone fall by only 70 percent. It is felt that the production and availability of estrone postmenopausally is by peripheral conversion of steroids mainly of adrenal origin.[8]

PROGESTERONE. This hormone is produced as a result of ovulation. It is not found in the postmenopausal female.

ANDROGENS. Androstenedione, testosterone, and dehydroisoandrosterone are the three androgenic substances that can be found both premenopausally and postmenopausally. It is felt that both the ovary and the adrenal glands contribute to the production of these androgens. Androstenedione is of particular importance since it can be directly converted to estrone and can also be converted to testosterone which can further be converted to estradiol. It is felt that the stromal cells of the ovary produce these androgenic substances and that this process probably continues postmenopausally. The circulating levels of these hormones do not change drastically from the premenopausal to the postmenopausal years. There has been some conjecture that the ovarian production of androstenedione and testosterone does not diminish through the menopause and that the ovarian stroma continues to produce these hormones postmenopausally.

VAGINAL BLEEDING

The manifestations of menopause are primarily the result of ovarian dysfunction and not uterine in origin. The cessation of menstruation or more properly, vaginal bleeding, is evidence that the ovaries have stopped functioning. Cyclic vaginal bleeding is usually referred to as menstruation. There is controversy as to whether the term menses refers to any periodic bleeding or is confined to that which follows an ovulatory cycle. For the purposes of this chapter, the terms vaginal bleeding and menstruation will be used interchangeably.

It has been taught that the number of ovulatory cycles is minimal at the time of puberty, rising to a maximum in the 20's, and gradually diminishing in number until the menopause per se is reached. Recent evidence has shown that although the number of ovulatory cycles diminishes as menopause is approached, anovulation, as determined by the temperature chart, is infrequent. Unless a basal body temperature is taken, it is difficult to determine which cycles are ovulatory since vaginal bleeding continues to occur at more or less regular intervals.

The most typical bleeding pattern that is noted is a shortening of the menses and lengthening of the interval between periods as total cessation of menses is approached. Eventually there is no further bleeding and menopause has been reached. Indeed, for those women who are sexually active, this type of bleeding pattern provokes anxiety. Pregnancy is always a consideration when the menses have either been missed or are very light. Pregnancies have been reported in women in their 50s. It is therefore mandatory that adequate contraceptive measures be utilized until the diagnosis of menopause has been firmly established. The rhythm method of contraception cannot be practised effectively because of the loss of cyclicity, regularity, and rhythmicity of the cycle. On occasion, the menses appear to be regular until total cessation of bleeding occurs. In these instances, the periodic rhythmicity of the cycle is maintained. Bleeding at the time of the period is reported as either normal or slightly lighter. The menses cease abruptly and menopause has begun. This is not seen as frequently as the scanty irregular period but is another variation of normal.[4]

Infrequently, other forms of vaginal bleeding are encountered. This may manifest itself as a heavier period. Clots may be noted. Prolonged and even profuse bleeding may occur once in a while. Bleeding, spotting, or staining may occur midcycle or at unexpected or unpredicted times. In addition, postcoital spotting may be noted.

Bleeding is usually called "dysfunctional" when no etiology for the abnormal occurrence can be found. It is thought to be the result of a hormonal imbalance. Progesterone, the hormone that is produced as a result of ovulation, matures the endometrium (the lining of the uterus) so that the contents are shed at the time of menstruation. In the absence of this hormone, or if it is produced in inadequate quantities, an irregular shedding of the endometrium may occur accounting for some of the abnormalities listed above. In addition, other causative factors of unusal bleeding include cervical polyps, endometrial polyps, cervicitis, and vaginal infections. Appropriate diagnosis and treatment of the lesion involved will usually correct the irregular bleeding pattern. These are benign conditions that are usually not harmful to the patient.

In any instance of abnormal bleeding (heavy menses, prolonged periods, intermenstrual or postcoital bleeding), the main consideration and concern is for the small number of women who have either a cervical or uterine malignancy. In order to reassure the patient that cancer is not present, a dilatation and curettage (D and C) is performed. This will provide optimal care by allowing early diagnosis and treatment to be instituted. On occasion, the D and C is curative of the bleeding even in the absence of a definitive diagnosis.

Once the diagnosis of menopause has been established, any form of bleeding is not normal. Genital tract malignancies are the prime consideration but not the prevalent etiology. Other causative factors are inappropriate and prolonged usage of hormones, vaginitis, and atrophic vaginal mucosa.[5]

VASOMOTOR INSTABILITY

This term refers to the lability of the blood vessels that occurs during the perimenopausal years. It is manifested as hot flashes, flushes, episodes of perspiration, or attacks. It has been described as the sudden onset of a feeling of warmth that pervades the upper part of the body. The face becomes flushed and reddened, and patchy red areas may appear on the upper chest, back, shoulders, and upper arms. This may be accompanied or followed by profuse perspiration. As the body temperature readjusts to its surroundings, the woman may feel cold and clammy. This is one of the most common signs of approaching menopause with up to 75 percent of women noting it to some degree. The frequency with which this symptom occurs is variable: weekly, monthly, daily, or even every few hours. The length of time that the flash lasts will vary from individual to individual and from time to time for any one woman. The duration may be anywhere from a few seconds and mild to over half an hour and quite intense. Moreover, approximately 20 percent of women will be symptomatic 5 years postmenopausally if left untreated. In general, the onset is gradual and sporadic and may go unnoticed for several months or years. As the actual time of menopause approaches, the flashes become more frequent and more intense. This then wanes in the postmenopausal period.

The etiologic agent in the production of hot flashes is unknown. They are probably hormonally mediated, although anxiety, stress, and excitement may precipitate and aggravate an attack and increase and prolong the discomfort.[3]

Chronologic time does not seem to affect the exhibition of these vasomotor symptoms. Hot flashes or flushes may occur during the day or at night. In general, those women who experience hot flashes at night also experience similar episodes in the course of the day. A change in dress style in daytime apparel, with the clothing taking on a layered appearance, may provide more comfort since it permits one to acclimate to the sudden elevation in body temperature by shedding a jacket at a moment's notice. At night, the flushes may be sufficiently disturbing to disrupt one's sleep. In rare cases, the perspiration is sufficiently profuse that night clothes and bed linens may need to be changed. This may cause interruption and disturbance of sleep for the entire family and may be sufficient to cause a tired, fatigued, and irritable household the next day.

Traditionally, vasomotor symptoms have been thought to be a consequence of the ovary's failing production of estrogens. Replacement therapy with estrogen will alleviate the symptomatology in most women. And yet, other disease processes in which estrogen levels are low, such as stress amenorrhea and anorexia nervosa, are not characterized by hot flashes. The role of the hypothalamus and/or the pituitary gland and the elevated levels of the hormones that they produce has yet to be clarified in this process.

ATROPHIC CHANGES

The skin, the subcutaneous tissue, and the mucosal linings of the body undergo atrophic changes as a normal progression of the aging process. This wasting process begins many years prior to the onset of menopause. There is a loss of elasticity and tissues appear to hang loosely and droop. For example, the round, firm, high breasts of the adolescent begin to sag and hang well before the climacteric. The entire skin surface no longer appears taut but hangs loosely, a condition that is particularly noticeable on the upper arms.

With the hormonal changes of the menopause, the natural moisture of some tissues is also lost, accentuating the atrophic changes. As a result, some dryness, reduction in lubrication, and thinning of tissues is noted:

Skin. The tissue appears wrinkled and shriveled from the aging process. For the woman who has always had difficulty in moisturizing her skin, the menopause and postmenopausal era may increase the dryness, and pruritus (itching) may develop. The woman with oily skin may not be as cognizant of these changes. Skin creams and lotions may provide temporary relief from the dryness and itching.

Nasal Mucosa. An unpleasant smell or odor may be created when dryness of the mucous membrane in the nose occurs. Estrogen replacement therapy may be necessary to control this condition. This is not one of the common sequelae to menopause.

Eyes. When the tissue in this area shows evidence of drying, the tearing process may be disrupted and the normal moisture of the eyes is lost along with the inability to cry with tears. Since moisture is essential to prevent eye damage, estrogen replacement therapy is warranted if this disorder arises. This is an infrequent result of the climacteric.

The Cervix and Uterus. This organ system shrinks in size. The cervix no longer produces any mucus. One is usually totally unaware of these changes except for the inability to reproduce and the absence of menstruation.

Ovaries. With the failure to produce ovum and the resultant diminution in estrogen and progesterone production, the ovaries decrease in size. The woman is usually not cognizant of the ovarian size change.

Vagina. This area is mucosal and will show the atrophic changes of aging as well as the hormonal changes of the menopause. It becomes thin and dry, and does not stretch or expand as effectively as it had. Intercourse may become painful because of these changes as well as because lubrication during sexual excitement is not produced as rapidly or in as great a quantity as was the case prior to menopause. A greater amount of foreplay may be necessary to produce adequate lubrication and prevent dyspareunia. In some cases, local application of estrogen cream may be necessary.

If coitus does not occur at all during the menopausal years, the vagina may actually shrink and become a small, semirigid tube that is no longer distensible. If sexual relations are resumed or initiated postmenopausally, dyspareunia may be marked. Gradual dilatation of the vagina with dilators may be required in addition to the local application of hormonal preparations.

The altered hormonal balance changes the pH of the vagina thus modifying the bacterial flora of the vagina. An increased incidence of vaginal infections is the end result. "Senile vaginitis" is the descriptive terminology associated with this entity. The usual therapy for vaginitis may not be as effective postmenopausally because of the altered vaginal flora. In repeated, persistent vaginal irritations, local hormonal therapy may be of value.

Perineum. The labia majora, the labia minora, and the mucosa covering the clitoris, urethra, and introitus will all undergo atrophic changes. A decrease in size of the labia majora prevents them from protecting the urethra and the vagina. These orifices are then exposed to and unprotected from outside influences. Even soft underwear can cause abrasions and irritations to these sensitive areas. Extra care must be taken so that inflammation and secondary infections do not occur.

Prolapse. The mixture of aging and hormonal changes leads to a loss of elasticity and thinning of the tissues in the pelvic area. Specifically, the vagina, urethra, bladder, uterus, and rectum no longer have good support structures. The resultant marked relaxation causes a prolapse or falling of these structures into the vagina. In extreme cases, the descent of these tissues may be beyond the vaginal orifice.

Stress Incontinence. A mild form of relaxation of the tissues will lead to minimal prolapse but still allow enough laxity to distort the normal relationships between the bladder and the urethra. The end result is an involuntary loss of urine which can occur during one's usual daily activity. It is most embarrassing and humiliating to the woman afflicted with it. Coughing, sneezing, laughing, or exertion may evoke some urine loss. This may vary from a few drops to copious fluid at one's feet. The urinary odor may be constant and pervade the clothing and habitus and be most distressing. Exercises to strengthen the muscles and tissue may be sufficient in mild cases to effect a cure. Frequently, surgical repair is necessary.

Urinary Tract Infections. Changes in the anatomical structure that occur following menopause may alter the position of the urethral orifice. It may now point directly into the vagina. Constant exposure of the urethra to the bacterial flora of the vagina can lead to recurrent urethritis and urinary tract infections. In addition, mechanical irritation of the urethra during intercourse occurs because of the loss of subcutaneous tissue between the vagina and the urethra. This may mimic urethritis and give the same symptoms. It may also aggravate a preexisting inflammation.

A cystocele (relaxation of the tissues around the urinary bladder) can lead to incomplete emptying of the bladder. Stasis of fluid can be influential in the development of infection. It is sometimes difficult to determine whether a woman's urinary symptoms are a result of infection, mechanical irritation, cystocele, or all three.

Constipation. The smooth muscle at the intestinal wall may relax along with other tissues and prevent the intestines from working as efficiently as they have in the past. This process promotes the development of constipation. Dietary changes and stool softeners may be necessary to alleviate the problem.

OSTEOPOROSIS

This disease process is characterized by a loss of calcium from the bones. The increased porosity that occurs from this process leaves the bones soft and capable of being compressed. This is of particular importance in areas where the bones bear pressure or have muscles pulling on them. The spinal column, specifically the vertebrae, are the most common structures to be affected. The collapse of the vertebrae leads to the shortened, stooped stature of the aged. Common complaints associated with this are chronic back pain and muscle spasms. The final outcome of the shortened spinal column with weakness and relaxation of the muscles of the back, is a stooped, bent-over, hump-backed, uneasy-gaited person who is more prone to tripping and falling. The loss of calcium leaves all the bones brittle, allowing them to break easily and frequently. Tripping or minor falls may result in fractured bones. Bed rest and immobilization of the affected area or broken limb causes increased demineralization which enhances and compounds the problem.

This is the end result of an asymptomatic process that probably began around age 40 years. It is usually difficult to make the diagnosis until the process is very extensive and well established. One must rely on radiologic evidence of calcium loss. This does not usually occur until the disease process is far advanced. This will frequently be in a woman who is 60 or 70 years old and well past the menopause. Clinical diagnosis by symptoms alone is not possible. There are no specific complaints that are pathognomonic of this disease process. The signs and symptoms may mimic and be the same as many complaints that deal with low back pain: overexercising, bruises, muscle spasms, and vertebral fractures.

The reasons for the excessive calcium loss is unknown. A degree of calcium loss is seen in both men and women, although severe osteoporotic changes are much more prevalent in women. The loss of ovarian hormones coupled with inadequate adrenal steroids is one of the postulates for the etiology of this disease. Estrogen replacement therapy will slow down the process of demineralization but not halt it completely nor will it recalcify the bones. Increased dietary intake of calcium will decrease the rapidity of the demineralization but will not remineralize the bone once it has become osteoporotic.[2]

Depression

Emotional disturbances have been reported in 10 to 30% of women who are menopausal. These difficulties probably have little to do with the altered hormonal balance. It has been shown that 50% of those women who have had emotional difficulties in the past will have an exacerbation of these problems around the time of the menopause.

This is one of those areas in which many factors interplay making it difficult to delineate a single etiologic factor. Along with the loss of estrogen goes the ability to reproduce. This is about the same period of time that children begin to express their need to be independent and frequently leave home. In addition, communication problems between partners that have been present for many years become apparent. Job and financial security may be threatened as young, bright, eager employees come looking for new positions. These problems may only be enhanced by emotional lability and instability, crying spells, apprehensiveness, nervousness, fatigue, irritability, depression, insomnia, decreased memory, and inability to concentrate. Estrogen replacement therapy may give a feeling of euphoria and well being and benefit some women but does not cure the basic, underlying, psychiatric difficulty.[6]

CHANGES IN PHYSIQUE

The body configuration or contour changes with the menopausal process and with aging. Advancing age and decreased activity reduces the need for a high caloric intake. If diets and calories are sustained and continued and not modified and adjusted downwards, weight gain and obesity develop. Moreover, with the hormonal changes, there is an apparent and real distribution of fat. The hips broaden and the waist becomes thicker with the development of the middle-aged spread. Subcutaneous tissue from the upper arms decreases leaving a flabby appearance. Lack of exercise will further lead to loss of muscle tone and enhance the appearance of flabbiness.

The breasts, which had begun to sag premenopausally, lose some of their subcutaneous tissue. The breast tissue itself, therefore, appears smaller. The skin above it appears more wrinkled and makes the breast appear to hang more. Estrogen replacement therapy will not replace breast turgor.

Most distressing to many women is the appearance of coarse hairs around the chin line. This "beard" makes them poignantly aware of their loss of femininity.

OTHER SYMPTOMS

Headaches are probably unrelated to the menopausal era. Most often, this is a prior complaint that becomes exaggerated at this period of time. Initial occurrence of headaches at the time of menopause is extremely rare.

True insomnia has not been correlated with menopause. With the aging process, the amount of sleep that is required diminishes. One does not need to sleep long periods in order to be rested. If true insomnia becomes apparent and is distressing, it may be a symptom of other difficulties in one's lifestyle becoming manifest at this period in one's life.

Libido (sex drive) has been noted to change. It has been reported to increase, to decrease, and to remain the same. For the most part, those women who have had an enjoyable sex life, will continue to do so. Those women who have never enjoyed sexuality will probably not delight in this activity during or after menopause.

Chronic Illness

With the aging process, the menopausal female must also face an entire gamut of illnesses and maladies. Elevated blood pressure, stroke, diabetes, cancer, and heart attacks become more prevalent as one approaches and passes menopause. These diseases are independent of menopause and occur concomitantly. There is a real need for routine annual physical examinations; early detection and treatment of disorders will avert and possibly prevent fatal outcomes.

Surgical Menopause

The extirpation of the uterus at the time of hysterectomy precludes further vaginal bleeding. The term total hysterectomy refers to removal of the uterus and the cervix and does not include the ovaries.* Surgical loss of the uterus will result in cessation of the menses and inability to reproduce. The signs and symptoms of menopause will not appear immediately but, rather, will become evident when the woman reaches her 40s, or when she would have naturally gone through these changes.

In contrast to this, any procedure which leads to ablation of ovarian function, e.g., surgical removal of the ovaries with or without hysterectomy or radiation therapy to the pelvis, will trigger the abrupt onset of menopause. In particular, there is the sudden onset of vasomotor symptoms. The lack of gradual and insidious onset of these symptoms may make their appearance seem more intense and disconcerting. As the body readjusts itself to its new hormonal milieu, the hot flashes will gradually wane and eventually disappear. It is of interest to note that not all women whose ovarian function has been terminated artificially will experience menopausal symptoms. Some women report mild or no symptomatology. This is another area in which we do not understand the role of the hormones in the production of the usual earmarks of the menopause.

Treatment

The treatment of the menopause has been aimed at those symptoms which are thought to be a result of hormonal deprivation. The

*Editor's note: Not all physicians are in agreement with this definition.

most success has been achieved with the treatment of the vasomotor symptoms. Therapy has been aimed at the replacement of the missing hormones.

Estrogen has been given in a cyclic fashion in sufficient doses to control the hot flashes. It is usually administered daily for 21 days with a 7-day rest period following. Some physicians prefer to give the estrogen alone on an intermittent basis during the week. Other physicians feel that in the woman who is still menstruating it is more advantageous to give the cyclic replacement therapy with the addition of progesterone from days 14 to 21 of the cycle, thus mimicking the more natural cycle.

The advantages to giving estrogen replacement are that most women will have relief of the vasomotor symptoms. And, if in addition, dryness has been noted of the vaginal mucosa, the nasal mucosa, or the eyes, this will help lubricate these tissues. Moreover, hormonal replacement has been equated with a feeling of well being, euphoria, and an improvement in one's self-image. To balance this, the disadvantages of estrogen therapy are the severe medical complications that may arise from using this type of drug. Estrogens have been implicated in the development of phlebitis and secondary pulmonary embolus. A statistically increased number of women who have taken these hormones have developed endometrial cancer. Additionally, these hormones can initiate breast nodules and malignancies in experimental animals. It is thus important that this type of hormone not be used injudiciously, and the woman should be under medical surveillance.

Androgens, testosterone in particular, have also been given for relief of menopausal symptoms. This is usually utilized in those women who are unable to take estrogens. These drugs do not work as effectively nor in as large a percentage of women. A deepening and lowering of the voice and the appearance of coarse hairs and a hirsute appearance make these drugs less than ideal.

The use of tranquilizers in some women may bring some of the vasomotor symptoms under control and secondarily aid a coexisting depression. This treatment is the least effective of the modalities listed.

Many women do not wish to take any internal hormones or medications but are concerned about the dyspareunia. Local vaginal creams containing estrogen may be utilized and are very effective. Topical estrogen hormones can be absorbed systemically. This therapy should be instituted and maintained with the woman under medical surveillance.

Skin creams containing estrogen will not restore the firmness to the skin. In addition, when used in large quantities, it is possible for the hormones to be absorbed in sufficient quantities to raise systemic estrogen levels and cause vaginal bleeding, mimicking a malignancy. This is frightening to the woman and her physician and may lead to unnecessary surgical procedures in an attempt to determine the etiology of the bleeding.

It should be emphasized that most women go through their changes with minimal difficulty. In addition, a mild or modified symptom picture is more typical. The majority of the manifestations of menopause that have been described do not have an abrupt onset but rather are gradual in their appearance.

The menopause and the aging process are so intertwined that it is difficult to separate out the chronology of events and the specifics of each process. Knowledge is limited and minimal research has been done to date on this phase of life. It is hoped that future research will clarify issues, and more specific treatment and therapy will be made available.

REFERENCES

1. Beard RJ (ed.): *The menopause*. Baltimore, University Park Press, 1976.
2. Campbell S (ed.): *The management of the menopause and post-menopausal years*. Proceedings of an International Symposium, London. Baltimore, University Park Press, 1976.
3. *Clinical guide to the menopause and the postmenopause*. New York, Information Publishing, 1960.
4. Goldberg MB: *Medical management of the menopause*. New York, Grune & Stratton, 1959.
5. Greenblatt RB: Diagnosis and management of abnormal bleeding in the menopausal patient. *The Female Climacteric* 2(2):3, 1971.
6. Kerr M: Emotional/hormonal aspects of the menopause. *The Female Climacteric* 2(1):3, 1971.
7. Kupperman HS: Management of the principal symptoms in the menopausal patient. *The Female Climacteric* 1(1):3, 1969.
8. van Keep PA, Greenblatt RB, Albeaux-Fernet M (eds.): *Consensus on menopause research*. Proceedings of the First International Congress on the Menopause, La Grande Motte, France. Baltimore, University Park Press, 1976.

Chapter 25

Menopause

Pauline B. Bart and Marlyn Grossman

They call me Grace.
Yesterday I went
to the grocery store.
I had filled up
the cart
and was half way through
the check stand
before I realized
I had shopped for the whole family.
The last child left
two years ago.
I don't know what
got into
me.

I was too embarrassed
to take things back
so I spent the week cooking
casseroles.
I feel like one of those
eternal motion machines
designed for an
obsolete task
that just keeps on
running.

From *Voices*
A play by Susan Griffin

While there is substantial evidence documenting medical misogyny [1-4] the topic of menopause does seem especially to elicit such sentiments. This may derive from the conviction of nineteenth-century medical "authorities," such as prominent gynecologist Charles D. Meigs, who described woman as "a moral, a sexual, a germiferous, gestative and parturient creature."[5] Another physician pontificated that it was "as if the Almighty, in creating the female sex, had taken the uterus and built up a woman around it."[6] Indeed historian Peter Stearns observed that in 18th- and 19th-century Europe physicians thought women decayed at menopause.[6] Victorian physicians invariably characterized it as the Rubicon in a woman's life, and medical popularizers of the day

PAULINE B. BART, Ph.D. • Associate Professor of Sociology, Department of Psychiatry, Abraham Lincoln School of Medicine, University of Illinois, Chicago, Illinois 60680.   MARLYN GROSSMAN, Ph. D. • Psychologist, Madden Mental Health Center, Hines, Illinois; Women in Crisis Can Act, Inc., Chicago, Illinois.

"blamed the frequency and seriousness of disease during this period upon the 'indiscretions' of earlier life."[7] Kellogg remarked that the woman who transgressed nature's laws will find menopause "a veritable Pandora's box of ills, and may well look forward to it with apprehension and foreboding."[7]

No substantial changes in physicians' attitudes have occurred over time. It might be surprising to some, not familiar with the pervasive sexism in current gynecological writing[3] as well as with the traditional male ambiance in medical education,[4] to learn that at a conference on menopause and aging sponsored by the U.S. Department of Health, Education and Welfare (a conference uncontaminated by the presence of a female participant), Johns Hopkins' obstetrician-gynecologist Howard Jones characterized menopausal women as being "a caricature of their younger selves at their emotional worst."[8:3]

This invalidation of menopause as a normal life cycle stage is consistent with gynecologist Wilson's warning to women that to stay "Feminine Forever" they should ingest estrogen as long as they live because menopause is a "deficiency disease."[9] (Not coincidentally, Wilson's work was funded by a drug company). Another physician compared menopause to diabetes and went on to say: "Most women suffer some symptoms whether they are aware of them or not, so I prescribe estrogens for virtually all menopausal women for an indefinite period."[10] He made this statement after publication of studies demonstrating the relationship between estrogen replacement therapy and increased risk of uterine cancer,[11,12] and long after it was established that estrogen is effective only for hot flashes and genital atrophy.[8:3]

Thus, not only have women unnecessarily been prescribed hormones but they have also incurred the risk of cancer at the same time—a risk made doubly unfortunate in light of the fact that many of these symptoms are psychologically and sociologically induced rather than physiological in origin.

McKinlay and McKinlay, in a trenchant methodological critique of the menopause literature, suggest that the failure of physicians to be more circumspect in the administration of estrogen and the failure of medical researchers to investigate fully the side-effects of estrogen therapy as well as possible alternatives to it may well stem from "its apparent effectiveness in reducing the symptoms (and therefore the complaints) and [its] ease of administration." In general, they ascribe the paucity of research on menopause, and the poor quality of what little research there is, to the related phenomena of the stigmatization of menopause in Western culture (and the sexism of physicians which perpetuates this attitude) and the unreasonable power of and false accordance of trust to physicians which has served dysfunctionally to shield the knowledge and practices of the medical profession, including the quality of their research.

> Through such phenomena, clinical experience has assumed unparalleled legitimacy as a basis of knowledge and practice, regardless of its lack of objectivity and substantiation through further, adequately controlled studies. This reliance of physicians on subjective 'experience' is particularly evident with regard to the menopause.[13]

Among the many specific defects of available research which the Mc-Kinlays note are the problems with retrospective data, the existence of inter- and intracultural differences in the recognition and definition of response to symptoms, and use of differing definitions of menopausal status and symptomatology.

Parlee's survey of the literature on the psychological aspects of the climacteric found it similarly sparse and unsatisfactory.[14] (In our review, climacteric and menopause are used interchangeably to refer to the period of the cessation of the menses). Parlee noted that the psychological aspects of menopause have received even less attention than the physiological ones. She, too, noted the male physician's bias against menopausal women, which leads them to make statements having no empirical grounding. Similarly, Osofsky and Seidenberg state that psychoanalysts frequently view menopause as a time of "mortification and uselessness," since the woman's "service to the species" is over. The authors note that:

> In contradistinction to the male, female psychology is seen as being dependent on biology. Youth, attractiveness, sex and motherhood are viewed as the important roles for women. . . . This thinking has influenced the therapy offered for menopausal symptoms. Physiologic symptoms have been treated psychologically and psychologic symptoms, physiologically.[15]

Two psychoanalysts who did early work on menopause are Therese Benedek and Helene Deutsch. Benedek comments that the tasks of the life situation at menopause are complex and demanding: (a) children leave, (b) sons marry, and (c) there are changing sexual needs between husband and wife. Declining hormonal production also can bring physical difficulties. When the woman cannot respond to or relate to her difficulties the way she did in the past, "her ego alien emotional responses threaten her." Not all women, Benedek believes, experience menopause as a time of difficulty. For example, there is a difference in tissue degeneration between those women who have borne children and those who haven't; the latter have menopause earlier and with more intense reactions. Women who have had premenstrual depression and dysmenorrhea suffer again at the climacteric.[16]

The psychological symptoms which often accompany the menopause, Benedek asserts, are "motivated by the psychosexual history of the individual."

> The climacterium is different in those women whose adaptive capacity has not been exhausted by previous neurotic processes. When the cessation of biological growth releases psychic energy which was previously employed in the reproductive tasks, this gives the flexible ego of such women new impetus for learning and socialization. The manifold interests and productiveness of women after the climacterium, as well as the improvement in their general physical and emotional health prompts us to regard the climacterium in the psychological sense as a developmental phase.[17]

As might be expected from someone whose training focuses on the intrapsychic, Benedek neglects in her analysis the major impact of social and cultural factors.

Helene Deutsch considers menopause a critical period, and "mastering the psychological reactions to the organic decline is one of the most difficult tasks of woman's life."[18:436] The course is determined by the cessation of ovarian activity with a resultant derangement of the endocrine system. Like Benedek, she frequently makes the analogy between women's behavior during puberty and their behavior during the climacterium. Because of the "cutting the psychic umbilical cord on the part of the children" the woman must focus her emotional energy elsewhere.[18:439] There may be marked changes in behavior, individual manifestations greatly varying depending on the woman's personality. "Homosexual panic" is frequent, although unconscious, causing the breakup of old friendships. The yearning for the son becomes more intense as the increased need for him is frustrated.

> Almost every woman in the climacterium goes through a shorter or longer phase of depression. While the active women deny the biologic state of affairs, the depressive ones overemphasize it. . . . hypochondric ideas appear, which in an overwhelming majority of cases relate to the genital organs.[18:473]

These "normal" depressive moods sometimes disappear and sometimes develop into a more serious melancholia. Deutsch thinks that "feminine-loving" women have an easier time during climacterium than do "masculine-aggressive ones." (Bart's data contradicts this point. She found that women hospitalized during the involutional period had higher feminity scores on the MF scale of MMPI than the average woman.)[30:115]

Although Deutsch appreciates that investment in a profession is a protection against the biological trauma of the climacterium, she also warns that women who go this route run risks.

Successful psychotherapy is difficult for women at this age, she feels, since there is so little in the way of substitute gratification to offer her, "for reality has actually become poor in prospects, and resignation without compensation is often the only solution."[18:476-477] However, a motherly woman, if she has permitted her children freedom, may now not only have good relationships with them, but also have added satisfaction from her relationships with her sons- and daughters-in-law. Furthermore she may find the role of grandmother extremely gratifying.

Stern and Prados studied fifty women who had been diagnosed on the basis of a physical exam as having a menopausal syndrome. All were of low socioeconomic status. They ranged in age from thirty-three to fifty-eight, and half were experiencing surgically induced menopause due to partial or total hysterectomy. Thirty-two were sufficiently symptomatic that they saw a psychiatrist. Hot flashes was the only physiological symptom universally present. Eighty percent (forty-one), however, experienced depression without guilt feelings or anxiety. Seventeen were depressed by their marital situation, one by downward mobility, two because of loss of children, and three for no obvious cause. They described the observed depression as having had roots in maladjustment preceding menopause. Since in ten of the twenty-two cases of artificial menopause, the hysterectomy was preceded by a period of serious marital stress, they concluded that there were somaticizing features involved.[19]

McKinlay and Jefferys conducted a mail survey which included women from all socioeconomic groups in eight areas in and around London. Although they used a mail-in questionnaire, their response rate was over eighty percent. Except for the cultural differences to be found in an English rather than American sample, this study provides some representative information on the experience of menopause. The sample included 638 women between the ages of forty-five and fifty-four.

Seventy-five percent of the menopausal women in the sample experienced hot flashes. For twenty-five percent of the women whose menses had ceased for at least a year, hot flashes continued for five years or more. The other six symptoms which were specifically inquired about, headaches, dizzy spells, palpitations, sleeplessness, depression, and weight increase, showed no direct relationship to the menopause but did tend to occur together, each being reported by approximately thirty to fifty percent of the respondents. Frequency of symptoms was not related to employment outside of the home nor to domestic workload. Despite the fact that three-quarters of the women experiencing hot flashes found them embarrassing or uncomfortable, only about one-fifth sought medical treatment.[20]

SOCIAL-PSYCHOLOGICAL LITERATURE ON THE MENOPAUSE

Neugarten et al.,[21] studying women's attitudes toward and experience of menopause, found great variation. While in general women were eager to discuss the menopause, upper middle-class women in particular denied its importance. Older women who had experienced menopause were less likely to consider it a significant event for women than were the others. The authors interpret this to mean that the loss of reproductive powers is not as important a concern as had been thought.

Levit studied sixty-nine married women with one or more children, in good physical health, between forty-four and fifty-seven years of age, half of whom were past the menopause, and half of whom were in the menopause. Half of the sample was middle class. Projective measures and scales were used to measure level and focus of anxiety, sexuality, and motherliness. Women who were in the midst of menopause displayed no difference in anxiety level as compared with those who were past the menopause except on some subscores of one of the scales. Levit found that:

> When the sample was divided according to scores on the motherliness scale into three groups, high, medium and low, no difference was found between the anxiety scores of the high and low motherliness groups. *However, when high and low motherliness groups* were again stratified by menopausal status, *the high motherly women in the menopause were more anxious than the high motherly, post-menopause women* [emphasis added]. Thus the transition from childbearing to non-childbearing seems to be more stressful to women who are highly invested in the motherly role than it is to those women who are not so invested in this role. Scores on the sexuality ratings indicated that women highly invested in sexuality are less anxious during the menopause than women who are not highly invested in sexuality.[22:5]

Whether or not the children were living at home made no difference in level or focus of anxiety. While for middle-class women there were no differences in anxiety between the in-menopause and postmenopause groups, working-class menopausal women were more anxious than those past menopause.

> The major findings of this study support the position that menopausal status is not associated with measurable psychological effects regarding anxiety. That is, for women in general, regardless of the level of personality examined, this period of transition is not perceived as an upsetting event. As measured by these instruments, neither the physiological changes nor their psychological implications have any noticeably stressful effect on normal women. The evidence presented here, therefore fails to support the personality theorists who describe the menopause as an upsetting event.

Since in large part these theorists derive evidence from clinical cases its applicability to women in general must be questioned.[22:7]

Kraines studied one hundred white women between the ages of forty-three and fifty-one in good health, none of whom had had a surgical menopause. They were married and living with their husbands, and the mothers of one or more children. The subjects were divided into three classes: twenty-eight premenopausal, forty-one menopausal and thirty-one postmenopausal. Half of each group was middle class and half was working class. They were given two long focused interviews, four direct self-report instruments, and three rating scales. While menopausal women had more of the various symptoms on the "Symptom Check List" (a list of twenty-eight symptoms of menopause), menopausal status was not found to be a contributing factor in the self-evaluations of middle-aged women. Kraines found that women who were low in self-esteem and life satisfaction also were more likely to have difficulty during menopause. The relationship appeared to be circular, i.e., low self-esteem led to difficulty during menopause which in turn led to low self-esteem, etc. She discovered, as Benedek speculated, continuity between a woman's previous reactions to sexual turning points and her reaction to menopause, finding a significant relationship with previous health problems, difficulty with menses, and attitudes and reactions during pregnancy. She concluded that, contrary to many clinical observations, menopause in itself is not experienced by most women as a critical event. Her data indicate no differences between premenopausal, menopausal, or postmenopausal women. She suggests that women who seek medical help are different from most middle-aged women in their physical and emotional reaction to stress and in their life-style of reacting to stressful events.[23]

In a recent review article, Neugarten and Datan appear to uncritically accept those studies which find middle age to be a neutral and frequently positive experience, while downplaying the problems people with fewer resources and thus fewer choices have at that stage of the life cycle. They rely heavily on a study of professional and business middle-aged people for whom terms like autonomy, predictability, and choice have some referents in reality.[24] Wood, whose work is cited in that article, has since reconsidered and now believes that women may have been hesitant to complain about their family to strangers, especially since the cultural norms for the behavior of adult children do not support the women's dissatisfaction.[25]

All the writers who deal with the problem of preexisting personality or continuity in response to psychosexual turning points agree that such continuity exists and that the response to menopause is a function of the woman's premenopausal personality and life patterns. The menopause itself does not turn a healthy, functioning woman into an involutional psychotic.

The literature on the menopause is, in certain respects, similar to the literature on middle age. The clinical works are problem-oriented, while the empirical data suggest that the stage of the life cycle is not difficult for most women. This is, of course, to be expected since the menopause occurs during middle age (generally, for American women, between forty-eight and fifty-two). While it is clear that middle age is not a crisis for many people, there are structural and cultural factors (e.g., female socialization) in our society that can increase the likelihood of an individual's experiencing problems at middle age (keeping in mind that problems are not necessarily crises). It should be pointed out that a policy implication of the position which emphasizes that most people do not experience mid-life crises is that no changes in the society are needed to better the situation of the middle-aged.

CROSS-CULTURAL STUDIES

One way to examine the menopause, to tease out the sociocultural from the physiological, is to look at cross-cultural studies. Both Dowty and Bart have studied the menopause in this manner. Dowty worked in Israel studying five subcultures which she arrayed on a continuum of modernization, from the traditional Arab women at one end to the European-born Israeli women at the other, with Jews from Turkey, Persia, and North Africa in the middle. The relationship between social change and difficulty during the menopause was curvilinear: it was the transitional women, midway between traditional life styles and modernization, who suffered most. They had lost the privileges afforded traditional women, while not receiving those benefits that modernization confers upon women; thus they had the problems of both groups but the advantages of neither.[26]

Bart, using the Human Relations Area Files as well as ethnographic monographs, found that certain structural arrangements and cultural values were associated with changes in women's status after the childbearing years.[27:1-18] These are summarized in Table I.

Thus, a strong tie to family of orientation and kin rather than a strong marital tie, an extended family system rather than a nuclear family system, an institutionalized grandmother role rather than no formal grandmother role, a mother-in-law role, rather than no role for a woman in relationship to her son- or daughter-in-law, and residence

Table I. Factors Associated with Increased and Decreased Status after Menopause

Increased Status	Decreased Status
Strong tie to family of orientation (origin) and kin.	Marital tie stronger than tie to family of orientation (origin).
Extended family system.	Nuclear family system.
Reproduction important.	Sex an end in itself.
Strong mother–child relationship reciprocal in later life.	Weak maternal bond; adult-oriented culture.
Institutionalized grandmother role.	Noninstitutionalized grandmother role; grandmother role not important.
Institutionalized mother-in-law role.	Noninstitutionalized mother-in-law role; mother-in-law doesn't train daughter-in-law.
Extensive menstrual taboos.	Minimal menstrual taboos.
Age valued over youth.	Youth valued over age.

patterns keeping one close to the family of orientation, all seem to go along with improved status at middle age. It seems reasonable that an increase in status would increase the likelihood of feelings of well-being. Thus, even if there are physiological stresses experienced at this time, they are well buffered structurally in kinship-dominated societies. When this system begins to break down, as it is now doing in some Third World countries, problems similar to those faced by some women in our culture arise. For example, one Indian mother who brought up her children to live in the modern manner, that is, independently, was very lonely and commented: "I sometimes feel, 'What is the use of my living now that I am no longer useful to them (her children)!' "[27:13]

In examining our own society, it is easy to see why there is stress for some women in middle age. In each instance, except for the mother–child bond which in our society is strong but nonreciprocal, we fall on the right-hand side with the cultures where the woman's status drops. For the women whose lives have not been child-centered and whose strong marital tie continues, or for those whose children set up residence near the mother, the transition to middle age may be buffered. However, it is important to note that even child-centered women claim that the relationship is nonreciprocal, that all they are entitled to is "respect."[28:86] Thus, for these women who have emphasized the maternal role or the glamour role, middle age may be a difficult stage in the life cycle. Our emphasis on youth and the stipulation that mothers-in-law should not interfere can make middle age stressful for many women. By examining the question in a cross-cultural perspective, however, we can observe the multiplicity of possible roles for middle-aged women and appreciate the fact that middle age need not be a difficult time. Indeed, it can and should offer women its own unique rewards.

SOCIOCULTURAL FACTORS

While the cross-cultural evidence strongly suggests that the phenomenon of menopausal depression is not as much related to physiological changes as to social and cultural structures and factors, a study of specific depressed menopausal women in our society could shed a great deal of light on how these factors operate in American culture. Bart[28,29,30] undertook such a study using the hospital records of 533 women between the ages of 40 and 59 who had had no previous hospitalization for mental illness. These records were drawn from five mental hospitals ranging from an upper-class private institution to two state hospitals. The records were used to compare all the women diagnosed as depressed (whether neurotic, psychotic involutional, or manic-depressive) with those women who had received other functional diagnoses. Twenty intensive interviews were also conducted to flesh out the picture obtained from the records. The interviews included questionnaires used in studies of "normal" middle-aged women as well as a projective biography test which consists of sixteen drawings of women at different stages of their life cycle and in different roles.

Statistical analysis of the hospital records indicated that role loss, including impending role loss, was associated with depression. Housewives were particularly vulnerable to the effects of losing other roles. Various ethnic groups differed in vulnerability with Jews being almost twice as likely as non-Jews to be diagnosed as depressed.[30:111] When family interaction patterns are held constant, however, and all women, both Jewish and non-Jewish, who have overinvolved or overprotective relationships with their children are compared with women who do not, the ethnic differences almost wash out. You do not have to be Jewish to be a Jewish mother, but it helps! Overall, the highest rate of depression was found among housewives experiencing maternal role loss who had overprotective or overinvolved relationships with their children. Thus the lack of meaningful roles and the consequent loss of self-esteem, rather than any hormonal changes, seemed largely to account for the incidence of menopausal depression.

This hypothesis received further support from the results of the interviews. All of the women with children, when asked what they

were most proud of, replied, "My children." None mentioned any ac-
complishment of their own, except being a good mother. When asked
to rank seven roles available to middle-aged women in order of importance, the mother role, "helping my children," was most frequently
ranked first or second. When children leave home, however, the
woman is frustrated in attempting to carry out this role she values so
highly, and she suffers a consequent loss of self-esteem. It is precisely
to the extent that a woman has been socialized to the traditional norms
of seeking vicarious achievement and identity that she is vulnerable to
trauma when her children leave. Moreover, many of those women
then experience their life situation as unjust and meaningless because
the implicit bargain they thought they had struck with fate did not
pay off. In the words of two of the women:

> I'm glad that God gave me . . . the privilege of being a mother . . . and I
> loved them. In fact, I wrapped my love so much around them. . . . I'm
> grateful to my husband since if it wasn't for him, there wouldn't be the
> children. They were my whole life. . . . My whole life was that because I
> had no life with my husband, the children should make me happy . . . but
> it never worked out.[30:111]

> I felt that I trusted and they—they took advantage of me. I'm very sincere,
> but I wasn't wise. I loved, and loved strongly and trusted, but I wasn't
> wise. I—I deserved something, but I thought if I give to others, they'll give
> to me. How could they be different but you see, they be different, but you
> see those things hurted me very deeply and when I had to feel that I don't
> want to be alone, and I'm going to be alone, and my children will go their
> way and get married—of which I'm wishing for it and then I'll still be
> alone, and I got more and more alone, and more and more alone.[30:116]

WOMEN'S SELF-HELP RESEARCH

As we have seen, the social science and medical literature on
menopause is sparse, at times hostile, and often irrelevant. As the
women's health movement has spread, however, we have seen the
emergence of a self-help literature[31-34] and of self-help research
efforts. Two of the latter have been directed specifically at adding to
our knowledge of the menopause. Two women's groups, one in Seattle and one in Boston, used mail-in questionnaires in an attempt to
survey women's physical and emotional experience of the menopause.

The Seattle group, calling itself "Women in Midstream," had originally set out to investigate what the experience of menopause was
like for women who were middle-aged before estrogen replacement
therapy was available. Accordingly, they sent one thousand questionnaires to nursing homes but received only seventy replies. These older
women were similarly unwilling to talk about the subject in face-to-
face interviews. This experience is of interest because it suggests the

extent to which women have been indoctrinated to regard normal bodily processes and life experiences with shame and to hide them from public scrutiny. It also suggests that most if not all earlier studies of menopause may well suffer from the respondent's unwillingness to reveal to researchers the full extent of their actual feelings and experiences. It may well be that only now, when there is support available in our culture for women sharing these formerly private areas of their lives with other women, particularly other women who are also experiencing similar things, that we can really learn about the truth of these experiences in a systematic way. The Women in Midstream collected their sample from a highly motivated group who wrote or called in order to receive the questionnaire after they read about it in the newspaper or heard about it on the radio. Accordingly, they think that the respondents are probably heavily middle and upper class and have had a relatively difficult experience of the menopause. (Even so, half of the group described it as "easy" or "moderately easy.") The sample was overwhelmingly white, married, mothers of about three children, but living only with their husbands at this time. They ranged in age from 28 to 73 with two-thirds of the group between 45 and 55. Sixty percent were Protestant and eighteen percent Catholic. Half of the women consider themselves "in the midst" of menopause and 16 percent "all through." Two-thirds of the group was working outside the home.

One of the most striking facts about this group is that three-quarters of the women reported receiving hormone therapy, even though no more than 60 percent of the group sought physician's help for the only two conditions for which estrogen replacement therapy has been proven effective. A staggering 55 percent of the women were prescribed psychotropic medications. One wonders how much of this was in response to the women's needs and how much in response to those of their husbands and/or physicians.[35] Only 55 percent of the women reported satisfaction with their doctor's attitude and found him or her helpful. Of the 20 percent of the sample who consulted other individuals about their problems, 80 percent found these people helpful. Seventy-eight percent of the group discussed their menopausal problems with female friends or relatives and nearly half of these found this helpful. Sixty-nine percent discussed their problems with husbands, male friends, or relatives, and 46 percent of these found them helpful. While it is surprising that male relatives and friends are almost as helpful as female relatives and friends in these matters, the fact that fewer women chose to speak with males about these issues in the first place suggests that they may well be more selective when choosing particular males to speak with as compared with particular females.

In contrast to the regional and age-restricted sample collected by the Seattle group, the Boston Women's Health Book Collective attempted to sample the attitudes toward and experience of menopause of women of all ages in all parts of the country. Mail questionnaires were sent to friends and relatives of the Collective members as well as to all of the clinics and counseling centers which ordered *Our Bodies, Ourselves*.[33:327] (Thus neither the Seattle study nor the Boston one is a random sample of all American women.) Of the Boston sample only 65 percent are married (as compared with 81 percent in the Seattle sample) though another 22 percent are divorced or widowed. Less than half (46 percent) of the group are Protestant, 26 percent are Jewish, and 20 percent are Catholic. As a group, they have slightly fewer children (2.3 vs. 3) than the Seattle sample. About 36 percent of the respondents (N = 175) were menopausal or postmenopausal. Two-thirds of this group, as in the Seattle sample, were employed outside the home.

Sixty-one percent of the Boston menopausal sample received estrogen replacement therapy. While this figure is below the 75 percent in the Seattle sample, it is still surprisingly high for a group which probably is experiencing many fewer "menopausal" problems (given the ways the respective samples were gathered). Eighty-five percent of the women reported talking with friends about their menopausal experiences while 70 percent talked to husbands (just about the same percentages as was reported by the Seattle group, though the questions asked were not precisely comparable). About 70 percent talked to children or other relatives and 15 percent each to therapists and women's groups. Two-thirds of the women had friends going through menopause at the same time. Twice as many women reported receiving emotional support as reported not receiving such support. Those who had friends going through menopause at the same time were three times as likely to receive support as not.

The Boston questionnaire covers a great many other areas and the reader is referred to the latest edition of *Our Bodies, Ourselves* for a more detailed report.[33:336]

POLICY IMPLICATIONS

Middle age is the time when reality catches up with women's image of the future, and some women are confronted with the meaninglessness of their lives. Women have been scripted to believe that they can achieve "true happiness" by self-abnegation, by sacrificing themselves to their husbands and their children, and that to do anything for themselves as persons rather than as mothers or as wives is selfish. Some women are able to evade this script. Some women are able to continue to receive the vicarious gratification for which this life style prepared them—their husbands are still alive and well and attentive, their children have made proper marriages and/or proper careers, grandchildren have arrived, and significant others congratulate them on a job well done. But for others the story is different. These women are bewildered by their children's life-style which rejects the very values that they have worked so hard to attain, indeed not so much for themselves as for their children. They cannot understand why their daughters do not want to have the children that they were taught were their destiny, and why they are denied the grandchildren they so joyfully anticipated. Their husbands may have left them for younger women to bolster their waning egos and diminished potencies (the data indicate that the average age of the second wife is younger than the current age of the first wife).[36] For these women to seek a younger mate would be considered ludicrous, for they are invisible sexually and perceived as obsolete (though physiologically, unlike men, they are as capable of sex as they ever were).[37] Because so many of these events coincide with menopause, they are attributed to this physiological change.

Alice Rossi, analyzing recent census data, notes that maternity has become a very small part of the adult woman's life: for a woman who marries at twenty-two, has two children two years apart, and dies at seventy-four, 23 percent of her adult life will be spent without a husband, 41 percent with a husband but no children under 18, 36 percent with spouse and at least one child under 18; but only 12 percent of her life will be spent in full-time maternal care of pre-school-age children.[38] This projection dramatizes how dysfunctional the standard script is. It is important that women be given this message early enough to prevent them from being middle-age casualties of their culture.

As feminist behavioral scientists we believe that societal problems cannot be dealt with on an individual basis. Along with other feminists we believe that there are no individual solutions, although a few women may slip through by chance or special privilege. What is required for the situation of most women to change is the organized efforts of many women working together to structure alternatives for themselves and others. Some of this has started to happen. While there is most familiarity with the involvement of younger women in the Women's Movement and in the support they have received from consciousness-raising groups, it is less well known that there has been an increasing concern with the problems older women face. The National Organization for Women (NOW) has a task force on older women. *Prime Time*, a feminist magazine addressing itself to the situation of women in the prime of life and providing a forum for communication among such women, was published until recently. These sorts of efforts, in addition to the existence of rap groups for middle-aged women, will make both the physical and social experience of this period of life more positive for increasing numbers of women. (There is at least one documented instance of a woman participating in a menopause consciousness-raising group finding that her formerly uncomfortable hot flashes were now experienced as pleasurable.)[39]

One of the signs of successful impact of the Women's Health Movement is the fact that gynecological self-examination, once a revolutionary cry of a small group, has begun to be a part of routine office practice among some gynecologists. As women demand more participation in and control over the various elements of their lives, we expect that the heavy taboos on natural bodily functions will decrease. Thus the public embarrassment component of the hot flashes that most menopausal women experience, at least, will be alleviated without the use of dangerous drugs.

It is clear from the review of the literature that to say "further research is needed" is not the cliché it frequently is when appended to an article. There is a shameful lack of knowledge about an experience that every woman undergoes. (We wonder if there would be so much ignorance about an event in the life of every man.) We must transcend the patriarchal perspectives which have inhibited the collection and dissemination of knowledge in areas relevant to women.

There is much talk of the wider range of options available to middle-aged women. However, options are limited by often ignored external factors such as economic conditions, racism, and previous educational opportunities. We must work for a society in which racism, sexism, and poverty are not endemic so that all women can live full lives. Group support can enable women whose options are not so limited to use their new freedom to change their life styles and fulfill some of their deferred dreams. Former Ann Arbor City Councilwoman Kathy Kozachenko's poem expresses both the attempts at social control some women experience when they change their way of being-in-the-world as well as their ultimate triumph.

MID-POINT

She stored up the anger
for twenty-five years,
then she laid it on the table
like a casserole for dinner.

"I have stolen back
my life," she said.
"I have taken possession
of the rain and the sun
and the grasses," she said.

"You are talking
like a madwoman,"
he said.

"My hands are rocks,
my teeth are bullets,"
she said.

"You are
my wife,"
he said.

"My throat is an eagle,
my breasts
are two white hurricanes." she said.

"Stop!" he said.
"Stop or I shall call
a doctor."

"My hair
is a hornet's nest,
my lips
are thin snakes
waiting for their victim."

He cooked his own dinners,
after that.

The doctors diagnosed it
common change-of-life.

She, too, diagnosed
it change of life.
And on leaving the hospital
she said to her woman-friend
"My cheeks
are the wings
of a young
virgin dove.
Kiss them."

KATHY KOZACHENKO

REFERENCES

1. Lennane JK, Lennane JR: Alleged psychogenic disorders in women—a possible manifestation of sexual prejudice. *New England Journal of Medicine 288*:288–292, 1973.
2. Howell MC: What medical schools teach about women. *New England Journal of Medicine 291*:304, 1974.

3. Scully D, Bart PB: A funny thing happened on the way to the orifice: women in gynecology textbooks. *American Journal of Sociology.* 78:1045–1050, 1973.
4. Campbell MA: *Why would a girl go into medicine?* Old Westbury, N.Y., The Feminist Press, 1973.
5. Smith-Rosenberg C, Rosenberg C: The female animal: medical and biological views of woman and her role in nineteenth-century America. *Journal of American History.* 60:332–356, 1973.
6. Stearns P: Interpreting the medical literature on aging, lecture in Newberry Library, Family and Community History Colloquia: The Physician and Social History. Chicago, Oct. 30, 1975.
7. Haller JS, Jr, Haller RM: *The physician and sexuality in Victorian America.* Urbana, University of Illinois Press, 1975, p 135.
8. Jones HW Jr, Cohen FJ, Wilson RB: Clinical aspects of the menopause, in *Menopause and aging* (U.S. Dept. of Health, Educ. and Welfare Pub. No. (NIH) 73-319). Edited by Ryan, JK, Gibson, DC. U S Govt Printing Office, Washington, D.C., 1971.
9. Wilson RA: *Feminine forever.* New York, M Evans, 1966.
10. Medical sexism. *Healthright* 6:Winter 1975–76.
11. Ziel HK, Finkle WD: Increased risk of endometrial carcinoma among users of conjugated estrogens. *New England Journal of Medicine* 293:1167–1170, 1975.
12. Smith D, Prentice R, Thompson D, Heirmann W: Association of exogenous estrogen in endometrial carcinoma. *New England Journal of Medicine* 293:1164–1167, 1976.
13. McKinlay SM, McKinlay JB: Selected studies of the menopause: an annotated bibliography. *Journal of Biosocial Science* 5:533–555, 1973.
14. Parlee MB: *Psychological aspects of menstruation, childbirth, and menopause: an overview with suggestions for further research.* Paper presented at the Conference on New Directions for Research on Women, Madison, Wisc., 5/31–6/2/75.
15. Osofsky HJ, Seidenberg R: Is female menopausal depression inevitable? *Obstetrics and Gynecology* 36:611–615, 1970.
16. Benedek T: Climacterium: a developmental phase. *Psychoanalytic Quarterly* 19:(1) 1–27, 1950.
17. Benedek T: The functions of the sexual apparatus and their disturbances, in *Psychosomatic Medicine.* Edited by Alexander F. New York, WW Norton, 1950, pp 239–240.
18. Deutsch H: *The psychology of women: a psychoanalytic interpretation.* New York, Grune & Stratton, 1945, p 436.
19. Stern K, Prados M: Personality studies in menopausal women. *American Journal of Psychiatry* 103:358–367, 1946.
20. McKinlay SM, Jefferys M: The menopausal syndrome. *British Journal of Preventive and Social Medicine* 28(2):108–115, 1974.
21. Neugarten BL, Wood V, Kraines RJ, Loomis B: Women's attitudes toward menopause, in *Middle age and aging.* Edited by Neugarten BL. Chicago, The University of Chicago Press, 1968.
22. Levit, L: *Anxiety and the menopause: a study of normal women.* Unpublished doctoral dissertation, University of Chicago, 1963, p 5.
23. Kraines RJ: *The menopause and evaluations of the self: a study of middle-aged women.* Unpublished doctoral dissertation, University of Chicago, 1963.
24. Neugarten B, Datan N: The middle years, in *American handbook of psychiatry.* Vol. 1. Second edition. Edited by Arieti S. New York, Basic Books, 1974. (Datan previously published as Dowty); and Neugarten BL, Kraines RJ: Menopausal symptoms in women of various ages. *Psychosomatic Medicine* 27(3): 266–273, 1965.
25. Wood V: Personal communication, June, 1976; and Wood V: *Role change and life-*

styles of middle-aged women. Unpublished doctoral dissertation, Committee on Human Development, University of Chicago, 1963.

26. Dowty N: To be a woman in Israel. *School Review 80*:319–332, 1972.
27. Bart PB: Why women's status changes in middle age. *Sociological Symposium 3:* 1–18, 1969.
28. Bart PB: Depression in middle-aged women: some socio-cultural factors (Doctoral dissertation, University of California at Los Angeles, 1967.) *Dissertation Abstracts 28*:475–1B, (Univ. Microfilms No. 68.-7452), 1968.
29. Bart PB: Mother Portnoy's complaints. *Trans-Action 8:* (1–2) 69–74, 1970.
30. Bart PB: Depression in middle-aged women, in *Women in sexist society: studies in power and powerlessness.* Edited by Gornick V, Moran BK. New York, Basic Books, 1971, pp 99–117.
31. Boston Women's Health Book Collective: *Our bodies, ourselves.* Boston, New England Free Press, 1971.
32. Boston Women's Health Book Collective: *Our bodies, ourselves—a book by and for women.* New York, Simon & Schuster, 1973.
33. Boston Women's Health Book Collective: *Our bodies, ourselves* (revised edition). New York, Simon & Schuster, 1976.
34. Weideger P: *Menstruation and menopause: the physiology and psychology, the myth and the reality.* New York, Knopf, 1976.
35. Seidenberg R: Drug advertising and perception of mental illness. *Mental Hygiene 55*:21–31, 1971.
36. Bell IP: The double standard. *Trans-Action 8:* (1–2) 76–81, 1970.
37. Moss Z: It hurts to be alive and obsolete: the aging woman, in *Sisterhood is powerful.* Edited by Morgan R. New York, Vintage, 1970.
38. Rossi A: Family development in a changing world. *American Journal of Psychiatry 128*:1057–1080, 1972.
39. Weideger P: *Menstruation and menopause: the physiology and psychology, the myth and the reality* (revised and expanded edition). New York, Dell, 1977.

Glossary

These definitions pertain to usage in the text; they are not necessarily complete if used in another context.

Adenosis: Development of an excessive number of glandular elements without tumor formation.

Adrenalectomy: Removal of the adrenal glands. A procedure used in the treatment of late-stage breast cancer.

Alveoli: Clusters of cells around a space.

Autonomic nervous system: Aggregations of nervous tissue through which the viscera, heart, blood vessels, smooth muscles, and glands receive their motor innervation. It is divided into the parasympathetic and sympathetic systems.

Autosome: Chromosome other than a sex chromosome.

Bartholins glands: Glands located near the entrance to the vagina.

Carcinoma in situ: A growth disturbance in which normal cells are replaced by abnormal-appearing cells which do not show the characteristics of cancer, i.e., invasion and metastasis.

Cervical dysplasia: Abnormal development or growth of cells of the cervix.

Cervical stenosis: Narrowing of the opening of the cervix.

Chromosome: Fiber completely or partially composed of genetic nucleic acid.

Cilia: Thread-like parts of cells which protrude and beat rhythmically, causing movement of the cell or of fluid over the cell.

Clitoridectomy: Removal of the clitoris.

Colostomy: The creation of an artificial opening in the abdominal wall for waste disposal.

Colostrum: The first fluid from the mother's breast after the birth of a child.

Colposcopy: The technique of examining the cervix (and vagina) with a low power (magnification 8–18x) microscope having a strong light source with a green filter to bring out the blood vessel pattern.

With the colposcope, the operator can visualize the zone where the squamous epithelium is growing over the columnar epithelium on the face of the cervix. This is called the transformation zone and is thought to be the area where all squamous cervical cancers arise. The visual findings on colposcopic examination have been correlated to a statistically significant degree with the changes present in tissue removed and examined under the microscope. In most instances the colposcopist can examine the cervix and predict where the abnormal cells seen in the Pap smear are coming from. Without the colposcope, any suspicious or positive Pap smear would have required further evaluation by an operative procedure called conization which removes the entire area at risk for developing cancer of the cervix. Now colposcopy can be used instead, and in many cases no conization is necessary.

Columnar epithelium: The tall mucous-producing cells which normally line the canal of the cervix and may extend out onto the visible portion of the cervix.

Conditional reflex: A response based upon an instinctive reflex at first initiated by a particular stimulus and later elicited as a result of repeated association and training by nonspecific stimulus.

Consanguinity: State of being descended from a common ancestor.

Conversion: A defense mechanism whereby unconscious emotional conflict is transferred into physical symptoms, the affected part always having symbolic meaning pertinent to the nature of the conflict.

Cortical depression: Reduction of functioning of the cerebral cortex.

Curettage: A surgical procedure for removing the contents of the uterus by a scraping or suction device.

Cytogenetics: Study of the genetics of cells. Study of chromosomes.

Decorticate: Posture assumed when the cerebral cortex is not functioning.

Denial: A defense mechanism, operating unconsciously. Used to resolve emotional conflict and allay anxiety by disavowing thoughts, feelings, wishes, needs, or external reality factors that are consciously intolerable.

DNA (Deoxyribonucleic acid): A type of nucleic acid which constitutes the genetic material.

Diuretics: Drugs that promote water excretion.

Dysplasia: Atypical growth that may be precancerous under certain conditions.

Ectopic pregnancy: A pregnancy located anywhere outside of the uterine cavity, most commonly in the Fallopian tube.

EEG (Electroencephalogram): A record of changes in electrical potential associated with the activity of the cerebral cortex, as detected by electrodes applied to the scalp.

Endogenous: Inherent, self-contained.

Endometrial: Referring to the lining of the uterus.

Endometriosis: The presence of endometrial tissue in abnormal locations, including the uterine wall, ovaries, or extragenital sites.

Enzyme: Protein catalyst of a metabolic chemical reaction.

Epididymis: The portion of the seminal or sperm duct which is connected to the testis.

Epithelium: The layer of cells that lines a surface.

Excision: Cutting out of a part or a growth from an organ or tissue.

Fascia: A band of fibrous connective tissue, often separating structures from each other.

Fibroadenoma: A benign tumor of the breast, containing some glandular and some connective tissue elements.

Fluorescent staining: Use of quinacrine derivative stains to produce unique banding patterns which enable the identification of each chromosome.

Follicle: The structure in the ovary containing the developing egg.

Gene: Smallest, independently functional unit of genetic material.

Hemoglobin: Oxygen-transporting protein in red blood cells.

Heterograft rejection: An immune phenomenon by which the tissue taken from one individual is repelled by the tissues of another individual to whom it has been grafted.

Heterozygous: Carrying two (or more) different alleles of a single gene.

Histology: Microscopic cell structure.

Homologous: Genetically corresponding.

Homozygous: Having identical alleles at two (or more) corresponding loci.

Hypertonic saline: A solution containing a high concentration of salt injected into the uterus for purposes of effecting termination of pregnancy in the midtrimester.

Hypophysectomy: Removal of the pituitary gland.

Hypothalamus: The portion of the brain which controls adult reproductive ability through its effect on the pituitary.

Hysterotomy: Major surgical operation for evacuating the uterine contents by way of an incision into the uterus.

Ileal loop: The use of a loop of the ileum, a portion of the small intestine, to replace a part of the genitourinary tract.

Incompetent cervix: Inability of the cervical opening (os) to remain closed during a pregnancy, thus potentially causing spontaneous abortions (miscarriages).

Infibulation: Fastening a ring, clasp, or frame to the genital organs to prevent copulation.

Irradiation: Treatment by photons, electrons, neutrons, or other ionizing radiations.

Leukocyte: White blood cell.

Limbic system: A part of the cerebral cortex thought to control various emotional and behavioral patterns.

Lobotomy: Surgical interruption of a part of the brain, usually frontal lobe.

Locus: Site in the chromosome occupied by a gene.

Lumpectomy: Surgical excision of a tumor mass.

Luteal phase: A phase of the menstrual cycle also called the progestational or secretory phase. During this phase, which occurs after ovulation, the glands of the uterine lining become distended and tortuous, providing blood supply for the potential implantation of a fertilized ovum (egg cell). In the ovary, the corpus luteum develops. It is composed of the tissue remaining in the ovary which surrounds the ovum. After ovulation it enlarges. If pregnancy occurs it secretes hormones to help maintain the pregnancy.

Malignant: Cancerous.

Mammogram: A diagnostic procedure for the detection of breast cancer, using X ray.

Mania: A mood disorder characterized by excessive elation, hyperactivity, agitation, and accelerated thinking and speaking. Sometimes manifested as flight of ideas. Mania is seen most frequently as one of the two major forms of manic-depressive psychosis.

Metaplasia: Transformation of one form of adult tissue to another such as the replacement of one type of epithelial (lining) cells by another type.

Metastasis: The spread of tumor to distant sites as from one organ to another.

Metastatic: The capacity to spread to distant sites, a capacity of malignant tumors.

Multifactorial: Polygenic quantitative trait due to the action of many gene pairs.

Mutation: More or less permanent, uncoded, change in the kind, number, or sequence of nucleotides in genetic material.

Nulliparous: Having never borne children.

Oncologist: A physician specializing in the treatment of tumors.

Oophorectomy: The removal of an ovary or ovaries; also called ovariectomy.

Ovulation: Egg production by the ovary.

Pap smear: A preparation of cells that have been peeled off an organ (usually the cervix) and placed on a glass slide. These cells are then preserved, stained, and examined with a microscope to detect changes which might indicate cancer.

Perimenopausal: Around the age of the menopause. The average age of a woman at menopause is now approximately 51. Greater than 90% of women will experience cessation of menses at 51 years ± 5 years.

Perinatal: Pertaining to the period of childbirth and shortly thereafter; usually beginning with the birth of a fetus of twenty weeks or more of gestation and ends 7 to 28 days later.

Phenothiazines: A group of drugs used extensively for the treatment of psychosis and other psychiatric syndromes.

Pituitary: The portion of the brain which responds to stimulation by the hypothalamus and controls egg production from the ovary.

Placental tumors: Rare abnormal growth form of placental tissue in which no embryo is formed and the placenta may have the characteristics of a cancerous growth (troph-oblastic tumors).

Polygenic: Multifactorial quantitative trait due to the action of many gene pairs.

Positive nodes: Lymph nodes invaded by neoplastic cells, in particular the axillary lymph nodes between the upper chest and arm.

Primary irradiation: Refers to the use of radiation therapy for the treatment of cancer as the primary source of treatment rather than as an ancillary treatment to surgery or chemotherapy.

Primipara: A woman bearing her first child.

Products of conception: The growing fetoplacental unit, at any age.

Prolactin: A hormone, secreted by the pituitary gland, that controls lactation.

Proprioception: Appreciation of position, balance, and changes in equilibrium on the part of the muscular system, especially during movement.

Psychodynamic: The study of human behavior from the point of view of motivation and drives, depending largely on the functional significance of emotion and based on the assumption that any individual's total personality and reaction at any given time are the product of the interaction between his genetic constitution and the environment in which he has lived from conception onward.

Puerperium: The interval following delivery, usually designated 6 weeks, during which healing, recuperation, and return of all organs and tissues to their prepregnancy state is accomplished.

Resistance: A defense mechanism characterized by the individual's inability to bring repressed material to light and to give up habitual patterns of thinking, feeling, and acting to take on newer modes of adaptation.

Sensate focus: The couple are each asked to touch each other and to communicate in this way in order to increase their sensual pleasure.

Sex chromosomes: Chromosomes that differ in number or morphology in different sexes and contain genes determining sex type.

Somatic nerves: Nerves supplying somatic structures such as voluntary muscles, skin, tendons, joints, and membranes.

Spermatogenesis: The phenomena involved in the production of spermatozoa (sperm) in the male.

Spina bifida: A type of birth defect involving maldevelopment of the spinal cord.

Squamous epithelium: The smooth tissue which normally lines the vagina and covers most of the cervix. It is composed of flat plate-like cells called "squames" from the Latin word for plate.

Stage IV carcinoma: Carcinoma with widespread metastasis and local invasion.

Tail of Spence: An extension of breast tissue toward the axilla (armpit).

Transference: The unconscious transfer of the patient's feelings and reactions originally associated with important persons in their life, usually family, toward others, perhaps a therapist or analyst. The feelings may thus be positive or negative.

Zygote: The fertilized egg before it implants in the uterus.

Index